C000063189

Sex Life:

This book includes: Taboo Sex Stories, How to Talk Dirty, Sex Positions for Couples, Tantric Sex, Femdom, Kama Sutra for Beginners

Taboo Sex Stories:

Erotica Seductive Sex Fantasies for Adults. Threesome, GangBang, BDSM and Femdom

of information contained within this document, including, but not limited to, — errors, omissions, or inaccuracies.

Table of Contents

Blind Pleasure

Catherine, a hesitant wife, gives in to Rich, her husband's greatest fantasy: He wants to see her fucked by other men. Yes, men—as in plural. He wants to watch her gangbanged while he enjoys watching every single moment of it, but she's not so convinced. She is nervous about what to expect but soon finds that she doesn't have to be so afraid of what is to cum, over and over again. She goes off to the local swinger's club with him for a night she will never forget—and may even want to repeat some time.

"Catherine."

The sound of my husband's voice sent a shiver down my spine, and the skin on my arms began to prickle into goosebumps. I knew what he wanted. I kept my eyes planted firmly on my reflection as I finished getting myself ready to his standards. Eyeliner, heavy and winged into the perfect cat-eye. Black, smoky shadow was blended onto my eyelids. My eyes, the most indistinctive shade of flat brown, looked bigger, and I could see my own hesitation in them.

"Catie."

His voice was quieter and more urgent. More needing. I felt his hand on the small of my back, and it sent a quick shock shooting within me. I loved his touch—I couldn't deny that. It was everyone else's that I was hesitant about. Still, I kept my gaze planted on myself, putting the finishing touches on my face. My lips, a deep pink, almost red against my naturally pale skin. My brown hair was straightened and lay almost pin-straight down to my shoulders, curving in just slightly toward my cheeks to frame my narrow face.

"It's time."

His hand slid off of my back, leaving the place that he had touched, feeling almost uncomfortably cold, vying for his touch again. His fingers wrapped around my wrist and pulled, beckoning me to turn, and I did to look at him.

My husband, Rich, was conventionally attractive. Between the two of us, he blew me out of the water. He had a perfectly sculpted jawline, strong and masculine, with just a hint of 5-o-clock shadow across it, and a strong brow. His eyes were bright blue and his hair, almost black and trimmed to create a taper cut. He was wearing a tight, black t-shirt and a pair of tight jeans that betrayed his large bulge in his pants. I looked over him and couldn't help it. Just the sight of him, all ready to go was enough to make me wet. He smirked at me as I looked him over, satisfied.

He grabbed my hand and took me outdoors to the car. We drove in a heavy silence to the club we were going to. We had never done anything like this before, and while I had agreed to do so, it was more because he wanted to than anything else. He wanted to see other men fuck me; he had said one day when we were showering after a night of X-rated passion. His cock had quickly hardened at the suggestion as he watched me, slowly washing away the sweat from the night. I had agreed to do it for him, but I couldn't say that I was particularly excited about it.

"You'll change your tune real quick, hon," he had replied when I shrugged my shoulders. "Think of all the men that are there—to please *you*. They're there to have fun with you." And so, here we were, preparing to enter a swinger's club for the first time. Rich had figured everything out on his own; he arranged for the night, for the reservations that we apparently needed, and for the people that would be there.

Before I knew it, we were parked outside of a nondescript building. I never would have guessed that inside was a club, apparently full of people that wanted to trade partners. It looked like a simple brick building without a sign, and if it weren't for the cars parked all over it or the fact that I saw another couple entering the building, I'd have assumed we were in the wrong place. I was expecting something a bit... More flashy? This was certainly not.

Rich squeezed my hand and brought me back to reality. I turned to look at him and was immediately met with his lips on mine. His tongue danced over my bottom lip, waiting for me to open mine, and I quickly obliged, feeling his tongue against mine. His hand slid up my arm and to my breast, giving it a quick squeeze. When he came up for air, breaking the kiss, he smirked at me again. God, I loved that smirk. "Don't sweat it, hon. You're going to love it; I know you will." He kept massaging my breast, playing with it, but this time, he let his finger linger over my nipple, pressing in.

I gasped, feeling myself begin to get wet, and my clit twitched, beginning to swell, and I leaned in for another kiss. My hand snaked around to feel his cock, so big in his pants and so trapped that I just *had* to free them from their cage. I unbuttoned the pants and undid the zipper, reaching in to pull it out. It was at full attention and ready to go. My hand ran over it, and I felt his body tense as he moaned against my lips. This time, it was my turn to smirk as I slowly rubbed his cock, up and down. Up and down.

He reached down to touch my pussy, slipping underneath my little black dress and right past the little black thong that I had worn to match, his fingers expertly finding my clit. He rubbed on it, and my legs spread open for him, granting full access. I ran my hand over his cock, feeling the shaft get harder. The car smelled of our passion as I quickly undid my seatbelt and leaned over to take him in my mouth, but he protested, quickly pulling his hand away from me and leaving me wanting.

"Slow down," he said with a dark chuckle. He was watching me with amusement as he took his fingers into his mouth, sucking off every bit of liquid that I had left on him. "We have plenty of time for that later."

So off we went, into the club, and we picked up a few shots, followed by a cocktail each, on our way, to "ease our nerves," Rich had said, but I knew he just meant mine. I was watching the way that his clothes clung to his body, and especially to his crotch, watching that bulge that remained there. No one batted an eye as we walked through the club. There was music, low, pulsing, but nondescript in the background to fill any silence, and couples and groups were talking quietly amongst each other as they sipped their drinks and looked at each other like chunks of meat. It almost made me nervous until I realized that I was looking at my husband in exactly the same way. With our drinks in hand, my husband led me to a private room in the back. When we entered, I saw that it was decorated like a hotel suite; there was a bathroom connected to it and a queen-sized poster bed.

The lighting was dim, and I finished my drink, placing the drink on a nightstand. The alcohol left me pleasantly buzzed, and Rich grinned. He could see the flush on my cheeks, even in the absence of light. He made his way over to me and roughly pushed me onto the bed, gripping at my breasts with both hands for a moment before they both slipped into the top of my dress, His fingers pinched at my nipples, delicately at first and then with more fervor as he nibbled at my neck before slamming his lips against mine. I could taste the alcohol on his breath and it just made me want him more. I spread my legs and thrust my hips against his, rubbing myself on his hard cock. I reached my hands down to undo his pants, but he stopped me, grabbing my wrist and then attaching a strap around them. I stopped, blinking in surprise. We had played with the restraints every now and then at home and I recognized them as the ones that we used. The restraint went around one of the posts on the bed and then another came out for the other hand.

Before I could protest, he had pulled out a pocket vibrator, placing it against my clit first and then teasing the slit of my pussy. My hips bucked upwards at the jolt, and a moan escaped my lips. He left it there as he placed a tie around each of my ankles as well, leaving me spread-eagle on the bed. I was enjoying the vibrator so much that I hardly noticed.

He reached back up for the vibrator, taking it slowly from its position and back up to my clit and then turned it off just as I was really starting to get into it. I could feel myself starting to drip, and I was certain that I had already left a wet spot on the bed. Before I could beg for more, I felt Rich's lips kissing me. His tongue flicked across my clit, making me gasp and shudder. He licked with a bit more force, one hand snaking up to grasp my chest. He pinched and pulled at my nipple as he licked, his tongue expertly tracing my clit until he moved downward, licking at my opening as well. He let his tongue tease the entrance just a bit longer with a quick "Mmm..." against me.

"Rich, fuck me," I managed to moan out as I felt my body flex. I tried to reach down to grab his head, but the restraints held me back. I felt him laugh against me. I was desperate to get that cock inside me, and he knew it. He knew how much I longed for it. He climbed atop me in the bed and pressed himself against me. He smelled like me, a faint, almost pungent scent, and he looked down at me. I leaned up to rub against him some more, but he pulled away.

"Oh, believe me, you'll be fucked plenty," he practically purred as he pulled something else out of his pocket. It was a black blindfold, and it was very quickly wrapped around my head. I couldn't see anything, and for a moment, I felt a hint of anxiety, but that was quickly forgotten when I heard a zip and felt his cock enter me.

It was slow at first, just the tip, and immediately, my body tensed up in pleasure. I felt every inch of him as he slid into me, and I squeezed against him, moaning softly. I tried to reach out for him, but my hands were restrained. "Good girl," he said softly as he thrust harder and harder. His balls bounced against my ass, sounding like slaps, and my pussy got even wetter than I thought was possible. I felt his hands clawing at my chest as if trying to tear away the dress that I was wearing. The restraints held me back, and it was almost hotter that I couldn't see what was happening. I was in total ecstasy as he rammed into me and I heard him grunt in equal pleasure.

"Fuck me harder, Rich," I moaned out, and he obliged, but just as I was about to orgasm, he stopped and pulled away. I was left in shock and utter silence. "... Rich?" I called out, only to hear him chuckling from across the room.

"Have fun," he said, and then I knew it was beginning.

Within seconds, I could smell a new man near me; he smelled of aftershave, woody almost. My heart was pounding in my chest, and I was almost afraid to speak when I realized what was about to happen, but all apprehension melted away as soon as I felt another vibrator rubbing against my clit as a finger slipped into my pussy.

"Mmm... Nice, wet, and tight," the voice said, almost breathy as the man that I couldn't see felt me up. He felt good. Maybe it was the alcohol and lack of inhibition, or the fact that Rich had been driving me crazy all night, or the fact that I had complete permission to fuck a strange man with him watching, but those first seconds were better than I expected.

Before I could say a word, I felt his fingers probe into me again, holding the vibrator in place with what I assume was his palm as his other hand squeezed my ass, pulling at my cheeks. His fingers teased my asshole, and my entire body tightened up in pleasure. I moaned as the vibrator was replaced with a face that felt clean-shaven—there was none of the prickling I usually felt with Rich. I felt him sucking, kissing, and licking at my clit, slowly at first, tantalizingly teasing me. "Such a bad little girl, look how much she wants it," he murmured between my lips. The feeling sent shivers down my spine. "Do you want it, you hot little slut?"

I moaned again, practically unable to speak as he continued to suck away. I felt him pull away and heard another zip as he undid his pants and the rustling of clothing. His cock felt different—it was wider than Rich's as it rubbed at my slit, teasing my swollen lips as he did so. I thrust my hips up, trying to get him to enter, but he pulled back, laughing. "She's ready to go, Rich!" he called out, and I heard Rich chuckling. I could hear the pleasure in his voice—it was low and almost urgent. He was enjoying every moment of this, so why shouldn't I?

I heard footsteps approach me as the strange man's cock continued to tease me, moving up and down, sometimes, sliding across my clit and sometimes circling my asshole, leaving me breathless with anticipation. My senses were on overdrive; I could hear his own breathing change as he enjoyed himself as well. Suddenly, I felt a mouth on my neck, and I smelled another scent—this one was citrusy.

"She's definitely a looker, isn't she?" said another voice, and I felt his hands lightly brushing over my arms. I shivered at the touch, moaning as the first man, the one who smelled of sandalwood, finally thrust into me. His cock was longer than Rich's too, it felt like, as it slid deeper and deeper, slowly penetrating me until I felt his balls against my ass. He held it there as I felt the other man pull down my dress, leaving my breasts bare. I knew

14

my nipples were perfectly erect at that point, and I could feel a faint breeze over them. It was warm. Was it his breath? His head must have been awfully close to them, and citrus man gently touched each one. Then, he pinched a bit harder, leaving me moaning again. I couldn't do anything; I was stuck exactly in place, but I really just wanted to ride the cock that was inside of me.

I felt the man who was next to me lower his head down to take my nipple into my mouth, and he bit down on it, hard enough to send a shiver down my spine but not so hard to hurt. The cock that was in me thrust harder, and I cried out, but not in pain. I felt the man inside of me squeeze at my ass and then suddenly smack it hard enough to sting. I cried out but felt myself get wetter against him, and I clenched against every inch of his girth, feeling it fill me. His cock pulsated against me as he pulled it out, never quite all the way, before slamming back into me, all the while I felt the man's fingers clawing at my ass more and more.

"I want more," I managed to gasp out, and in response, I got another slap across the ass, a bit more forceful this time, and I yelped in response. This brought another slap quickly, followed by another.

"You want more, you little slut?" Sandalwood said, his breath starting to hitch as he kept slamming into me. I moaned in response as I felt another slap. I'm sure my ass was red by that point, but I was too lost in passion to care. "Yes, please give me more," I managed to moan out between breaths.

Then, I felt another hand on me suddenly. This hand was different. It was rougher. Stronger. More confident as it caressed over my body. Three. There were three pairs of hands on me now, and strangely, I didn't mind. In fact, I loved every moment of it. One pair held me in place as Sandalwood continued to thrust with as much force as he could muster, and I lifted my hips so that my clit would

15

rub against his pelvis. Citrus continued to knead and suck at my breasts and nipples, and this new pair of hands was slowly exploring my body with his hands. I heard more zipping, and very quickly, a rock-hard cock was shoved in my face.

"Open," I heard a gruff voice command, and I did so, turning my head toward him. He shoved himself into my mouth so hard that I gagged at first, tears springing to my eyes. I let my tongue roll over his dick, lingering on the frenulum before pushing it deeper into my mouth.

I could hardly take it. Every nerve in my body felt like it was on overdrive as I was pleasured from three different men, and I could hear my husband's own breathing, almost ragged in the corner. Was he jerking himself as he watched? The thought of Rich's face, enjoying watching his wife become a toy for all of these men, was enough for me, but he loved it.

I knew I wasn't going to be able to last much longer. I could feel my own pleasure building and building until I could hardly take it anymore. My own moans had grown louder, and I could feel my body taking control, moving and grinding into Sandalwood harder and harder. Citrus was sucking harder than before, so hard that it would have hurt, but in the moment, I loved it.

Right as I was about to cum, I felt Sandalwood pull his dick out of me and leave me thrusting my body upward, searching blindly for him. He wasn't there, but I could hear him chucking. I could feel the warmth of his body radiating off of him, just outside of my reach.

"Beg for it," he said.

My mouth was full of another cock, licking and sucking on it, and I whined. I tried to open my mouth to pull away to speak, but the man held me in place roughly, twisting his hand in my hair to keep me right where I was. I got it
16

then—I wasn't going to be allowed to finish until they were each satisfied. I sucked on his dick with as much passion as I could muster. I could feel his shaft twitching and bulging in my mouth as I continued to slurp at it. He held me in place and slammed himself into my mouth, letting himself go down my throat to make me gag. He didn't let up, going harder and harder until I tasted him. The salty, hot liquid shot down my throat, burning and making me gag as I felt him cum into my mouth. His cock twitched and pulsated in my mouth as he held me there to his own pleasure, and when he pulled out, I moved to spit, but he held my mouth shut.

"Swallow it," he told me. I did, shuddering as it went down my throat, leaving its aftertaste in my mouth. I wasn't normally a swallower, but nothing about this situation was normal. It was strangely erotic to be ordered around, and at this point, I think it would have been impossible for me to get any wetter. I could feel my own juices dribbling down to my ass as I was spread out, and the sheets right underneath me were soaked. The whole room smelled musty, of sex and men, and I *loved* it.

"Please," I said breathlessly, thrusting my pelvis up, looking for Sandalwood. He had to have been there somewhere. But then, another dick was shoved in my face. I sucked it in greedily and tasted myself all over it, and that woody smell of the man who had, only moments prior, been thrusting into me was standing over me. He shuddered as my lips wrapped around his shaft, licking myself up and savoring the taste. He was so hard, and he was so wide that my jaw was opened up almost uncomfortably far as I took him in, gently, slowly, sensually using my tongue to caress his head and shaft.

Then, I felt something else beneath me. Was that Citrus? I couldn't smell him near me anymore, I realized, and that must have been why. He was underneath me now, rubbing his own cock against me. He started up on my clit, making me moan against Sandalwood's dick as he did. It was a gentle touch, but it was enough to drive me crazy with desire. I wanted him, and I wanted him *then*.

I thrust my hips up just right, taking the cock into my body as I continued to suck on the first one. I groaned in ecstasy as I felt the length of him enter me. He pulled my legs up as much as he could with the constraints and thrust his way into me as hard as he could. I cried out, only to have my head thrust back onto the cock in my mouth, and I continued to suck on it.

Citrus was a much more sensual fucker than Sandalwood had been. He entered me and gyrated his hips, allowing himself to touch more of me. He angled himself just right to shoot toward the top of my vagina, rubbing against the walls and leaving me hotter than before. As my body got closer, and I felt more of my own wetness dribble out and down onto Citrus, I felt him pull away, just like before. I wanted him so badly, but I knew what was happening. I needed to finish off Sandalwood first.

I sucked on Sandalwood harder, craning my neck as far as I could until he pushed himself toward me. My nose was against his groin. It was unshaven; I could feel the hairs tickling against my face as I took as much of him in as I could, letting my lips tighten around him before pulling away. "That's right, you little slut," he managed to hiss out as I pulled away, letting the tip of my tongue trace along his shaft as I did it. I smiled until the next thrust from Citrus made me moan, almost losing myself in the pleasure. Sandalwood's hand, yanking my hair, brought me back to reality, and I repeated that motion, again and again, getting quicker and quicker until he was shaking. I teased his head with my tongue. I could feel his dick getting firmer. He was getting close, and I could taste the precum on the tip as I flicked it with my tongue. I shoved him down my throat as hard as I could manage without gagging and sucked, and then I felt him jolt, thrusting himself into my mouth as again, I was rewarded with the taste of cum shooting down my throat. His was slightly

18

less pungent than the first man's, and I sucked it down greedily, licking along his shaft as his body continued to be rocked with enjoyment. I grinned. Mission accomplished. Now, there was nothing standing in my way.

Citrus slammed deeper than before into my body, and I felt his weight atop me as he climbed into the position that he wanted. I could smell him as he fucked me, and I moaned out, craning my head to kiss him as he continued to slam into me. I was searching for him, yearning for his mouth, but before I could find it, it was back on my nipple, flicking it with his tongue, sending my whole body convulsing. I was so close. "Fuck me harder," I managed to whisper between gasping breaths, my mouth now gloriously free from cock as I leaned up, placing my head into the crook of his neck.

He obliged instantly, shoving his dick harder into my body, and I lost myself in the moment. I cried out and rubbed myself against his pelvis as he continued to thrust, and almost immediately, all of the frustration and tension was released in ecstasy as I *finally* got the orgasm I had been waiting for. I felt my pussy clench around his dick harder and harder as he thrust, cumming within me to the feeling of my walls tightening. It was so intense that I lost myself, unaware of everything in that instant. I collapsed against the bed; all energy thoroughly drained from my body. I couldn't keep going even if I wanted to.

When I regained my wits, I realized it was almost silent, but I could hear someone shuffling around. I sat there in my post-sex haze, utterly exhausted and uninterested in what was going on around me, and I suddenly felt the restraints loosen and fall off and then felt my blindfold removed.

The room was surprisingly empty. I could see Rich staring at me with a look of arousal, admiration, and satisfaction all in one. He was thrilled to have seen me do what I had

19

done. I was totally exhausted on the bed, and even freed up, I was not sure that I wanted to get up and do anything.

Rich smirked at me as I laid there in my post-sex high. "You ready for another round?" he murmured, running his hand up and down my body, sending a shiver down my spine.

I laughed as he got on top of me to kiss me unabashedly, his tongue dancing in my mouth as he savored the taste of others on my lips. His own cock was pressed against me, bare and rubbing against my thoroughly fucked, swollen pussy. I kissed him back. Surely, round two wouldn't be so bad. It was the least I could do to repay him for the fun I had.

Variety Is the Spice of Sex

Lindsey loved fucking new people. For her, fucking was something exciting and new, and while she loved fucking her husband, she wanted more. She wanted the act of exploring new bodies and getting new sensations and new connections. Her husband, Matt, has always seemed uninterested in the threesome or open relationship life, but for his wife, he's willing to try anything once. They open up a to their neighbor, sexy Delilah for some threesome fun to try to accommodate Lindsey's needs, and spend a day fucking harder than they have ever fucked before, leaving both Matt and Lindsey thoroughly satisfied.

I was bored.

I was being fucked by my husband, but I was completely bored out of my mind. Sex had grown dull. Sure, we could bring in toys. We did that a lot—I had toys of every kind imaginable. Rabbit vibes and cock rings and dildos galore, but none of them could keep my attention for very long at all. I wanted *more*. I wanted something else that would keep me happy. I wasn't sure what I wanted yet, but I knew that whatever it was, it wasn't this.

I pinched and kneaded at my nipples as my husband fucked me from behind. He grunted and groaned and unleaded within my pussy, collapsing onto me as he did. I could feel his heart pounding in his chest as he rested there for a moment before he turned his head to kiss me. He smiled at me, but it quickly faltered. "Again?" Matt asked with a hesitant frown.

I averted my gaze, almost ashamed that I was unable to enjoy the moment. We had tried everything that I could think of. We had done some of that teacher-student roleplay. It wasn't for me. We tried some light bondage, but I didn't care for that, either. I was just *bored*. This was the first relationship that I had been in for longer than a few months, and I almost thought that what I needed was something fresh. Fresh meat to enjoy or something. It was exciting to explore new bodies sometimes, and I felt like I hadn't been able to do that. I loved my husband, sure, but sexually? I was an explorer. I wanted to get out, fuck my brains out, and fuck as many people as I could. I had given up that life when I got married, but a part of me couldn't help but think that that was what I was missing.

"Is there anything I can do?" asked Matt.

I shook my head. It would be another night for the vibe in the bath with a glass of wine for me. I didn't need to make him feel worse or more inadequate about it.

"Do you want to fuck other people?" he finally asked me. I could hear it in his voice. It was almost breaking him to suggest it, but he loved me, and he wanted me to be happy.

I hesitated, but he must have seen the excitement that I tried to hide in my face. I saw his shoulders fall.

"What about a threesome?" I suggested suddenly.

He looked at me, confused.

"I don't want to fuck someone on my own," I told him. "I want you to join in. Wouldn't you want another toy to play with?" I winked at him and slapped his ass, enjoying the quick bounce as I did, squeezing and kneading the muscle. His ass was firmly toned. He, for one, did not skip leg day, that was for sure.

Matt sighed. "Lindsey, I don't know..." He looked at me with mixed emotions swirling in his green eyes.

"You'll love it," I promised him, giving him a quick kiss and nibbling on his lip. "It's fun."

He shrugged his shoulders. I was his only partner that he had ever had; he had wanted to save himself for marriage. He wasn't religious or anything, but he hadn't wanted to, shall we say, play the field; he wanted to keep sex something special for himself. But let's be real—a quick fuck is so much fun.

I grinned. "Trust me?"

He sighed again and nodded his head. "But no dicks. I'm firm on that one."

"Fine by me!" I said with a grin. I slapped his ass again, giggling as it bounced. There was a pink print on his cheek now as I clenched. I saw dick start to harden again as I did it, and I smiled at him, genuinely excited. I pulled him forward, kissing him, and he kissed back, ready for round two.

I did all of the work from that point on. I screened out options that would be interested in a bit of rough fun with us. I looked for women only, knowing Matt's stance, and I didn't mind myself. Sometimes, all you want is an extra pair of tits to fondle that aren't your own. Eventually, I had found the perfect person: The young neighbor that had just moved into the apartment next door.

Delilah was a perky, young 19 years old. Perfect tits, double-Ds on her hourglass figure. Her skin was a deep olive color, and her hair was down to her waist, black, thick, and I could only imagine pulling it myself as I played with those perfect little nipples that I made sure to check out and sample before choosing her to be the perfect partner. She was *gorgeous*. She was kinky, too—she had shown me her collection of restraints and even a few leather floggers, and I knew that we would be in for fun.

She knocked at the door, and when I opened it, she looked shy; she was almost too nervous to enter. I grabbed her wrist brusquely, immediately feeling a thrill as I pulled her in. This would be fun, and I was determined to enjoy each and every moment of it. The thought of a fresh, new body made me wet; I could feel my pussy twitch as I led her in. She looked at Matt and blushed a bit, but it just made me want her more.

Matt was sitting on our bed, naked and almost lazily stroking his own cock, displaying it for Delilah to see. He seemed a bit hesitant but was willing to give it a shot.

I took off my robe that I had been wearing to open the door, revealing that I was perfectly naked underneath and looked at Delilah. She was eyeing my husband's cock with a mixture of being impressed and desiring to get her own hands on it. I could see that look in her eyes—the look of lust. The look of her lips parting slightly as she inhaled. The shine of her eyes dilating as she looked at him. She wanted him, and that was enough to make me happy.

"You ready?" I purred as I reached over to pull Delilah's shirt over her head. She nodded her head and turned her eyes to me, taking in every inch of my body. I instinctively straightened out, pushing my chest outward more, and Delilah reached up to grab them. She ran her fingers over my nipples, pinching and rubbing at them, and I gasped at the feeling. Her fingers were so soft and warm as they worked their magic, the touch of a woman who was clearly experienced with the female body.

I leaned in to kiss Delilah, watching Matt's reaction as I did. He watched us intently, and I could see the way his cock twitched when I did it. I smiled against Delilah's lips as my tongue parted them and made its way into her mouth, tasting her. She tasted sweet, almost like a cup of wine. Had she had to drink a glass of wine to loosen up? I chuckled as I nibbled on her lips, and I led her to bed to join Matt.

24

Matt grinned as we did and opened his arms to us. I settled in on the left side of him, and Delilah was on the right. I pulled her in again to kiss, both of our breasts resting against Matt's chest as we did so. I moaned as I kissed her, and I felt Matt reach up to grab my breast and touch it. He touched my nipples with his own fingers. They were rougher than Delilah's; I immediately noticed. He flicked his fingers over them and was just a bit tougher than I was.

I reached down for Matt's hand on my breast and removed it, guiding it over to feel Delilah's as well, and I immediately felt him tense up, his breathing picking up. Then, I pulled away from Delilah's lips, pushing her down to kiss Matt as well.

He reciprocated, his cock twitching as he did. I reached down to stroke it, running my nails gently up and down the shaft, making him shudder as he continued to kiss Delilah, with more fervor as I continued to play with him. He bit her lip, and I could hear him groan as I lowered my head down to lick him. I used just my tongue at first, running it up and down just as I had done with my nails. I saw his hips shift upward as he sought out my mouth, or any other wet hole he could get his cock in, and I obliged, taking it between my lips and hearing him moan against Delilah. After all, this had to be just as enjoyable, if not more so, for him than for me if I wanted him to feel like he wanted to do this again. I was in for the long haul, and I didn't mind sharing my new toy.

I turned to look at Delilah, who was shifting to straddle him now, his hand both reaching for her breasts, kneading, tugging, and rubbing them between his hands. I could smell her wetness between her legs as she continued to kiss him, and I shifted down a bit to let her make her way downward. I pulled her hips, guiding her perfectly round ass down to him. I lined her up and took Matt's cock, still wet with my saliva, and put it into her. As soon as it felt her lips, it thrust upwards, and she moaned, throwing her head back.

Then, he thrust again and again. He was watching her intently, watching those perfect breasts bouncing on her chest, nipples pointed out, and still shimmering with saliva. He turned his attention back to me then and reached out with his hand to grasp my breasts as well. Mine were just as big, but age had already started to weigh them down. He didn't seem to mind as he greedily tugged and squeezed at them. His fingers glossed over my nipples, and I felt myself get wetter, my own clit starting to swell in anticipation of my turn for fun.

I watched as Delilah rode Matt harder and harder. She started to really moan and whine. "Oh, Matt!" she groaned, her head thrown back. "Fuck me harder!"

I slapped her ass, seeing the red mark appear almost immediately, but she only moaned louder. I grinned and slapped her again and again. I could feel myself starting to drip down my legs as they continued to fuck, and before they could get too into it, I interrupted the fun. I pulled Delilah up and off of Matt, pushing her down next to him. She gasped, looking up at me, almost in surprise. I could see the wetness from their fucking glistening between her thighs. Her pussy was perfectly waxed and hair-free. Perfect.

I looked over my new toy and forced her legs open. She was caught off guard, but she obliged, and I quickly buried my face between her lips, feeling that one little nub that seemed so hard for so many men to find. She gasped and shuddered as my tongue ran over her. I positioned myself just right on my knees, head down, and ass raised. Matt watched as I continued to lick at Delilah and seemed to get the idea as I shifted. He could enter from behind.

Matt quickly got into position and slammed into me quickly. "Lindsey, you're so wet," he groaned as he slid all the way, stopping only when his balls slapped my ass. I chuckled at him as I continued to lick Delilah's clit, feeling her shift at the feeling. She moaned as she continued to get licked. As I felt her getting closer to cumming, I slapped her ass suddenly. It surprised her, judging by the yelp, but judging by the gush of fluids in my face, she loved it. I slapped her again and reached up to take her breast in my hand.

Matt continued to fuck me from behind, and I kept my composure, sucking on that little nub. I slide my fingers into Delilah, one at first, then another. Then, I angle them just right, reaching around to get to that magical g-spot, and as soon as I reach it, I hear her moan, her hips shooting up as soon as I touch it. I grin to myself, knowing that I have reached it.

I played with that little spot inside of her a bit longer, listening to the change in her breath and feeling the fluids soaking my hand as I continued to lick her. Within seconds, I could feel her whole body spasm, and her vagina tightened and clenched on my fingers over and over again.

I pulled my hands away from her, knowing that she'll be far too sensitive for the next few moments to be of much fun. Instead, I turned to look over my shoulder at Matt. He was watching us intently as he thrust deeper. He had kept pace deep and slow while I tongued at Delilah, but now that I was done with her, he sped up, harder.

"Spank me," I managed to moan as he pushed deeper and deeper into me. I reached down between my legs to touch my clit, swollen and soaking wet, as he obliged, pulling out just long enough to slap both of my ass cheeks in quick succession. The sting felt so good, and just as quickly as he had stopped, he slammed himself into me again and again. I felt his hands tangle into my hair and pull my head back—it was uncharacteristically rough for him, and when I looked up at him, I could see his gaze fixated on me. He was completely in the moment, enjoying it.

"Play with her again," he said gruffly, shoving me down toward Delilah, who was watching us with heated passion.

I grinned, feeling wetter at the thought of my husband, my usually so sweet and gentle husband, getting rough and hot and bothered by the idea of me fucking another woman. I could live with that. "My pleasure," I told him as he slowed down his fucking to let me keep my own balance.

I pulled Delilah closer to me, and she smiled up at me, her eyes begging for round two. I lined her up underneath me so that I could grind on her pelvis while I leaned down to kiss each of her perky little perfect nipples before taking one in my mouth.

I heard Matt's breathing pick up as he watched me, and I knew I needed to put on a show. Arching my back just right to bring my ass up for him, I leaned in to tug on Delilah's lips before I reached over to the nightstand next to our bed. I pulled out a toy—a large vibrator , which I quickly placed against Delilah's clit before settling my own right onto it as well, starting it on low. I gasped at the feeling, gliding my clit atop it as I watched Delilah's delicious expression on her face. It was perfect in that moment—she was so hot with her fuck-me eyes as she leaned up for a kiss, moaning against me. Matt's own tempo increased a bit, and I could feel his desperation as he fucked me harder. I heard him getting closer and closer and I pulled away from Delilah's mouth just long enough to look over my shoulder at him, making eye contact as he watched me. I turned away to suckle at Delilah's nipple again, but just as my lips grazed over the tiny little nub, he yanked my hair back.

"You'll look at me now," he practically growled, and I smirked at him. He thrust into me again, and my mouth

28

opened, head back as he took me harder. I pushed harder against the vibrator that was underneath me, reaching down to turn up the speed.

Immediately, Delilah cried out in pleasure, and I pinched her nipples a little bit harder that time, never looking away from Matt as he continued to fuck me. Any time I started to close my eyes to enjoy the moment, he pulled my hair harder and forced me to keep my eyes on him. My pussy clenched his cock tighter as he forced me. Who knew I was into him being more dominant. It wouldn't be long—I knew I wouldn't be able to last out much longer as he continued to ride me.

"You don't cum until I tell you to cum," he told her, never letting up the intensity in his gaze or his fucking. All I could do was nod in response as another wave of pleasure threatened to throw me over the edge. The vibrator was too strong for me to be able to resist for too much longer, and I shifted off of it, leaving it in place for Delilah, who was practically in her own little world, enjoying herself. As soon as I was off of the vibrator, she took it with her free hand and plunged it into herself with a moan, her back arching, and eyes closing tightly.

Matt let go of my hair, and I looked down at Delilah, grinning at my handiwork, but before I could do much more, he thrust into me again, so hard that I could hardly stand it. I whined as he got deeper and deeper, and I knew he was challenging me. He *wanted* to make this hard for me, and could I really blame him? He was reclaiming his confidence—he *needed* to do this.

I tried to fend off the impending orgasm, but before I knew it, my vagina was tightening in waves of pleasure all down his shaft, and I felt him thrust harder into me and groan as well. I rode the waves of pleasure before collapsing onto Delilah, who smiled knowingly at me before she reached up to toy with my sensitive nipples.

She didn't get to for very long before I felt Matt's hand wrap around my arm, flipping me over. "You didn't listen," he told me, his eyes shining in dark amusement. I couldn't quite tell what he thought as he looked down at me.

"Sounds like I'm in need of a punishment," I replied coyly.

"Someone's a bad girl," purred Delilah with a giggle as she gently rubbed the vibrator along my clit. It was almost too sensitive to be enjoyable in the moment.

"Are you going to help me punish her?" asked Matt, looking at Delilah. "You'll get your reward when you're done."

This new side of Matt was so incredibly hot, and in that moment, I realized that this is exactly what we were missing in our own sex life. We were missing that carnal, intense, uninhibited pleasure that we were enjoying right that moment.

Delilah giggled sensuously as she lowered herself. "It's my turn to do the licking, I think," she murmured as she ran her tongue from my nipple all around my areola before lowering herself to lick at my stomach as well. She was so gentle, and her face was so smooth, in stark contrast to the looming form of Matt as he looked over his handiwork. My entire body was glistening with sweat, and my hair, once perfectly put in place, was tousled and knotting. He loved ravaging me and he loved looking at the ravaged body he left behind.

As Delilah slowly worked her way right back up to the other nipple, I moaned in pleasure. I could feel myself getting primed for another round already. My clit was twitching to attention, and my pussy ached to be filled again. I wanted this—I wanted to be dominated and controlled.

Matt watched as Delilah played with me. He watched the young woman's perfect figure move to straddle me, placing her clit against mine before rubbing. He watched as I gasped at the sudden shift and as my back begin to arch. His own cock was already hard and ready for round two, and he rubbed it slowly to keep his hands busy as Delilah's danced all over my skin. She was everywhere as she touched me; her hands never lingered too long in any place as she rode me, watching me. I felt myself getting wetter and more eager to continue playing the more that she rode me. I felt myself vying for her, and my own hips thrust upwards to meet her.

"No," Matt said.

I looked at him in surprise. No, what? He answered my silent question almost immediately.

"Don't move, or I'll have to tie you up."

I was shocked at what he said, but it only made me hotter. It only made me want to move to make him do it, but I found myself obeying. I didn't move as Delilah continued to ride me. I fought the urge to move, and she seemed to take it as a challenge to make me fail. She removed herself from me and lowered herself down to lick my slit, tasting the amalgamation of our juices that coated me as she did. Her tongue penetrated into me, and I gasped, but still managed to avoid moving. She licked me harder and harder, quickly taking the vibrator and turning it on as well, placing it against my clit. Her other free hand squeezed my ass, her nails digging into my skin just enough to pleasantly sting as she did so.

"Mmm..." I heard myself moan, and I looked at Matt in the eyes. He admired the work that was being done above me before lowering himself down. He took Delilah in front of him, positioned her just right, and thrust into her. The motion pushed her deeper into me and I could hear her gasp as he took her. I looked up and saw them

31

fucking. He pulled her hair back, just as he had pulled mine, exposing a neck that he leaned down to nibble on before he sucked deeply onto it. I could hear the slurps as he sucked on her neck, marking her. I took a moment to catch my breath and reached down for the vibrator.

"Don't move," he repeated as he pulled Delilah back and fucked her harder. I obliged and sat there, watching him thrust his cock deeper into her, watching his balls bouncing and watching the ripples in his thighs as he held himself up and balanced them both. He was on his knees, as was she, her back arched so that he could reach her chest and her neck all at once. She moaned, eyes closed as she enjoyed the moment, and Matt maintained perfect eye contact with me as he took the vibrator that I had tried to use, turned it on, put it in place on Delilah, and finished the job.

Her head was thrown back in pleasure, mouth wide open and eyes squeezed shut. I could see her thighs tighten and contract as she came, and as soon as she was done, Matt let her go, shifting right back over to me without missing a beat or breaking eye contact.

"Don't move," he reaffirmed one last time as he watched me. "And you don't cum until I tell you to. Do you understand?"

"Yes," I breathed, watching him. My legs were quivering on their own, aching for his touch, and as soon as he spread my legs himself, I felt my breathing quicken almost immediately. I didn't move, and he thrust into me with abandon. He did not look away as he continued.

Before long, he yanked me up. "Turn around," he commanded, and I did so immediately. He pulled me into that same position to take me from behind, and got in deeply, pushing and thrusting as hard as he could into me. He pulled my hair and bit at my ear as he did so. I felt my breath gasping and felt his hands around my throat, not hard enough to completely cut off breathing, but just enough to put some pressure down as his cock reached deeper than ever before into me.

He grunted as he thrust, quicker and quicker, his shaft pulling out all but the tip of his head before thrusting it back in. "You're mine," he whispered into my ear gruffly as the pressure on my neck suddenly loosened. I had completely forgotten all about Delilah at this point, and quite frankly, I didn't care whether she was there or not. Matt shoved me down on the bed, slapping my ass with actual force behind it, so hard that I yelped, but that yelp of pain very quickly became a moan of pleasure as he buried his cock in me again, all the way to the balls. At this angle, they slapped against my clit just right, and he slammed into me, quicker and quicker.

"Cum for me now, or not at all," he told me suddenly, and he didn't have to say anything twice. As he buried his load in me, I felt myself clench all around him. I felt each thrust as he came before collapsing against me in a sweaty, exhausted heap. He pulled himself out of me and looked me over. My ass was red from the slaps, and my hair had gotten even worse. Delilah had apparently taken her leave while we were in the throes of abandon, but I was pretty sure she looked almost as disheveled as I did. I sighed, thoroughly fucked, thoroughly satisfied, and thoroughly ready for a nap.

"So, when's the next time?" Matt practically purred, running a hand up and down my arm, watching as I shivered in response. All I could do was laugh in response.

Clara's Experiment

Clara has never known what she wanted out of life. She was never very satisfied, and even though she always tried to enjoy herself, she decided that she wanted to try something new—she wanted to be dominated, and she wanted to do it with someone that she would never have to see again. Armed with the power of the internet, she finds someone to dominate her and goes for a night that she will never forget, meeting sexy, alluring Anthony in the penthouse suite of a hotel for a night of dark passion and submission that introduces her to a lifestyle she's not likely to forget anytime soon.

I looked down at my phone and saw an unbelievingly handsome face looking back at me. It was the profile for the man that I was heading to meet that evening, and I felt a pit of apprehension in my stomach. He looked like he was... Well, experienced, and it made me nervous. I had spent the night prior looking into doms online. It turns out; there are dating apps just like that. I'd never tried anything like that before, but a quick one-night stand seemed like an ample opportunity to get to know whether I'd like it or not.

The man's face was very serious. His skin was tanned, but not dark, and his gaze, intense. His profile picture showed that he meant business, I noted—it was that of someone who knew what he wanted and was not willing to let anyone else prevent him from getting that, and that was exactly what I wanted. I was curious, vaguely, about the sub life, but had never had the guts, or the opportunity, to experiment with it myself. That was, until that night.

I stood at the bottom of a tall hotel, looking up at it, my phone still in hand. It was maybe 9:30 pm on a Friday night, and I was all dressed up. My makeup was expertly applied, and I wore red pumps with a short, form-fitting red dress that was stretched practically taut over my body.

Underneath, I wore nothing—no bra, no panties, just as I had been told to do. I had to be careful when I leaned over or sit down or I'd run the risk of flashing someone, but that was a small price to pay for the pleasure I hoped to get that night. I was eager to give this a shot, that was for sure. I just had to get out and make it happen.

I took a deep breath. "Clara, get it together. You can do this!" I told myself, tightening my grasp around my phone before I stepped into the building with purpose. My head was held high and confident, despite feeling the exact opposite. I went up to the penthouse. I typed in a quick message into the dating app, informing him that I was on my way up, and I marveled at the fact that I would be setting foot into the area that would be deemed "high-class" or whatever else people say of the presidential suites in hotels. I had no idea what to expect as I made my way up the elevator to the room.

The elevator doors opened and revealed the man, Anthony, staring back at me. He was leaned against the wall, arms crossed casually, head back, and eyes glancing up and down as if trying to determine if I was worth the effort on that very night. He must have decided that I was, as he straightened up as soon as I stepped off the elevator. Did he think that I'd chicken out, maybe? Maybe he thought I'd just get right back on it and leave. Who knows? Whatever it was, though, I knew that I was in for a unique time. I had never seen anything like him before—his gaze was intense, but something in it was reassuring. I immediately felt at ease, something I had never experienced with a man before, certainly not a strange one that I had never met.

He looked at me and smirked. I was no longer standing tall—I was standing with my body relaxed as we walked. My arms were pulled in slightly... Almost submissively. He placed a hand on the small of my back, and I felt a thrilling jolt through me. I hadn't expected that at all, not that I could complain. It was nice.

Very quickly, we were inside the room, behind a closed door, and I stood, not really sure what to do next. I wasn't sure where I should be, and I looked around myself nervously. Thankfully, I didn't have to bring myself to ask. We hadn't yet exchanged a single word.

"Sit," he said. It wasn't a request—I could hear that. He wasn't yet looking at me, too busy rustling through a few things. I nodded my head to myself before moving to sit down on the bed. My head was spinning, but I obediently sat there without a care in the world. I was almost shocked at the fact that I was there without a protest, but I chose not to say a thing.

"Did you prepare yourself?" he asked. Anthony had given me several instructions—I was to be clean-shaven and without underwear when I arrived. Again, I nodded my head without a word.

He looked up to me briefly, almost questioningly. "I didn't hear you, Ellen."

Hearing my name on his lips brought a quick shiver down my spine. "Yes," I replied quietly. My voice quivered.

He stood up to full height as he looked over me, his dark eyes almost disapproving for a moment. "This is your first time," he said suddenly.

"Yes." I turned my gaze away from him.

He blinked, clearly taken aback by that. "You're... New and you were looking for partners on a dating app?" Something about the way that he said that made me feel a bit embarrassed. Had I made a mistake already? I had hoped to get everything just right.

"... Yes?"

He ran one hand through his hair, his gaze lifting off of me and focusing on something behind me as if considering something. "Look, had I known..." he began before I had to interrupt him.

"I want to learn."

"You need to learn some manners," he said with a smirk. I could see his hand tense at his hand, as if he had resisted the urge to smack me across my face. I shrank back slightly at the thought, but at the same time, I felt myself starting to get wet. I hadn't expected that, at all, but I was interested in seeing where things would go.

"I'm sorry," I told him contritely, looking at him.

"Look away," he commanded me, and I obeyed. "You have a lot of learning to do. Are you sure you want this?" In the corner of my eye, I could see that he was hard. He wanted to punish me. He wanted to discipline me and teach me what I should and should not do. But, he also didn't want to get me in for more than I expected. After all, from everything I've read, this is about consent. Consensual abuse, basically. Or at least, that's how I understood it.

"I do want this," I told him, keeping my gaze planted firmly on his feet. It felt comfortable to look there, and I was looking at his brown shoes. They looked like leather, quite nice from what I could see.

"Okay," he replied simply after a pause. "Then let's begin. Safe words..."

With all of the niceties figured out, he grinned at me. It was a dark grin on his face, one that showed that he's more interested in using me than anything else. "Strip," he told me.

I nodded my head and grabbed the hem of my dress to pull it up. As soon as it was over my head, he swatted my now-bare ass swiftly with his hand, and I yelped at the sting. It started, but it was almost... pleasant? "What's that?" he practically purred, "I can't hear you."

"Yes, sir," I told him quietly, using the manners that he had just gone over with me.

"That's better."

He watched as I removed the dress, tossing it onto the bed. I was standing there, bare naked, aside from the red heels I had on. Red was his choice—he liked his gifts wrapped in red, he had told me. I looked at his feet a bit longer, watching as they walked in a circle to get a good look at his prize for the night. I got the feeling that I was being hung up for display, like a piece of meat, but somehow, the thought of being used like that only made me even more eager to please. He pushed me over the bed to take a look at me and pulled my lips and cheeks apart, viewing my pussy. He must have grinned—I couldn't see his reaction, but he gave each cheek a slap.

"Such a naughty little whore you are, aren't you," he practically purred, running a finger over my little nub, trailing down the outside of my lips and back again.

I gasped at the touch. I hadn't expected it so quickly, and yet, there it was. His fingers were gently, delicately, tantalizingly rubbing along my inner lips, careful to avoid the slit itself. He didn't want to move too quickly. I could feel myself begin to leak more, and he chuckled behind me. He was clearly fully satisfied, and he gave me another slap on both cheeks, harder this time. I yelped, and he let go. The sound of his footsteps said that he was leaving the area and I looked tentatively over my shoulder to see what he was doing.

Anthony had gone over to get something from a drawer, and I had to admit, I was a little afraid to see what he'd bring back. Quickly, I found that he had brought back a
38

little riding crop. It smelled of leather as he put it down next to me. "You are to obey me and only me," Anthony said as he put down what looked like a strand of beads as well, and a toy that I couldn't quite tell what it was for. He grinned, but I hesitated to make eye contact with him.

"On your knees," he said suddenly, and I obliged. "Lean forward," he demanded.

I sat on the bed, on my knees, leaning forward so that my head rested against the bed. My ass was up in the air, and I felt the beads teasing at my pussy, a little at first. "Mmm," I purred as he let them go in, one at a time, inside of me. He let them all enter me and then quickly pulled them out. The feeling was shocking and unexpected and almost as good coming out as going in. I felt my pussy clench between my legs at the sudden absence of stimulation, but before I could protest, I felt him probing my asshole, gently at first.

"Have you ever had anything up here," he asked as he used what I assumed was his finger at first to poke at me. I was tight and clenching it in nervousness. I shook my head no, biting my lip and squeezing my eyes shut in anticipation for what I assumed was about to happen. "I don't hear you, slut," he said with a quick slap against my upper thigh.

"N-no, sir," I replied through clenched teeth. That had hurt, and yet, I felt myself grow wetter. I wanted this, I realized.

"Do you want it?" he asked me, and I saw him reach for the leather crop next to me.

"Yes, sir," I told him, and he snapped the crop against me. It stung, but just as quickly, he gently pulled it across the reddening skin, almost delicately, and I felt myself gasp. It moved slowly, moving to tenderly trace the outsides of my lips before gently tapping at those too. It was just enough to bring feeling there, barely brushing over them and I gasped at the sensation.

"Good," he growled, leaning over me to cup a breast that was hanging down on the bed. My nipples were brushing the sheets as he did it, and he reached up to bring them between his fingers, rolling them about until I moaned my pleasure. I loved it. I wanted it. I wanted more, and without saying a word, he obliged. He placed a couple of nipple clamps onto me, bringing a sudden gasp out of me. It was borderline painful, but another few traces around my lips and clit were enough to make me forget the pain in the moment.

He pulled my hair back, and I could see him watching me from the corner of my eyes. "Is this what you want, bitch?" he asked her, and I could see the steely amusement in his eyes. It was exactly the look I didn't know I wanted to see from him.

"Yes," I told him. He gripped my head harder. "Yes, sir!"

Anthony then took a moment to shove those beads, the beads that I had all but forgotten, into my ass, one at a time. Each bead that popped in made me gasp and shudder. Two... Three... Four... Five... My thighs were quivering, and I was barely holding myself up. The feeling was so foreign, but the weight within my ass was pleasant. I clenched around it.

"Good girl," he said with a slap, sending me gasping again. He flipped me over to look at his handiwork, and I laid there, palms up and at my head, turned to look at him from the side, and he grinned. "Good," he said, watching as my breath heaved in and out rapidly. My mouth was agape and I could feel the pressure within me building.

Without a word, he plunged his fingers inside of me, reaching up to find my g-spot, pressing against it. I shut my eyes and whined at the feeling, unable to help it as my
40

thighs shot upwards in response, begging and pleading wordlessly for more than I had already gotten.

He chuckled darkly at me. "You think you're ready for this? For me?" he purred, leaning closer. He swatted at me with the crop just under my rib cage with a smirk. He was enjoying every moment.

"Y-yes, sir," I managed to just barely breathe out. I couldn't help it. I was spilling all over his bed; I could feel the wetness when he pushed me right down onto the mattress roughly. The sight only made him hotter, and I could see his dick hardening in his pants. He released it, revealing a solid seven inches—larger than average but not overwhelming. He rubbed it along my lips, his head tracing them, but never diving into the opening.

The feeling was enough to make me shudder and hitch my breath in my chest. My nipples were aching wonderfully under the weight of the clamps, and I reached toward his hips without thinking about it, preparing to pull him in.

Anthony pulled away, swiftly swatting both hands with his crop, leaving me crying out as pain met pleasure. "You do not touch me unless I tell you to," he told me curtly. "Do you understand, slut?"

"Yes, sir," I squeak out, rubbing my hands.

"Since you can't control your hands, I'll have to control them for you. Over your head, slut," he told me, and I obeyed as he walked around me, unwilling to give me the pleasure of feeling him against me by reaching over. He clenched both of my wrists and bound them together, putting them above me and into a bond to keep them from moving. The bond clipped to something on the headboard—I couldn't quite see it, but I could feel that it pulled my arms tightly. I tried to shift up to relieve some of the pressure.

"You stay here," he told me as he walked back to the other side of the bed and between my legs, pulling my hips back down toward him. I winced at the feeling of my wrists being pulled tightly but resisted making a sound. "Good girl."

As a reward for my obedience, he shoved his dick right into me, just as I had been waiting for. He pushed every inch in quickly, not giving me the chance to adjust to his length or his girth as he slammed against me. I caught my breath in my chest and whimpered as he did it again. His balls slammed into the beads in my ass, and I couldn't help but pull away a bit, only to meet his hands roughly holding me in place.

"You will stay here and take my cock like a good girl, do you understand me?"

"Y-yes."

"Good." He pushed in harder and harder, lifting the crop to tap it against each of the nipple clamps, evoking a scream from me as my hips slammed up to meet his as he thrust again. "Good, slut, take every inch of me."

"Give me every inch," I mewled in reply, breathing heavily. I was in heaven—I could feel the pressure of the beads within me rubbing pleasurably against the pressure of his cock as he continued to whip along me. It was so good... I was getting wetter within him, and I felt myself clench up around him.

"You are not to cum yet, do you understand?"

"Yes..." I breathed out between moans of pleasure. My head was back, eyes short, but I could hear him grunting as he sped up. He kept the rhythm, hard, fast, and deep, for a moment, his own breathing starting to hitch within him as well. He sounded so sexy in the moment as he used me like the toy that I knew I was meant to be. I

42

wanted him to have me, and I let him pound me so hard that I thought I might tear under his pressure.

He groaned in pleasure as I felt his hips buck against me, leaving his load inside of me. He remained there, pushing against my hips for a few moments before he finally decided to pull away, looking at me like a piece of meat. He took a moment to catch his breath, his cock half-hard still, and shining in the dim light.

Wordlessly, he climbed up over me and dropped his balls in my face. "Lick them clean," he told me, and I obliged immediately.

I licked up every last drop of me from his balls and from his shaft, slowly and tenderly removing it. He was fully hard again by the time that I was done sucking on it and playing with it. "You have five minutes, suck me off, or you will be punished." Without a word, he set a timer and removed the restraints that had held me against the bed, though my hands were still together.

I obliged immediately, leaning down and taking as much of his girth as I could into my mouth. I lingered on the tip for a few moments, sucking it until I felt it twitch, and then I moved on to the shaft. Without my hands, I'd have to make do with just my mouth. I ran it into my throat as deeply as I could manage without choking and let my tongue squeeze against it, quickly pulling it out of my mouth and licking it from the balls up to the tip again and again.

The more that I sucked on him, the more I felt him twitching in my mouth and tried my best, but the timer came and went, and he flipped me over onto my back. He swatted me with the crop four times, hard this time, and I cried out at the feeling dancing. I was certain that the skin was welted at that point. "Nice try, but you failed," he told me as my eyes watered from the smarting welts underneath me.

"I'm sorry, sir," I told him, wincing. All I wanted at that point was to finish. I was going insane, feeling the weight of the beads within me, and I was getting desperate.

"Your punishment," he told me, "is that you will be fucked without being allowed to cum, do you understand me?"

"Yes, sir," I said back, despite feeling like I wanted to protest. It was almost like my body and mind wanted two different things. He slammed his cock into me again, once again hard, and he worked me up, slamming in harder and harder. He could feel me getting close and pulled out just before I was able to cum, leaving me collapsing against the bed, frustrated.

"What's wrong?" he asked, leaning over me with that same smirk on his face. "Frustrated?"
"No, sir."

"Oh, I see," he said, prying my legs apart. He lowered his head to lick at my clit, his tongue dancing gently around the protected little nub. He licked up and down it slowly, sensually, watching as my body tensed up in response. He lowered his tongue to dance on the outside of my lips, teasing the entrance just barely with a flick of his tongue before bringing it right back up to the top again. He sucked on the little nub, his tongue dancing on and around it as he did. His finger snaked up to penetrate me, slowly pushing into me as he did. He looked up at me from his place, eating at me and watched as my back arched and I moaned loudly in pleasure. I couldn't take it... I felt the pressure building up, and I didn't think that I could hold it back anymore...

And he pulled away. He looked at me from his position and stood up over me.

"The little slut doesn't deserve to finish tonight after failing me," he told me with a quick swat of the crop
44

against my skin, leaving me wanting desperately without anything to relieve myself. I groaned as I fell down onto the bed, and he smirked again.

"Then again... You are a new little slut, aren't you? Do you want to beg for release?"

"Please," I said suddenly, my voice pleading. My pussy was dripping and empty, and I wanted something—anything—in it.

"Please, what?"

"P-please fuck me," I cried out in desperation.

"What's that?"

"Sir, please, fuck me sir!" I moaned, fighting the urge to reach for him. My body couldn't take the buildup any longer, and before I could say another word, he pushed himself into me again. I gasped, shuddering at the feeling. It was exactly what I needed, and I writhed on the bed, thrusting my body against his.

"Cum for me, slut," he commanded firmly.

I felt my body oblige immediately. I felt the clench of pressure in my pussy as it gripped against his dick. I felt the waves of release that I had been waiting for all evening, giving way around him, over and over, for what felt like forever as he finished within me. I felt his release alongside mine, and he pulled himself out of me.

My breathing was heavy, and I was exhausted beyond belief, eyes still closed. My whole body ached pleasantly under the strain and release. I felt the nipple clamps release off of me, and I looked up to see Anthony watching me. He smirked self-satisfied. "Now, get out of my sight, you slut. I'll see you tomorrow."

He didn't even have the courtesy to ask—just assumed that I'd be back again. He wasn't wrong.

Amelia's Punishment

Amelia is a housekeeper that has a strange job. Every
week, she's asked to come over and clean, wearing a
skimpy outfit for a man that rarely ever says more than a
word or two to her at a time. She cleans the spotless
surfaces for the money but finds herself getting paid more
than she ever thought she could ask for when she
accidentally drops a crystal glass and needs to be
punished for her transgressions by her sexy boss, Mr.
Erikson, who wants nothing more than to rip her skimpy
little outfit off of her and ravish her body.

Even though the area was always immaculately clean, I
was still always asked to come over every week to dust,
wipe, and polish anything that I found on the shelves. It
was mildly humiliating; Mr. Erikson required me to wear
this skimpy little maid's outfit that barely covered my ass
cheeks, but let's be real here for a moment—I *loved*
having my cheeks hang out. Sometimes, if Mr. Erikson,
the fine specimen of a man that he was, was looking my
direction, I'd intentionally stand up on my tippy toes to
reach out to some imagined hard to reach area *just* to give
him a flash of my ass. No panties. That part was all me,
not him. I imagine that he'd get hard at his desk, hidden
behind the wooden surface, as I reached up. I imagined
that he'd let his eyes slowly take me in as stretched. I
imagined that he was an ass man, based on the fact that
mine was just barely covered, but to be fair, my dress
barely covered my tits either—it pushed them up, almost
uncomfortably tight, to create a huge cleave down my
front as they were smashed together. I looked good, that
was for sure, and I always had to wonder if he only
wanted me here so that he could have some eye candy.
After all, there were rarely any real messes for me.

I was busy scrubbing some invisible splotch on the wall,
over and over, slowly just rubbing my towel on the wall.
Sometimes, I'd sit there and sensually begin to clean

objects, suggestively running my fingers up and down the length of an ornate crystal decanter filled with amber liquid. It was rum, maybe, or brandy or whiskey. I never opened it up, but I did know that the amount of liquid in the bottle was always changing from week to week when I did my rounds, so it must have been for more than just decoration.

That day, I could feel Mr. Erikson watch me with mild disinterest as if I weren't there. His gaze would drift over to me, and I'd feel tension in the air, but he must have been distracted. It was like he saw right through me as his eyes caressed my legs, lazily going up and down their lengths, but his mind was clearly elsewhere. I'd have to try harder if I wanted him to actually look at me. The idea of a challenge made my pussy twinge in anticipation. We never fucked or anything. In fact, we never even touched or said more than just a few terse words to each other, but the tension in the air was palatable. I bet Mr. Erikson could have cut the tension with his dick. I knew he liked watching me; the bulge that he had in his pants the few times he walked by, unabashedly unconcealed, told me that much.

I'd have to try harder; I told myself if I wanted to win that day. I wanted that sexual tension to build up so much that I could hardly take it. I'd never actually initiate; the job paid too well to just be eye candy. But, I'd be lying if I said that I didn't regularly think about throwing myself on the desk and begging him to take me on more than one occasion.

As I worked on cleaning up the wall, then, I let the rag slip out of my hand to the floor. Honest mistake, right? I bent down, keeping my knees straight, revealing myself to Mr. Erikson. Considering the clattering of his pen that I heard, he must have seen it all, and I smirked, feeling another twitch in my pussy. My clit was starting to swell, and I could feel the fluids beginning to soak everything. Slowly, I straightened up without a word, discarding the rag and getting a clean one, and I moved on to polishing

48

the glasses that matched the decanter. They were smooth and felt hefty in my hand, the cool crystalline surface shining brilliantly in the light of the office. The office was kept dark most of the time, curtains drawn and warm lamps on creating just enough light for Mr. Erikson to do whatever it was that he did at his desk. I wasn't sure what he did—I had never thought to ask him, nor did I really care. We didn't talk much. My job was to clean everything and I was not allowed to leave for the whole two hours that I was paid to be there to clean it. At first, the two hours seemed to drag on forever, but our unspoken game made the time fly by when I wasn't paying attention to it. I gently placed the glass back down and picked up the next one, polishing that one as well. I would imagine that they were his cock, hard and smooth in my hand, as the towel rubbed up and down, polishing even the bottom of it. My fingers would linger, rubbing sensually on the crystal surface. I'd do them one by one before putting them perfectly down where they had been before. As I reached to put the last glass down, it slipped from my hand and clattered as it fell onto the ground, thankfully onto a rug. I froze when I realized what happened.

"Amelia?" I heard him speak—he never spoke if he could avoid it.

"Yes, sir?" I managed to force myself to say, my voice shaking. I was shocked that I had made such a mistake—I was usually so careful with what I did. It was highly abnormal for me to make mistakes like that. Everything was calculated and planned out, but I had gotten careless.

I heard Mr. Erikson's chair move out from behind his desk, and I could hear the rustling of his clothing as he stood up. He was looking right at me, but I couldn't bring myself to even look at him. I had done it now! I knew I'd be fired on the spot—I'd heard rumors in the house that he was always firing the house staff if they didn't exceed his expectations! I groaned inwardly.

49

"Amelia." He was firmer this time as my name escaped his lips, sending a shiver down my spine. Despite the concern for being fired, I *still* wanted him. Hell—half of me hoped he'd bend me over the desk and spank me for my punishment and let me get back to work.

I forced my eyes to slowly shift over to him; my gaze slowly drifting across his body from the ground up. When I made it to his cock, my eyes widened, seeing it swollen and bulging against his pants, threatening to destroy the zipper if it wasn't freed soon. His pants were black, crisply ironed and somehow, without a single wrinkle in them, despite working at a desk. He was toned—or at least, I assumed he was toned by the shape of his arms when he'd work, bulging and rippling. He clearly exercised regularly. When I finally raised my gaze to meet his own icy cool one, I was greeted with the sight of a barely perceptible smirk. If I didn't know him better, and to be frank, I barely knew him at all; I'd say that he was giving me bedroom eyes—you know the kind that says that you're ready to throw the person onto the bed and fuck their brains out kind of eyes.

And it made me so hot.

"You've been a naughty girl, Amelia," he said, his voice quiet and in control as he looked me over. I was shrinking into myself, making myself as small as possible. My arms were crossed in front of me, pushing my breasts up further in their skimpy little covering that could hardly be considered covered in the first place.

"I'm sorry sir," I managed to squeak out in response.

And he chuckled. It was a dark chuckle, sensuous as he looked me over like he was considering something. "You better be." Something about the veiled threat sent a thrill running down my spine. "Do you know what we do to naughty girls around here, Amelia?"

"N-no sir." I had some high hopes, though.

"They are punished according to their crimes. Do you know why that glass is always here?"

"No..."

"No, what?"

"No, sir."

"Good girl." He smirked, one brow raising up as he did. He was checking me out. "That was my late father's set. It is irreplaceable."

I hadn't realized, and suddenly, I felt bad. It wasn't broken; somehow, it had managed to land on a rug and didn't break, thankfully, but I still felt *awful*. "What is my punishment, sir?" My gaze was firmly on his feet at this point. I couldn't explain it, but all of my confidence that I had had just moments prior had all melted away.

"You need a spanking, Amelia." I heard him cracking his knuckles then, and I looked up at him in surprise. His dick was harder than ever, judging by the fact that his pants had somehow become even tauter than they had been just moments prior, and I looked at him in awe. Was he going to fuck me? I kind of hoped he did. My fear melted away as he beckoned for me to move closer to him, and I did it without a single protest.

Suddenly, I felt his hands wrap around my wrist and pull me close. I could smell his aftershave; he smelled clean and strong with a hint of subtle spiciness, and I loved it. His fingers on my skin were strong and warm, firm, but not painful, and he placed his other hand on the small of my back, wordlessly telling me to bend over, and I did, my body resting atop his desk. He was strong and firm; I couldn't help but want to obey, even as I felt the first sting of his strong, warm hand hitting my bare ass. I squealed in surprise, bucking back at the sudden surprise of the movement, sending a pen holder clattering to the ground. I tried to pull away, but he firmly pressed into the small of my back. He wanted me to stay there.

"You've been such a naughty girl," he practically purred in my ear, his voice low and husky. I could hear the desperation in it. He wanted this just as much as I did. I didn't protest as I felt his hand slowly rubbing over my ass, giving it a firm squeeze as he did. Then both hands groped at me, pulling my cheeks apart. "You have such a tight little ass," he marveled under his breath. "I'm going to make it mine."

I gasped as he pressed his cock against me. It was hard and larger than I had thought in his pants. He leaned over me, letting his hands slide up my whole body from my ass, up my back, and sliding around my waist and up higher to grasp my tits, squeezing them tightly. He fondled them, letting his hand squeeze a bit tighter than I had expected. With the weight of him atop me, I felt my heart pounding in my chest, and I gasped. I fought the urge to turn my head to kiss him. I was so wet at that point. I'm sure it was soaking through his pants as he continued to grind his cock against me. I could feel myself practically dripping between my thighs as he kneaded at my nipples, slipping his fingers into the tight top of the dress. He didn't even bother fighting with it; he just tore it off, literally tearing down the front, and I didn't say a word. It was almost hotter to see the display of strength as he did it.

With my breasts free, he pulled at them before pulling back. Then, unexpectedly, I felt another slap against my ass. It was strong, and it was painful, almost immediately. I cried out at the sudden impact, but it was more in shock than anything else.

"What a naughty, dirty little slut you are," he breathed in my ear as he leaned over me again. "You're dripping." His breath on my neck sent shivers down my spine, and I

52

turned my head just slightly, granting him access to do whatever he wanted to it, and he obliged. His lips fell on my neck and I felt his tongue dance across my skin before he nipped and nibbled. He wasn't rough enough to hurt, but I was sure I'd need to wear a scarf for the next few days.

He pulled back, and again, I felt another slap on my ass, but this time, he didn't pull his hand away. He let his hand linger against my skin. "Do you like your punishment?" His fingers slid closer to my slit, close enough to feel my wetness all over them.

"Yes, sir," I breathed out, tensing up and pushing my ass out just enough to try to encourage him to enter me. He pulled his fingers away from me, teasing the lips with the lightest of touches. He wasn't going to let me enjoy things that easily.

"Good. I don't tolerate little dirty sluts that don't know their place. You're going to learn your lesson tonight, do you hear me?"

"Yes, sir." I felt him let go of my ass and slap me again, and I cried out at the strange immersion of pain and pleasure as he did it.

Mr. Erikson flipped me over onto his desk and lifted me up as if I weighed nothing, setting me down atop it to get a full view of his handiwork. He looked at my breasts, no longer covered up by the black fabric that was in tatters around my waist, as if considering something, and then tore it all the way off. "You don't need this, do you?"

I shook my head breathlessly, in awe at the strength of the man in front of me. He leaned over me, his hands resting on either side of my legs, his nose so close that I could have touched it just by leaning forward. The urge to kiss him grew harder, and I leaned in to do it, only to feel his hand pulling my hair back to stop me. I squealed and looked up at him.

"You do not touch me. I touch you. You are here for me."

"Yes, sir," I said, trying not to struggle against the tugging on my hair.

He released my hair and pushed me down onto the desk, unzipping his pants and releasing the largest cock I had ever seen. No wonder his pants looked so tense against the heft of it. He pushed it against me, and I could feel it, hot and pulsating against my thigh. He rubbed it on me, up and down, and I could feel it gliding over me. The rubbing on me seemed to turn him on more, and he suddenly rammed it straight inside of me without hesitation.

I felt his big cock fill me up until I felt like I couldn't possibly expand any further, and yet, he kept pushing it in, forcing it deeper until I wondered if I would split in half. He held it there, tense and deep within me, and I realized he still hadn't gone all the way.

"Your wet pussy is so tight," he growled in my ear. He gyrated his hips just enough to press against my inner walls, and I moaned in pleasure. It was a tight fit, but that made it even better. I clenched against him as he slowly pulled himself out, and he thrust in again and again. "I will ravish this pussy tonight, do you hear me?"

I could barely manage to speak at the feeling of his cock rubbing against me. It was like a dream come true—I had fantasized about this moment so much, and here it was, happening.

"Amelia. Do. You. Hear. Me." He thrust in deeply between each and every word he said, making me moan every single time. I was breathing heavily, looking up at him, my mouth agape. I could hardly control myself enough to speak.

"Y-yes, sir," I managed to breathe between thrusts. His cock was better than I could have possibly imagined.

"Do you want me to take this pussy?"

"Yes!" I cried out, throwing my head back, bracing myself against the desk. He reached out and grabbed my breasts, weighing them in his hands. He was rough, but not hurtful as he ran his thumbs over my nipples, tracing circles right around them with the pads of his thumbs resting right onto them. My eyes were shut, enjoying the sensations of my body as he continued to thrust within me. I could feel the tension building up in pleasurable waves as he occasionally flicked and twisted at my nipples between thrusts.

I could feel myself getting close, and my breathing hitched in my chest as he continued to thrust inside of me. He would go faster and slower. Sometimes, he would almost tenderly and slowly pull it out and push it back in, other times, he would thrust his cock into me so rapidly that he had to hold me in place so I wouldn't fall off of the desk.

More items clamored to the floor, landing near the torn and discarded maid's costume. Just when I thought I wouldn't be able to take it any longer, he pulled out of me, looking at me in dark amusement. He was enjoying taking charge. "You're not cumming 'til I tell you that you can," he informed me as he flipped me over and pushed me back. I was standing on the floor now, on my tiptoes, and my arms and torso were stretched out across the surface of the desk. He spanked me again, hitting atop an area that had already been swatted earlier, and it stung enough to make me hiss in pain, but before I could protest, his cock was right back inside of me, making me forget all about the stinging.

He stayed there for just a moment or two, and as soon as I could feel myself getting close again, he stopped. "You're such a dirty little wench, aren't you, getting close already? Control yourself." He took my hand this time and led me to a door in the back of his office that I had never entered before. As soon as he opened the door, he revealed that there was a large, walk-in closet, but it was entirely devoid of any hangers or jackets, or even office supplies. Instead, there was a large, thick pole that went from wall to wall, and there were restraints suspended for it, thick and black and appearing strong enough to hold someone up. I hesitated, looking at it, but felt Mr. Erikson's cock against my back, wet and chilled by the ambient air. It pressed against me firmly, ushering me to enter, and I did, slowly turning around to look at him. Now we were in uncharted territory for me, but I wasn't sure that I really cared. I wanted this man's cock in me as hard as it could be to get me off as soon as possible and he seemed to sense that based on the fervor with which he wrapped his fingers around my delicate wrists and tied me up. It wasn't so bad; I told myself as I felt the restraints. They were tight against my wrist, but they didn't hurt. They held my hands right above my head and kept me from being able to move them too much, but it was okay with me. I didn't mind—until suddenly, he tightened the restraints and I felt my arms being yanked upward. I had to stand on my toes to keep the pressure from getting to be too much for me.

Mr. Erikson looked over my body carefully, eyeing my tits and my hips and the dip between them. He spread my lips between my legs and smirked as he did. "You've quite the body here. Why have you teased me so much with it?" His gaze flitted to mine for a fleeting instant, and I saw that intense desire burning within them. I smirked back, but just as quickly as I did, I felt a quick stinging across my thighs as he slapped them. I could see the handprints welting immediately.

"Did you want me?" he asked me after a moment.

56

"I did, sir," I replied, licking my lips slowly. I could see him watching me do it. I wanted him to want me right that moment so that we could fuck more. I stood up taller, thrusting out my chest, hoping that he'd give in and take me right then and there.

He ran his fingers up and down my thighs before slipping them between my legs, reaching up to touch that tiny nub folded away in my lips. He touched my clit, and I felt my legs immediately begin to quiver. I moaned softly at the contact, my hips thrusting. I felt his fingers trail further downward, and he traced my slit, pushing against it, but never actually penetrating me. His fingers slid further back than that, too—his fingers danced around my asshole, pressing on it. His finger, still wet with my juices, penetrated just slightly, slowly making its way into me. "Have you ever been fucked here before?"

"N-no sir," I gasped out as he pushed his finger deeper into me. I felt my muscles contract around his finger, and he put a second finger in as well, moving it in and out. After a few moments, he added in a third as well, gently penetrating just enough to get the muscles used to it. I felt myself starting to relax as he continued, and the sensation excited me further. The feelings of pleasure bloomed, and I found myself loving it, and then his fingers pulled out altogether.

I felt a dildo, larger than his fingers, thrust into my slit, pushing and twisting it deeper and deeper, and I felt the pleasure begin to build up even more. My pussy was swelling with anticipation as the sensations grew stronger, and he pulled the toy out, immediately pressing it against my ass again before slowly easing the toy in. "We'll have to work up to my cock. I wouldn't want to tear you in half," he said with a smirk as he slid the toy into me. I was on my tiptoes still, desperately trying to keep my legs from giving out underneath me as the pleasure threatened to overcome me, and just as quickly as it had started, he pulled it out and removed the restraints. I practically collapsed under the weight of myself, but he caught me and lowered me to the ground, positioning me on my hands and knees with my ass in the air. He pumped his cock into me a few times, lubricating himself with my own fluids, of which there was no shortage, before easing himself into my ass. His cock was massive, and I didn't think that it would fit, but still, it plunged deeper and deeper. I threw my hand backward with a moan of pleasure, and he wrapped his hand around me, reaching for my throat. He put pressure on it as he fucked me harder, not enough to cut off my windpipe, but just enough to elevate the sensation as he continued. He thrust harder and harder into my ass, and I could feel him getting harder inside my tight ass until finally, he groaned in pleasure, thrusting deeply and holding me there as he released his cum into me before pulling out slowly.

"Hold that cum in you. Don't let a drop fall out," he told me as he stood up, straightening out his tie and fixing his pants. I stayed on my hands and knees as he cleaned himself up, clenching my ass and feeling endlessly frustrated. He flipped me over. "Now, I can see that the dirty slut didn't finish with my cock, is that so?"

"Yes, sir," I told him, feeling the ache growing more than before. I wanted to fuck still, but he had other plans. He smirked at me. "Make your dirty pussy cum for me, but don't lose a drop of what I left in you," he commanded, crossing his arms and leaning back. I was taken aback by the command, but it wasn't the worst thing in the world. It would be the perfect way to entice him back for another round later. After all, I worked there several times a month.

I reached around, still on my hands and knees, using one hand to gently touch myself. I felt just how wet I was; I was practically dripping. My ass was still up in the air, and Mr. Erikson got the full view of my fingers, gently caressing my lips and rubbing on my clit as I did. I ran my fingers over the opening slowly at first, then pressed them

58

in, one at a time, moaning sensually as they penetrated me. I reached in deeper, angling my fingers upward, touching at my g-spot within me, and I felt my hips thrust themselves in pleasure. I ran my fingers in deeper and deeper into myself, feeling every clench of my inner walls, every time I tightened and every shudder, and finally, within moments, I felt the pleasure welling up within me. I could feel the climax peaking, threatening to erupt, until it finally exploded, sending my hips and my vagina into spasms around my fingers, tensing up tighter and tighter, over and over again.

As the pleasure subsided, leaving my body pleasantly buzzing, I slowly pulled my fingers out from within me and looked at Mr. Erikson, who was watching with great interest, and I slowly licked my fluids off of myself. I sucked them clean, never breaking eye contact with him, even when I could see his pants start to tighten around his crotch again. "I can't wait for you to punish me again. I might have to even do some naughty things on purpose next time," I practically purred as I stood up to look at him.

He smirked back at me. "I'll just have to punish you harder next time."

Unwrapped Gifts

Nora loves her boyfriend and wants to give him a present for his birthday that he'll never forget, so she wraps herself up with her best friend for as long as she can remember, Becca, and sets herself up for some steamy action for Jared, happy to give him a day that he'll remember for years to come. Together, the naughty women enjoy themselves a little too much and leave him aching for more and looking for as much of a fuck as he can get. The lucky guy gets to unwrap two presents at once and enjoy every moment of it.

It was Jared's birthday, and I had a big plan in store for him. It was going to be the greatest birthday of his life, and he had no idea yet. I grinned at my friend, Becca, who was next to me. She was drop-dead gorgeous. She had naturally auburn hair that fell in waves and the greenest eyes that I had ever seen, and her lightly tanned skin was dusted with freckles right atop her perfectly sculpted cheekbones that sat high. She was wearing sultry makeup that day, her eyes shadowy and perfectly done, and she had a skintight, short dress with a deep v plunge, showing off the perfect cleavage she had.

Becca was my best friend and had been for years. She was someone that I was willing to share just about anything with—and I mean *anything*. As we smirked at each other, we knew that we were in for quite the night. I reached out to touch her arm, and she looked at me for a moment. "Are you sure about this, Nora?"

"Of course! It can't be too bad, can it? Besides, don't you remember our experimental phase in college?" It was true—we had been quite willing to explore each other's bodies and the wonders that they brought with each other when we were roommates, especially after a few nights of too many drinks.

She smiled widely, her eyes sparkling. She knew I had a point, but it wasn't every day that you fuck your best friend with your boyfriend. She put a hand on my back gently, and I hugged her. We would have a good time, that much I was sure of. I just had to be willing to actually do it, and I was sure that, in the moment, the look on Jared's face when he realizes that his birthday gift is literally his dream, being able to fuck two women at once, he would love every moment of it.

"What do you say we pre-game a bit?" asked Becca, looking at me through her lashes, her lips tugging upwards just slightly. She raised one brow as she did, waiting for my response. That didn't sound like that bad of an idea, I told myself. Besides, watching me get it on with a girl was another one of his biggest fantasies, and he was due to be home any time now.

I leaned in toward Becca, planting a kiss on her lips gently, and as I pulled back, she dove in for more. She pulled me in greedily, savoring the taste of my lips as she bit onto them, her tongue skating across them as she sucked. Her eyes were closed as she enjoyed herself, moaning against my lips. Her hand snaked around my neck, wrapping itself into my hair to hold me in place tightly in her passion. We weren't in love or anything, but who said a couple of girls couldn't platonically enjoy their body together in peace?

I reached up toward her breasts, feeling them gently with my palms. Her nipples hardened underneath the weight of my hand, pressing against my skin, and I could tell that she liked it by the way she kissed harder. Her hands twisted in my hair and one of her hands dropped down to rub on the outside of my own dress, right on my crotch area. We were careful not to mess each other up too much—we were all dressed up for Jared to unwrap. But, we could still tease each other and that we were doing.

Becca's breasts were so soft under my hand. Seriously, women's tits were like nature's greatest stress balls. The more I played with her, and the more she rubbed up against me, the less nervous I became. I found myself stroking her thighs, up and down, letting my fingers skate across the smooth, perfectly waxed surface. I was on her inner thigh, feeling the softness and the warmth emanating from just above. I could smell her moistness, soft, sweet, feminine, and carnal all at once, and it just made me want to play with her more. I let my fingers sneak their way up her dress to rub against the thin fabric of her panties. They were lace, and they weren't doing much at all to contain the juices that were beginning to flow. They were damp already, and I was able to slip my finger around them to touch the waxed pussy that was waiting for me. She was so warm and so soft under my fingers, and as soon as I let them graze over the lips between her legs, I felt Becca's kissing grow more desperate. Her pelvis tensed and her hips thrust forward, and I felt her legs spread apart just enough to let my had have more access. I reached up to touch her clit, rubbing it gently and tracing circles around it. I could feel it twitching and throbbing under my finger, telling a tale of how much she was enjoying the moment. Her breath caught in her chest and suddenly, she was practically silent and still, feeling my touch.

I reached my other hand to knead at her breast, rubbing it in between my fingers as I did. She loved every moment of it, and she couldn't hide it, even if she wanted to. I smiled as I slammed into her lips again, letting my tongue slip between her lips to taste hers this time. My fingers rubbed up against her over and over again before finally slipping inside of her. Her pussy was so tight against my fingers as I pushed in, feeling her inner walls clench against me. She wanted me to push into her, and I did, over and over again. I pushed harder and harder until I could feel her practically writhing underneath the weight of my hand.

62

She was so tight with my fingers in her, and I plunged deeper, twisting my fingers within her. I could feel her body begin to tense up more and more until I made her cum with a loud moan, head thrown back and hair draped down, exposing her long, slender neck as the waves of pleasure shook her body.

I kissed against her neck as I waited for the waves to subside, and when they did, she looked at me lustily, grinning. Her hair was mussed, but it just made her look hotter. She leaned over me, pinning me to the wall, ready to return the favor as she pushed her fingers around the tiny black thong I was wearing and stroking my clit. The sensation zapped throughout me, earning a throaty moan, and she pressed harder. She was touching me harder, tugging at my hair with her other hand so that she could wrap her lips around my neck and suck on the skin.

Her fingers expertly stroked over my clit as it swelled and pulsed until a finger slid into me. She curled her fingers up, and I felt myself tightening up as she stroked the inside of my pussy walls. I felt myself gyrate my hips, pushing her hand deeper. "You feel so good," I whispered to her between deep breaths as she teased me more and more. I wanted her deeper as I pushed against her hand, and she obliged, reaching her other hand to grope at my breasts instead, teasing my nipple underneath her fingers. I was practically whimpering at that point as she continued to fuck me with her fingers. Her mouth nibbled and licked at my neck and my ears as her fingers continued to knead me through the cloth. My body was shaking underneath the weight of her body and before I knew it, I was cumming around her fingers, feeling the pleasure overcome me for what felt like forever.

When I finally regained my senses, I opened my eyes to look at Becca, only to see Jared with an awestruck face right behind her. He had dark hair and skin, and his eyes were nearly black, but in the moment, he was slack-jawed, and I could see the erection growing in his pants. Who knew how long he had been watching, but he had certainly liked what he had seen enough to let us continue, completely uninterrupted.

Becca, seeing my focus shifted somewhere else, turned around to see what had caught my attention and smiled her sexiest smile, leaning forward and putting her hands in front of herself, clasped together so that her breasts were squeezed and pushed up. "Happy birthday, birthday boy!" she purred as she leaned over to run a hand up and down his chest, just as we had planned.

"We've got a great day in store for you," I chimed in, leaning over and planting a kiss right on his face, letting my hands slide down to rub against his hard cock in his pants. I unbuttoned him right there. "I'll unwrap you first so you can unwrap your gift." His pants were quickly discarded, as was his shirt, leaving him there, naked and wonderfully toned, not unlike a Greek statue—the ones where every single bulge is in the right spot. But this statue had one extra part—a long, rock-hard cock that was ready for action. I touched it, feeling it twitch underneath the touch.

He looked at me and then at Becca, and it finally seemed to register. "Really, babe?" he asked, and I nodded in response with a sly smile. I was glad that he seemed eager to enjoy his gift, and I took him by the hand and led him to our bedroom. We had a king bed so there was plenty of room for anything that we wanted to do. We could both lay together there no problem, even with Becca. We weren't exactly big women by any means; we were both maybe 5' even and petite, in perfect contrast to Jared's 6' and muscular build.

As we got into bed, I felt Jared's hand slap my ass, and I squealed and giggled in response. We were definitely in
64

for a fun time. "What do you want us to do?" I asked him in my sweetest voice. "We'll do *anything*." I really emphasized that last word, letting it hang with a suggestive waggle of my eyebrows that got him to chuckle to himself.

"Anything?"

"Anything," we both replied, hoping that he wouldn't come up with some off-the-wall answer about what it was that he actually did want. We waited for him quietly, looking at each other.

"Striptease," came his reply after what felt like forever.

We grinned. We could do that. And so, we did. I reached over to Becca, letting my hand rub along her neck as I grasped the lining of her dress before pulling it over her head, revealing her naked body for Jared to see. I looked at her—she had gone braless, which explained exactly why I had been able to feel her nipples so easily, and I tossed her shirt aside, looking at the beautiful, pink circles in the center of her breasts. I wanted to suck on them, and I leaned in to plant the lightest of kisses on each nipple, watching them stand to attention after doing so before letting Becca do the same to me. My dress was also discarded, but my thong and bra were left on.

"Remove her panties with your teeth," Jared told me suddenly, and I'm not going to lie—that caught me off guard. But, I did it anyway, leaning in closely to Becca's leg and sensually rubbing along the skin before reaching up with my mouth to wrap myself around the lace. I could smell her arousal; she was dripping even more now than she was before as I pulled the panties down carefully with my teeth, getting a glimpse of her perfect bare ass. Seriously, Becca was a goddess of a woman.

"Play with each other some more," commanded Jared, and we both obliged immediately. After all, he *was* the birthday boy—what he wanted, he would get. We just had to be willing participants for his every whim. Becca took charge first, leaning over me on the bed. Her perfect, perky tits hung over my face, tantalizingly teasing with every movement she made. I reached up to caress her nipples, and she leaned down to remove my bra, tossing it to the floor with abandon. She leaned down, looking up at Jared and holding his gaze as she kissed each of my nipples and let her tongue snake out of her mouth, licking the areolas, careful not to ever touch the nipple itself. She teased around the nipple, leaving it erect and longing. It felt good, but I found myself desperate for her touch, my own arousal growing with each and every lazy circle around the top of my breast. She moved to the other, slowly circling around the nipple again, leaving me breathless. She let her breath linger over it, watching as Jared stroked himself to us.

He loved his private show, his cock hard and long in his hand as he slowly, almost lazily, went up and down its shaft. I watched him touch himself and felt myself get wetter at the thrill of knowing that we were driving him crazy with every movement we made.

Becca slid down, kissing my taut stomach as she made her way down to my crotch little by little, she kissed the mound at the top. She let her tongue taste me, but only tracing the outer lips of my labia, driving me insane. I felt my hips thrusting of their own accord, silently betting her to touch, and I could feel the wetness beginning to accumulate, and then be licked up greedily by Becca's swift tongue.

She teased me up more and more, knowing that she was driving me crazy. I always loved being licked up and down, and she knew that more than anyone else—but I still was denied.

And just as quickly as it began, it stopped as Jared came over to get between us. His cock was hard in his hand, and I could see the desire in his eyes as he looked at both of us, almost as if choosing which one of us he wanted to get to fuck first. His eyes rested on me as if waiting for my approval, and when I nodded my head, he turned to Becca and grabbed her shoulder, spinning her around. Her eyes widened for a moment, but she didn't protest as he pushed her to the bed.

He rubbed his cock on her clit, and I could see her pleasure clear as day as she moaned, head back before he pushed deep into her with a hard thrust. He was quick with his thrusts, going as deep as possible. His balls slapped against her ass over and over, and he let out a groan of pleasure as he reached forward to greedily paw at her breasts, holding them in his hand and squeezing.

Just as quickly as he started fucking her, he reached over to grab me and pull me over next to her. He pushed his hands inside of me as well, letting his rough fingers penetrate deeply and stroke my inner walls as he tried to please me as well. He had one hand on Becca's breast, his cock deep in her, and his other hand inside of me as I reached down to touch my clit as well, with another hand on my breast, tugging at my nipples.

He fucked harder and harder into Becca until her moans of pleasure became cries of utter ecstasy, so loud that if we had been in an apartment, I would have worried about neighbors hearing us. He fucked deeper and deeper into her, focusing on the sensation, his fingers slipping out from me and shoved into her face, which she happily lapped up, taking my taste into her mouth and sucking on them. He groaned again with one last thrust, shaking as he came deep in her. Judging by her face and sudden silence, she finished as well.

Jared pulled himself out of her and turned to me. "I'm not done with you yet," he told me with a sound that told me that he was serious. He leaned over me, towering over my small body. He grasped my breast and let his fingers return to my clit, gently grazing over the swollen little nub that was desperate for attention and release. My breathing got quicker as he touched me, and my hips thrust into him. I wanted him—bad. I pulled him against me, and he lowered his head to lick at my clit instead, first circling around it before finally flattening his tongue and pressing against it, rubbing and licking it until I couldn't take it any longer.

Just before I could get over the edge, he pulled away, leaving me ultimately disappointed as I looked up at him. He smirked. "Not so fast. I want to really enjoy my gift," he told me as he let his cock just barely touch the outside of my slit, driving me wild. I pushed up, hoping he'd give in, but he pulled back even further. He flipped me over onto my back and positioned me just right so that he could slam in from behind.

He thrust deeper and deeper into me, pushing further from behind. He was rubbing up against my inner walls. He pulled my head back, hooking my mouth with his fingers. I could taste myself on him, or maybe it was Becca on his fingers, either way, I let him pull me further and further back against him, letting myself get lost in the moment. I loved every moment of the fucking as his cock went deeper into me than I thought was possible.

"Do you like that?" he grunted as I moaned in ecstasy, pushing my ass up and slamming it against him to get him in me as deep as possible. I wanted him to fuck me harder.

"Yes," I gasped out between moans of pleasure. "Harder," I told him, and he obliged instantly. He let go of my head and slapped my ass, yanking my hair this time as he rode me. I felt him getting harder within me as he grew rougher. "Harder!" I cried out again.

He stopped and flipped me over again, looming over me, his cock ready for more action. He slapped at my thighs, leaving red welts on them before turning to slap me across the face. "I'll fuck your cunt harder," he told me as he thrust in deeper. I was in total ecstasy, feeling the waves of pleasure continue to rise up. He fucked and fucked until the lines between pain and pleasure were blurred, and I found myself succumbing to another wave of pleasure overcoming my whole body. I convulsed against his cock, once, twice, three times, and tightened up around him, moaning loudly. I could hardly think in the moment, and he pulled out.

"Done already?" He shoved his cock in my face. "Suck it."

I obliged, still trying to catch my breath. I sucked his cock into my mouth, tasting my cum all over it as my tongue slid down the shaft. I forced it down my throat deeply and sucked and sucked. I looked up at him and moaned against his cock, letting him feel my tongue near his head, and lingered on the frenulum. I lifted my hands to his cock and rubbed with them too, pulling down with my hands as I pulled my head and tongue back. I used the tip of my tongue to swirl around the head of his cock as I sucked, letting him hear my slurping.

He seemed to be loving it, as pretty soon, I could feel his hips starting to tense up. He wasn't going to last much longer. I watched him watching me and then reached over for Becca to get involved. I reached for her, beckoning her closer as I stopped sucking. I made space for her, and she quickly obliged, turning to lick his cock with me. We were on either side of his cock, sharing it as we licked, one at a time, on either side. I grabbed his balls, giving them a quick fondle and pressed against the perineum behind them, pushing up. His moans betrayed his pleasure and we could feel his cock starting to pulse against us harder. He was building up that fluid; he wouldn't last for much longer.

"How do you want to cum, birthday boy?" I purred for him, looking up with my best fuck-me eyes, and he smirked.

"On both of you," he said matter-of-factly between his breathing. His voice was low, husky, and sensual as he demanded it. He pushed against us with his cock, and we both started to lick at it again.

I sucked on his cock as Becca moved down for the balls, licking and sucking on them gently. We both kept going, feeling his cock swelling even more. He was just about to cum—we could both feel it as we tried to suck even more on him. It wouldn't be that much longer.

I felt his hand roughly grab the back of my hair, and I could see that he grabbed Becca as well, holding our heads steady as I kept sucking. His eyes were closed, head back as he thrust deeper and deeper into my mouth before he finally pulled himself out of my mouth, shifting to his hand.

He used his hand to keep jerking himself off, aiming his cock at both of us and finally, the strings of fluid came out of his cock, first on me and then onto her as well, spurting out in several streams as he groaned his pleasure, watching both of us as he did. He slowed to a stop after and looked at his handiwork. Both of our faces had strings of cum all over them, and the sight must have pleased him based on that satisfied smirk.

"Clean it off," he demanded, holding his cock to me, and I put the whole thing in my mouth, sucking and pressing my tongue against the bottom of his shaft to get the rest of that fluid out of him, swallowing it. "And each other, too," he told us.

I looked at Becca closer this time; she had it all across her lips and her cheek. Her tongue was already making quick work of the cum on her lips, but she couldn't reach on her cheek. I leaned forward and gently licked it away, letting my tongue linger as I did. When she was clean, she returned the favor, licking along my face as well. He chuckled to himself at the sight. "Good girls," he said huskily as he collapsed onto the bed, thoroughly spent.

"Happy birthday," we both told him as we curled up on either side of him without a care in the world. I didn't mind sharing with Becca at all, and in fact, it had actually been far more fun than I expected to share with her, and I wasn't quite sure that we'd never attempt that again. In fact, I would have loved to do that again in the future. It would be absolutely thrilling to get to fuck each other again, but not quite yet. I had had my fill. It was absolutely time for a nap before we decided on a round two.

Closer to the Edge

Erin is *frustrated*. She just wants a quiet home and a good, hard fuck that will leave her satisfied, and unfortunately, luck is not in her favor as she finds herself lacking both of those. She's woefully single with little desire to go out and find a one-night stand, and her neighbor loves to blast loud music to hide his own actions on a regular basis. Confronting her darkly sexy neighbor, Damian, to turn off his music, she finds herself tangled up in some sexy playtime that may be more than she ever bargained for, and she can't get enough of it.

I could hear the loud music pulsing against my wall in the apartment. It was loud and annoying, and I never wanted to hear that same bassline again. Of course, the neighbor never cared when I complained. I had tried telling him that his constant thundering about made it impossible for me to do my studying, and he laughed at me. I told him once that I couldn't sleep when he was listening to that loud music all night long and he told me to wear earplugs. When I tried telling him that he needed to learn to respect the people around him, he told me that all I needed was a good fuck because I was too uptight.

Now, I'll be honest; I hadn't had a good fuck in a while. But, that didn't mean that I couldn't think about things clearly. Besides, that's what my toys were for. I didn't need a dick to have a good time. And I clearly didn't need a dick to enjoy myself. I tried to ignore the music that was playing and went about my day. I couldn't read my book. I couldn't focus on the games that I was playing. I could even hear their music through my headphones, and no matter how hard I tried, I couldn't get away from it.

I tossed and turned around in my bed, desperate for some sort of relief; I couldn't get away from the noise, and eventually, I had had enough! I took my robe, tied it up around me, and stormed over to his door. I pounded on it and waited. Of course, no response. The neighbor had given up answering the door to me long ago, no matter how much I tried to knock. I ended up pounding again.

"DAMN IT, DAMIAN OPEN THIS DOOR RIGHT NOW!!" I shouted, slamming my fists against the door. "I'VE HAD ENOUGH WITH THIS MUSIC ALREADY! TURN IT OFF AND GET OUT HERE!"

I raised my fist to slam against the door again, but as I swung, he finally opened the door, and my hand connected with his chest. He stood there with a cocky grin on his face, one eyebrow, pierced, raised up, and arms crossed in front of him.

"Can I help you, Erin?"

I stared at him in shock. I hadn't expected him to open the door—and yet here we were. He was looking right at me, face to face, and I couldn't figure out what to do next. "Erin." He repeated himself. "Please take your hand off of me."

I realized that my fist was still against his chest and pulled away, embarrassed. "S-sorry. But seriously, Damian! I can't think with your music so loud! What is wrong with you?!"

"Nothing's wrong with me; I'm just having a good time. It sounds like you need some practice learning about what a good time means," he replied. He held the door open wider, inviting me in, and I hesitated, not totally convinced that I wanted to enter.

Damian was the stereotypical bad boy neighbor. He wore all black, and his current tank top was skin-tight and taut, revealing the abs underneath. He wasn't a bad guy—I knew that much. I saw him occasionally carrying up groceries for the elderly neighbors and saw him feeding a stray cat outside once. But, he was also highly annoying. He lived in a corner unit, and I had the only unit that connected to his, so lucky me, I got to hear all of his music in all of its annoying blaring that I desperately wished I could make go away.

"Don't be a buzzkill, Erin. Get in here," he told me with that trademark smirk.

I huffed but finally went in. Why not? Maybe, if I talked to him like a normal human being, he'd actually shut up and let me live in peace.

We went into his home, and thankfully, he *finally* turned down the music to a tolerable level. It was still annoying, but at least it was no longer unbearable as the bassline continued heavily, punctuated by all sorts of drums. I had never been in his home before, and looking around, I could see why. It was clean, but at the same time, I had not been prepared to see what was in there.

The living room was lined with sex objects. There was no shortage of beads and dildos lining up and down the walls, and there was what appeared to be a bunch of restraints in there as well. I looked around at everything and turned to look at Damian with a look of mortification on my face. He must have caught onto it because he smirked at me. "Problem?" he asked.

"N-no..." I managed to squeak out, feeling my face flush. I looked around for somewhere to sit, unsure I really wanted to sit down in the first place. Did I really want to touch anything in here?

"Do you like what you see?" His voice had a hint of edge to it, and he looked at me with that look I hadn't seen from someone in a long while. It was the look of someone wanting to consume what was in front of them. He was loving every moment of this, and honestly? The sound of his voice kind of got me going almost immediately, and I

74

suddenly became aware of the fact that I was really only wearing a robe with just my underwear underneath it and I flushed even brighter.

His cock was hard in his pants, and he didn't seem to care about it at all. He simply walked over to me to usher me to his couch and sat me down. I wasn't sure what I was thinking when I agreed to come in.

"So, Erin," he said, looking at me. He stood in front of me, and I was at eye level with his hard cock. "What is it that you came over here for?"

"Your music was too loud," I told him, trying hard not to look at his cock in my face. But, the harder I tried to resist from looking at him, the more that I really just wanted to. I was wet underneath my robe, and I prayed that he wouldn't be able to tell or smell it or anything else. I hoped that I'd be able to just sneak out and enjoy the rest of my quiet night.

"Really," he said, leaning in toward me. His face was right next to mine now as he leaned, and I could feel his breath on my skin. I wanted to slap him and kiss him all at the same time, and I could feel my clit at attention, ready for some loving that it had been so denied lately. It wanted to be touched. *I* wanted to be touched, but I didn't want him to know it.

"I can see how turned on you are right now," he whispered. "Your eyes... Your lips... I can smell it on you." He looked at my lips and bit his own, looking like he was ready to take them for his own. "You need to learn to lighten up, Erin," he purred to me. He looked at me closely, as if trying to discern my own interest. I could feel my own breath hitching as he looked at me, and I couldn't lie; the sexual tension was palpable between us. "I can teach you to lighten up."

"Really." I looked at him and scowled, crossing my arms in front of me.

"Yes, Erin, really," he told me. "Give it a shot. Besides, what's wrong with a little night of fun every now and then? Want a drink?"

I hesitated. Even though my mind wanted to say no, my body was begging me to give in. My body was begging for that connection and human touch. I needed it more than I have ever needed anything in my life, and I desperately wanted to accept in that moment. So I did something unexpected.

"Sure."

"Are you a wine kinda girl?" He looked me over as if trying to figure out my drink preference on his own.

"Whiskey, neat."

"Oho, big taste for someone so small, huh?" He smirked. "Coming right up."

He returned a few moments later with the drink in his hand and handed it over for me to sip at. I downed it, the whole two shots worth and handed him the cup back, proving the point. I wasn't some delicate flower, a special snowflake that wanted the world to cater to me. I just wanted some peace and quiet.

"So, Erin. Let's talk about boundaries."

"What kind of boundaries?" I glanced around his room and realized that we were in what was probably some sort of sex playroom, and suddenly, the loud music made sense. Was it there to drown out the sounds of fucking? That was honestly kind of hot, I realized, and my mind started to wander. Was every time the music got blasted a time when he was getting fucked? Was it possible that he was just enjoying the moment, or was he trying to hide the sounds of passion from me?

"What are you willing to do, and what are you not willing to do?"

"We'll get to that when we get to it!" I insisted, deciding to rush past that. I didn't want to talk about what I wanted and what I didn't.

"Fine, let's at least set up a safe word," he told me, and I started to worry a bit. Should I be concerned about what was going to happen? Safe words made it sound like it would be almost... violent. "Yellow for you're approaching a boundary. Red if you need to stop. I will respect those safe words. You can beg for me to stop, but unless you say, 'red,' I'm not stopping."

I nodded.

"Repeat the safe words to me, Erin."

"Yellow for slow down, red for stop."

"Very good," he replied. "Now, are you ready?"

"Yes." I looked at him and actually made eye contact without feeling feelings of rage for a moment. It was totally different than when we were fighting. I felt a strange mix of arousal, anticipation, and a bit of nervousness as well. What did the night have in store for me?

"Take off your clothes," he told me.

"That's rather forward, isn't it?"

Damian's hand wrapped around a flogger that he had in his back pocket, and he pulled it out. "I punish dirty little girls that don't listen to me," he purred, his eyes shining with arousal. He watched me closely, waiting to see if I said the safe words that we had talked about. I almost did, but I wanted to see where the night could go. Instead, I stripped as asked.

His eyes betrayed the surprise that I had only been wearing a bra and underwear underneath the robe, but he grinned at me, a dark, almost sadistic grin as he looked me over. "You've got quite the hot body, you little slut," he told me as his eyes rested on my breasts. "Take the underwear off, too. I want my toys to be completely naked. I'll be patient with you this time since you're new to being my little plaything, but I expect compliance."

Wordlessly, I started to drop the clothes onto the floor, and he suddenly swatted at me, making me squeal and pull my hand back in shock. I hadn't been expecting that. My hand, where I had been swatted, was already bright pink.

"You will respect me when I talk to you," he demanded. "You will say, 'yes, sir' when I tell you to do something. Do you understand?" His cock bulged and twitched in his pants.

"Yes, sir," I managed to say, rubbing my hand.

"Good. Now, strip."

"Yes, sir."

He tossed my clothes to the floor and inspected my completely naked body, nodding his approval. "Now, turn around. Bend over."

I was kind of shocked at the suddenness, but for some reason, I complied. "Yes, sir." When I bent over, he got to see my ass and lips in full view, and he chuckled to himself.

I couldn't see him, but I could feel his breath on my skin as he inspected my body. "It looks like you're already raring to go," Damian commented offhandedly, as matter-of-factly as you would expect someone to be over the weather. His finger traced the entrance of my pussy, picking up the liquid that I had already started to leak before sucking it off of himself. "This poor little pussy looks like it was neglected.

To be fair, it had been and hearing him say that only made me hotter for him. I felt my clit twitch, and he chuckled, putting his finger on it, rubbing it gently in soft circles that felt so good that I moaned. It had been so long since I had been touched by someone else that way. He continued to circle around it, watching my reaction as I sat there and let him have his way with me.

"Today's an exercise in patience, do you hear me?" he growled at me as he continued to rub along my clit. "If you are patient, you will be rewarded. If you get impatient or you're a naughty slut that can't control that sloppy pussy of yours, you will be punished. And trust me, I don't take my job lightly. I hand out punishments that I intend to keep."

"Yes, sir!" I squeaked as I felt his finger penetrate into my slit, stroking the inner walls. I felt the flogger that he had used on my hand dangle above my back, tickling and exciting the nerve endings in my bare skin as he did. The leather was cool and soft to the touch when it was not swung to sting, and it further excited me. I felt myself clench around his finger, and just as it did, he pulled his finger out from inside of me. "Slow down there, little slut. Enjoy the ride. You need a lesson in patience." He swatted my ass with the flogger, and I cried out as it stung against me. It had caught me off guard, but after the initial shock, it wasn't so bad after all.

"I'm sorry, sir," I gasped out. I didn't want to tell him the truth—that I was just a desperate, lusty slut that hadn't

79

been fucked in far too long, so instead, I remained silent. I didn't say a word beyond that; I just looked over my shoulder, giving him the best fuck-me eyes I could.

He flipped me over and took my hand, leading me over to a bed, which he promptly pushed me onto. He was rough, but not hard enough to scare or worry me, and I went down as he wanted. He walked over to a drawer and pulled out a few different things, and when he came back, I saw this strange collar and a blindfold. I balked at the sight, and he hesitated for just a moment, giving me the chance to use those safe words if I wanted to, but when I didn't say a word after a few beats, he moved forward and got to work. He wrapped the restraint around me and before I knew it, my arms were tied to my neck and torso, and my legs were spread open. If I tried to move too much or if I tugged the leg restraints to put my legs back down, the restraint would tighten around my neck, forcing me to stay put, and the blindfold was added as well.

I couldn't see anything at all, but I could hear Damian moving around the room, and suddenly, there were headphones placed firmly over my ears, and the music was turned on. It was quieter music at the very least, but it was the same bass-heavy music that he normally listened to. I groaned my displeasure, but before I could remain irritated for long, I felt his cock at long last finally slide into my pussy and bring me that joy that I had been missing in my life. He slid right into me and I was shocked at how large he was. Holding my legs up at that angle actually made it better and the occasional tightening around my neck actually elevated the sensations of being fucked as Damian continued to go at it.

I felt myself starting to tense up, my poor, neglected pussy too weak to resist the desire to cum, and before I knew it, I was exploding with pleasure. It must have been just four or five thrusts before I had already finished, moaning out loud and momentarily forgetting the order that I had been given. As the orgasm ended, I felt Damian's flog hit
80

against my ass again, stinging and making me yelp in pain. He drew back and hit again and again, and I whimpered. The music stopped suddenly as the headphones were removed from my head. "You're in for a punishment now, Erin. You were a selfish girl and selfish girls get punished." And just as suddenly as the headphones were removed, they were replaced and the music was turned up a notch or two, growing more intense.

I was a bit concerned when I realized that I wasn't feeling anything at all. I couldn't feel him moving around and obviously couldn't hear or see him. It made me nervous, but there was nothing that I could do, other than maybe saying the safe word, but that would be admitting that he won.

My legs were starting to burn with the effort to keep them up, and I could feel them trembling. I swear, Damian was laughing somewhere nearby, even if I couldn't hear him, and suddenly, I felt him approach. The air shifted and I knew he was coming. I expected to feel another lash of the whip, but instead, I was pleasantly surprised; a vibrator was placed against my clit, and it was happy to jump right back to action. I felt it stirring to life again, willing to go for a round two. It had been so long that I may as well enjoy it again. My clit twitched underneath the weight of the vibrator and I moaned, feeling my hips lift of their own accord as it rested against my body. I grinded against it, enjoying the moment, but just as I started to really get going, feeling my pussy starting to soak itself, I felt the vibrator disappear.

I gasped as it was pulled away, and instinctively, I looked around, only to be reminded that I couldn't see or hear anything. I sighed to myself. Was this my punishment? Was he just going to be a tease? At the very least, it would still be fun, I told myself.

Next, I felt his mouth on my nipple, going around the tip with his tongue gently and carefully, not willing to do

81

anything too intense. He danced about my nipple, making me wetter than before. I moaned, my pussy feeling achingly empty, and there was nothing for me to push up against. I couldn't even clench my legs together to try to make myself feel better—all I had was waiting for him to come back to me and who knew when that would be? His tongue spun about my nipple again before letting go. He hovered just above it. I could feel his breath on the wet skin with every breath, driving me madder than before.

He moved to the other nipple then, but never quite touched it, keeping his lips tantalizingly above my skin so close that I could touch it, but not close enough to bring me to any sort of release. I could feel him, and it felt good, but it was making me desperate. My pussy was sopping wet now, and I could smell my fluids all throughout the room. I could feel the slight vibrations on the bed—he must have laughed at my expression of sheer indignation at the deprivation that I was facing.

Damian moved away; suddenly, the air was colder around me, and he left me there for a few minutes. All that I had to keep me company was the throbbing of the bass in the song, throbbing much like my swollen, tortured pussy that wanted to be filled up, and when I finally felt like I couldn't take it anymore, I felt his tongue on me. It was flat and hard as he pressed it against my clit, letting his tongue caress the little nub while his fingers danced just outside of my slit, greedily touching everything that they could.

He plunged his tongue into me, and I moaned, back arching as he did it. He was getting more and more creative with what he was doing to me, and he was making it perfectly clear that he had no intention of ever actually letting me get off. As I'd start to tense up again, he pulled back, just long enough for my aching, quivering pussy to slow down before starting up again. Just as he'd get a rhythm, sensing the impending release, he'd change it up completely, sending me crashing back down and needing to be worked up again.

I felt like crying with desperation as this continued. He shifted from his mouth to his cock for a while, fucking me deeply and hard, only to stop when he thought that I was getting too into it. He teased me silly, and the whole time, I couldn't do anything. I was at his utter mercy, and there was no way for me to do anything but sit there and take it and hope that maybe, he'd show just a bit of compassion and let me get off.

Of course, that never happened as he expertly played with my body like it was made just for him. Maybe it was with how well he was able to turn it on and keep it going—all I knew was that I wanted to fuck him silly, free of the restraints, but I knew that if I said the safe word, it would all be over.

He pulled out again, this time, squirting his load all over my chest as he did, leaving his sticky cum all over me as he licked it up, little by little off of me. He rubbed around my breasts, but never touched the nipples as he ran his hands over me. And finally, he lifted up the headphones, making it possible for me to hear his voice in my ear.

"You have something to be mad about now, you dirty slut," he whispered as he released the bonds and removed the blindfold.

I sat there in shock as I looked at him. He looked satisfied with himself as he looked at the massive puddle that I had left on his bed. He looked over me as I stared back at him, and he waited for me to do something.

"That's it?" I finally managed to say, frustrated.

"That's it," he confirmed. "Naughty girls aren't rewarded in this house. You didn't hold out for me, and you didn't get rewarded any further." He leaned over, planted a kiss atop my head, patted my frustrated pussy, and handed me my robe. "Don't worry, Erin, I'll keep the music down lower for you," he said with a wink as I picked up my clothes and put them on, in shock. As frustrated as I was, I had to admit that he had been the best lay I had had in a very long time. When I was ready to go, he held the door open politely. "I'll see you again very soon," he murmured as I walked by, smirking.

I scowled, both frustrated with the end result of our encounter and the fact that he was right—he *would* be seeing me again in the near future. There was no way I could resist that cock again, and I'd have to be more disciplined next time to actually enjoy it.

Shut Up and Fuck Me

Krissy is a secretary that often feels like she doesn't get appreciated enough. She hates when she is stuck working late on Fridays when she's waiting for her boss to finish working so she can wrap everything up, and so one day, she decides to spice things up. Horny and with nothing else to do while she waits for her boss, the CEO of a financial institution, to finish up, she fantasizes about fucking him, or rather, him fucking her, while she has some fun with herself. Is it possible that the fantasies could become a reality when he walks out to her with her fingers inside of her?

I closed the laptop in front of me and sighed to myself. I had all this work to do, but I only had one thing on my mind: Hard, thick cock. More specifically, hard, thick cock slamming into me over and over again to get me off. I was so wet and horny as I sat there at my desk. I was all alone in the office, save for my boss, Mr. Roberts, in the room behind a closed door. He didn't like to be bothered while he worked, and he was scheduled to be on a conference call for another twenty minutes or so. I sighed again, letting my hand slide over my arm as I did. I wanted that release—no, I *needed* that release, and I didn't know how I could expect to get it. I needed to find some way to release all of that pressure that had built up within me, but it seemed so indecent to do it at work, knowing that my boss could open the door at any point in time to ask me to do something.

But for some reason, the idea of him opening the door only made it seem hotter than before. The idea of getting caught actually made me hotter than anything else. I imagined the scenario out in my mind. I was touching myself, probing at my innermost bits and feeling my wetness, groping my breasts, hair askew, and nipples poking out of my shirt for easier access for my wandering hands. I was moaning to myself in joy, and the door opens. Instead of getting up or apologizing or trying to cover myself up, I would stare my boss in the eyes as I continued to finger fuck myself, giving him those eyes that would dare him to come over and get involved as well.

He would get involved in that scenario in my mind. He would be so overcome with desire at the sight of his secretary fucking herself that he would throw himself at her, putting her up on the table and fucking her silly. His cock, I imagined, would be long, hard and thick, and it would fill me up so much that I would worry that I would tear. His hands would be needy as they ran over my body, tugging desperately, and his breath would be heavy in my ear as he whispered into it that he wanted to fuck me more than anything else.

The image of him plunging himself into me over and over again was almost overwhelming. I found myself gasping at the sight, and I realized that my fingers were wet—I had already slid down my skirt and was fingering myself. I glanced at his door—still locked, and I could hear his occasional roaring laugh as someone that he was trying to woo into a business deal said something that was probably not the least bit funny, but he laughed anyway in hopes that it would lighten the mood. I imagined the look on his face if he were to walk out right that moment—it would be shock and instant arousal as he did and I imagined the bulge in his pants that would grow as he did. It made me hotter to think about all of this, and I felt myself get even wetter as my fingers touched my insides. I rubbed against my inner wall almost lazily as my mind wandered.

What if instead, he threw me over the desk and fucked me silly from behind? His cock would be so hard and so satisfying as it pushed within me, deeper and deeper, as he demanded that I let him ravish my body, and I would not have a care in the world. I didn't care that we were at work and that he, or I, could lose a job over it. I imagined the sheer carnal pleasure at fucking someone without

86

inhibitions, just enjoying each and every moment as it happened. I imagined the joy that I felt, letting him slam into me. It was so hot.

I felt myself let out a little whimper, biting my lip as I let my fingers dance around my clit. I felt myself feel a bit more desperate for that release, but I also didn't want it to end so quickly. I wanted to savor the moment. I wanted to live vicariously and dangerously, and right now, sexually explicit behaviors right in front of my boss's door seemed like a great way to make that happen. Maybe I was fucked up, I thought if I thought that the idea of potentially getting caught fingering myself was hot, but I didn't care, not in the moment.

My other hand reached over my breast, tantalizingly stroking the smooth skin. I reached down my shirt and let my fingers graze over my nipple. It felt so good as my nipple immediately responded, hardening underneath the touch. I licked my lips as I let my fingers trace the slit beneath the clit, but never entering me. Fuck, I needed to bring a vibrator to hide in my desk, or even in my purse, I told myself. It could be hot having someone find it in my desk, or having the security officer that has to check our bags make eye contact with me, blushing when he realizes that I'm carrying around a sex toy. It's not illegal, so he can't confiscate it, but he can think all about what I'm going to do with it later on.

I let myself tease myself a bit longer, running along the inner labia before I finally plunge my fingers in to rub at my inner walls. They are tight now from all of the buildup and tension that I have made as I continued to play with myself, and I looked over to the door. Still nothing, but he had to be getting close to wrapping up that business call now... and sure enough, I saw the light on the office phone turn off, signaling that he had hung up.

It was now or never, I told myself, looking at the door. Did I stop, or did I push my luck and see what would happen next? I decided to take my chances, drawn by the heady hormones coursing through my body and the feeling of excitement that was growing more and more tantalizing by the second the longer that I touched myself, and sure enough, I heard the click of the lock and the door handle opening up. I looked away from the door, throwing my head back in pleasure and pretending that I didn't see him coming out.

The door opened as I continued to finger fuck myself, and there was a moment of silence. I realized that touching myself was feeling even better, but it was not a cock in my vag—that's what I wanted more than anything else.

"Krissy?"

I heard his voice. It was bewildered at the sight. It was shocking, and possibly even a little turned on by the waver that I heard as if he was hesitant to stop me from the sexual release that I was so clearly enjoying. Head still tossed back in enjoyment; I opened my eyes to meet his gaze, slowly pulling my fingers out of my mouth and licking my fingers, one by one. I watched as his eyes widened slightly in response, but he never looked away. I could see his pants tighten, and I smirked. Instead of waiting for him, I stood up and walked toward him.

"I need you to fuck me right now," I told him in a low voice, looking at him through my eyelashes and pushing out my chest. One of my nipples was poking out for him to see, and I picked up his hand in my own, placing it on my chest. I pushed my hips against him, grinding on his rock-hard erection in his pants, and I pushed him toward his office without another word. He shockingly didn't fight back, considering that he was so much larger than I was. He seemed willing to comply with whatever I was going to ask him to do.

He probably thought that it was his lucky day; I told myself with a satisfied smirk as I felt the ache in my pussy

88

grow more intense. I pushed him toward his chair. "I want you to do exactly what I say, do you understand me?" I told him without waiting for much of an answer as I pressed against his chest, urging him to sit down. He did, and I straddled him, rubbing myself against his cock that was still trapped in his pants. It was about as big as I had been hoping, I realized, and that was absolutely fitting for a man of his stature. I whined to myself as I felt his hardness underneath me and I grinded against it harder.

"I'm going to tie you up and have my way with you. I need your rock-hard cock in me so bad right now. You don't even know how badly I need to feel you within me," I told him, looking around for something—anything—that I could use to secure him behind me. I settled for some zip ties that I found in his drawer and put them on him, just behind the back of his chair. It wasn't much, but it would be enough for me to have my fun. A part of me was shocked that he was not protesting, but that only made it better in my book. I felt myself getting wetter, and I looked my boss over. He was the CEO of a major financial firm, and here I was, tying him up and getting ready to fuck both of our brains out, totally in control of every single moment of it.

Satisfied with how secure he was, I looked at his face. He was silent and watching me, but I could see the pleasure shining in his eyes. Did he get off on being dominated? I smirked, unzipping his pants and releasing his cock. It was still just as rock hard as it had felt inside of them as it sprang to attention, and I ran my fingers up and down over the length, enjoying the twitches that I got in response. He was turned on by that, too, it seemed. I chuckled to myself as I lowered my head onto his cock to suck on it. I didn't want to just throw myself onto him without first letting him warm up. He needed to be nice and ready, and the harder that he was, the better.

As I sucked on his cock, I heard him groan in pleasure, thrusting his cock closer to me as he did. He pushed up toward me, and I chuckled on his cock, letting my tongue linger as I let go of it. "Someone's ready for a good fuck," I purred as I looked up at him from his cock, my lips still touching it right around the frenulum as I spoke. His hips thrust forward as I did. "Aren't you going to say anything at all?" I asked him as I licked at his frenulum some more.

"You are fucking hot as hell," he managed to get out between heavy breaths. "I've wanted to get you over my desk ever since I hired you."

I laughed, rubbing over his cock. "Well, who's got whom now?" I asked as I took off my shirt, revealing my toned stomach and perky, D-cup breasts. I lowered them around his cock, letting him rub it between the soft, warm skin as I held them together and kneaded at my nipples for even more pleasure than before. I loved every moment of what I was doing, and from the look on Mr. Roberts' face, he did too.

I felt his dick getting harder as I rubbed him down with my breasts. "Oh, Mr. Roberts," I moaned, looking up at him, "Don't cum already. I've got so much more in store for you than this." Just saying that as I rubbed my tits over him got him cumming, and he squirted all over my tits and my face.

He seemed almost embarrassed that he had cum already, but he didn't say a word.

"Uh, oh, someone made a mess," I purred, using my finger to clean up every last drop of cum from my skin and licking it up, enjoying the taste in my mouth. I leaned forward to suck the last of it from his cock, too. There was no use in wasting the good stuff when I was right there and more than willing to suck it up if there was nowhere else to put it. I licked it up and looked at him with a smirk. He was watching me in awe, as if he had never seen someone do that before. His cock stayed mostly hard, even after he had spilled so much. As it started to soften, I

90

sucked on it and licked at it, trying to keep the blood flow there. I rubbed myself on it, getting back onto his lap and straddling him. I removed my panties and left the skirt on, letting myself rub up on him over and over to bring him back to life. I put my tits in his face for him, letting them bounce with every motion that I made to try to wake his softening dick up again for more.

He leaned over and took control then. He sucked on my left tit first, licking desperately at it and then finally pulling the whole thing into his mouth, his tongue spinning all around it as he did. He was rough, but not hurtful as he tugged at my nipples. He licked and sucked on them carefully, and the more that I rubbed on him, the closer to finishing that I got. I couldn't hold out for much longer, I realized. I needed to fuck him soon, or I wouldn't be satisfied, but his cock was still woefully unready for that.

Instead, I chose to let myself grind on him longer, waiting for that refractory period to end. I lost myself in the moment, rubbing the tip of his cock against my clit and letting his shaft rub up against the lips. Up and down, up and down I went, and I used my other hand to play with my other nipple as well. I lost myself in my mind again, imagining what would happen if I were to undo his ties right that moment. Would he bend me over? Would he fuck me raw? What would he do for me? I wanted to know.

I imagined him taking me from behind, his cock reaching the deepest part of me while his balls slapped at my clit with every thrust, fucking me to the best climax that I had ever felt. I imagined him flipping me over and fucking me silly on my back, his hands on my breasts and mouth on mine as he fucked harder and harder. His cock was large enough to make that happen; I had to admit that much. It looked like it would be exactly what I needed to finish myself off that night. All I needed to do was get it back to hard again.

I rubbed harder against it, desperation in my aching pussy apparent as I did it more and more. I felt him finally starting to respond, and as his dick swelled against me, I came atop him. My whole body betrayed me, with me rubbing harder and harder against him as my hips gyrated atop his own as I did.

He chuckled at me as he continued to suck on my tit. "Someone's enjoying themselves," he murmured, the sensation of his lips moving making me realize that even after a spectacular orgasm, I wanted *more*. I wanted to be selfish.

"You're going to fuck me," I told him, getting off of his lap and clipping the zip ties off of him so that he could get up. He rubbed his wrists as he regarded me with lust shining in his eyes and dick, pointing at the ready to keep going.

"I can do that," he replied, his hands suddenly on my hips as he turned me around and bent me onto his desk, sending items clattering to the ground. Neither of us paid any attention to it as we did, and I felt his hand on the back of my head, pushing it down and then shifting to my hips to line himself up just right. "I'll fuck you so hard that you won't be able to walk those pretty little legs out of here," he growled in my ear before he thrust into me.

He wasn't kidding. And I was all the happier for it. I wanted a good, hard fuck, and if he was willing to give it to me, I was happy. After all, all I had wanted was a hard cock inside of me one way or another.

I felt him thrust so deeply into me that I let out a guttural moan of pleasure, my back arching on its own accord as he did. He let his cock linger there inside of me, letting me finally enjoy what I had wanted more than anything. He let me clench against it tightly as he lingered there, and I was happy to do so. I clenched all around it over and over again, letting myself enjoy it.

92

Slowly, he pulled his rock hard cock out of me, and I tightened up again as if I could prevent it from leaving if I tightened up enough. It slipped out, leaving just the tip keeping my lips apart so that he would be able to thrust in again when he was ready. He let it rub against me, moving his hips in a circle to tease those sensitive, swollen, needy lips of mine, and it was driving me *crazy*. I wanted that cock back inside of me so bad.

I wanted it so bad that I shoved my ass toward him, plunging his cock right back into me without him being able to protest. I rode it harder on my own this time. I fucked it standing up, pushing myself onto him over and over again. His cock felt so good to ride as it glided in and out of my wet pussy, and I needed it so bad.

I pulled away and turned around to face him, pushing him to the floor. He obliged, laying across the thin carpet as I had requested, and I straddled him, preparing to ride him as hard and long as I wanted to. I pushed myself around him, letting his cock deepen, pushing my whole weight down to sit on him as I moaned in pleasure.

He reached around to play with my ass, placing his hands on either cheek before he started to guide my movements. He pushed up and pulled me back down to his own rhythm, and I was more than willing to oblige as we did. I felt myself getting hotter and tighter around him. His mound of fur around his cock was glistening with my juices and the smell of sex, hot and heady, filled the room as we fucked harder and with reckless abandon. I rode him gleefully, head tilted back as I did. I bounced harder on his cock, letting it get deeper and deeper into me as I did. I put his hands on my boobs to hold them in place as I looked into his eyes. He was watching me with an impressed, turned on expression as he rode me harder and harder. He wanted to fuck me just as much as I needed him, it seemed.

He let me have my fun before flipping me over, pulling my hair as he thrust deeper into me. He had one hair in my hair and another clawing at my chest, clenching down on my breasts tightly. His nails dug into my skin, just hard enough to avoid breaking the skin. He left his hands there, smashing his palm into my nipple and teasing me harder.

"It's my turn to do the fucking and the leading," he whispered in my ear. "And I want you to be a good girl and cum when I tell you to. Do you understand me?" His voice was breathy in my ear as he spoke, slamming into me as hard as he could.

I could barely speak as the pleasure began to build up again, and I nodded my head to him.

"Good girl. Now I'm going to ride your little ass hard until you cum when I tell you to." He wasn't joking, either. He fucked me so hard that all of the fantasies that I had been having, all of the visualization that I had been doing, was gone. He fucked me so hard that all I could focus on was the feeling of his cock inside of me, ramming me harder and harder.

He stopped suddenly, and I gasped at the sudden lack of sensation, suddenly flipping me over.

"I thought you were going to ride me?" I asked between heavy breaths with a smart ass smirk on my face.

"Oh, I will. But we're going to do something else first. He laid down on the floor and pushed my head toward his cock, soaked with my moisture. "Lick it."

I obliged, tasting the sex on his skin with a long moan of pleasure. It was so hot to taste our fluids combining. He pulled me closer and positioned me just above his face, and suddenly, I felt his tongue on me as well. He was tonguing me as I blew him, and I moaned on his cock

94

again. I kept my grip on him tight. I could see that his balls were starting to tighten up, and I could feel the tension in his cock the more that I sucked him off, and I knew that if I kept it up, I'd be able to get him to cum.

But more importantly, he was licking me so much that I wasn't sure that I'd be able to hold out. His tongue skated across the tip of my clit as he slammed a finger into my pussy, reaching for the g-spot as he tongued me, and the feeling was so intense that I almost came right then and there. I was getting desperate as my poor, aching, soaking pussy craved to be filled up, and I stood up suddenly as I felt myself approaching the point of no return. I slipped past the grip he tried to use to hold me in place, and I got on his cock as quickly as I could, letting the pleasure build up even more until I could no longer take it. With a cry out that would make anyone blush, if they heard it, I came on that hard cock just as I felt him thrust up into me. We both moaned in pleasure, enjoying the ecstasy of each other's bodies as we came, our bodies spasming to each other in almost perfect harmony as we both finally got the big moment.

It felt like it went on for ages as my body, desperate for that release, clenched against him again and again until finally, spent and exhausted, I collapsed against his chest, sweaty, breathing heavily, and hearing his heart thundering against my ear. We weren't going to cuddle, but I took the moment to enjoy myself before getting up and straightening myself out. I cleaned myself up, taking a moment to glance in the mirror to see that I was looking quite disheveled.

Wordlessly, I put my clothes on and tried to make my appearance as appropriate to going out into the real world as I could. When I was satisfied, I turned to look at Mr. Roberts for a moment. He was reclining back in his chair, arms behind his head and looking fully satisfied himself as if it were not just his cock that had been stroked, but his ego as well. "I'll see you Monday, Krissy," he said with a smirk and a knowing look that said that this would probably become a regular thing.

I smirked right back at him as well. "See you on Monday," I replied cheerfully with a wave as I left, fully aware that my walking was not quite right. It seemed he had kept that promise after all.

Description

Warning: This book is for adults that are looking for something to drive them wild.

Are you looking for something to spice up your night? Look no further—this book features seven highly erotic stories that will tickle your fancy while you tickle something else. If you're into taboo, sexy stories filled with subjects that would make your mother blush, you're in the right place. Open this book and find something to get your panties soaked today. You'll find stories that are rough and sensual at the same time, tickling taboo fancies and wetting panties, such as:

- **Blind Pleasure:** A woman exploring a swinger's club with her husband getting a night that she'll remember forever after the sexy, sensual experience that she has with more than one man. Who knew so many different hands could feel so good?
- **Variety is the Spice of Sex:** A woman who is bored with her married sex life decides to bring in some reinforcements to relive her days of not being beholden to just one body, spending some sexy, sensual time with both her husband and their neighbor to spice their bedroom life up a bit more than they realized they needed. Variety is the spice of life—and sex!
- **Clara's Experiment:** A woman exploring her interest in being submissive learning what it really means to be bound and used like a toy for the thrill of someone else, being truly at the mercy of someone else, and discovers that she loves every single moment of it.
- **Amelia's Punishment:** A young, hot housekeeper makes a mistake that deserves to be punished. After all, what good is it to have housekeepers that can't do what they're told when

they're told to do it? Sometimes, you need a firm hand to teach you what needs to be done, and her boss is not afraid to teach that lesson if he has to. In fact, he's more than willing to and teaches her a lesson she'll never forget.

- **Unwrapped Gifts:** If gifts are meant to be opened, does that mean that our clothes are just gift wraps for when we give ourselves to someone else? In this story, a woman and her best friend present themselves as the ultimate gift to her boyfriend for a celebration of a lifetime.

- **Closer to the Edge:** Noisy neighbors can be the worst—but what if they're also smoking hot and you're desperate? This story takes you alongside a woman who confronts her noisy neighbor, only to be in for a night that she'll never forget. Let's just say he gave her something to really be frustrated about.

- **Shut up and F*ck me:** Sometimes, when you have the urge, you have to satisfy it, and this hot secretary knows that better than anyone else. But, she wants to take things one step further and make her fantasies a reality when she knows that her boss is in the room next door, finishing up a business call. Can she convince him to give her what she wants?

How to Talk Dirty

Transform Your Sex Life & Spike Up Your Libido. 200 Real Dirty Talk Tips to Drive Your Partner Wild. Make Your Partner Your "Sex Slave"

of information contained within this document, including, but not limited to, — errors, omissions, or inaccuracies.

Table of Contents

Introduction

Dirty talk: It is something that too many people feel awkward about. So many people find that even talking about sex in a normal way is just too much. There are people that are embarrassed to talk about what they want or how they feel. They are embarrassed to use words to describe what they enjoy or what they dislike, and unfortunately, that embarrassment of talking about what is wanted is linked to a lack of intimacy as well.

What makes sex good? For some people, it is intimacy. For others, it is the raw, unadulterated passion. For others still, however, it is the simple act of communication. It is the communicating of what you want in bed; it is the idea that you can tell someone else precisely what it is that you want so that you can get it. If you want mind-blowing sex, then you need to know how to tell people what you want, and until you can do that, you will never have sex that is as good as you would like it to be.

There is an easy answer to being able to manage your sex life and make sure that you are getting that mind-blowing finale that you have been wanting. You can learn to make your partner want you more than ever just by learning how to communicate better in ways that are both erotic and informative at the same time. The answer is with dirty talk.

Dirty talk is talking about the acts that you would like to do with your partner in a way that is arousing. It does not need to be demeaning or violent—but it certainly can be if both partners are in agreement. For some, being called a slut in the context of dirty talk can be highly arousing—it can elevate the experience that is being had. For others, that is not okay. It is important for you to understand what it is that you can and cannot say to someone else to keep them hot and bothered, and this book will be your guide.

As you read, you are going to learn all about how you can introduce dirty talk into your bedroom. You will learn how you can drive your partner *wild* for you with just a few simple words and learning to understand what it is that they want to hear. We are going to be going through what dirty talk is and how it serves as a sort of foreplay for your relationship. We will go over dirty talk for both men and women, as well as a guide to sexting and digitally talking dirty to your partner. We will consider what *not* to do when you want to talk dirty, and we will finally look at some bonus tips that you can use to help spice up your bedroom with minimal effort. You will drive your partner crazy for you, and all you have to do is learn how to talk to him or her.

Remember, keep an open mind as you read. You are not trying to learn to say things that make your partner feel bad; you are saying things that will bring your partner pleasure and enjoyment. Yes, you may be saying things that are offensive in the moment if you and the other person were in any other situation, but oftentimes, in the moment when you are bent over, or have the other person bent over, it can be incredibly erotic to be called a name. It can be erotic to tell someone to suck your cock in the right context, or it can be horribly offensive.

Dirty talk does not come easily for everyone, and some times, it can be more difficult to use than people would expect, but you can usually work through it and become an expert at turning your partner on with just your words. You can use just those simple words to bring the other person to their knees, maybe even literally, just by knowing all the right things to say.

Keep in mind that this book is, by no means, supposed to make you an expert at sex, nor is it a medical guide to try to up your performance. It is here as a reference with all sorts of suggestions that will help you spice up your sex life and drive your partner crazy. Will all of these suggestions work on each and every individual person? Probably not—but they are worth a try.

Chapter 1: Introducing Dirty Talk

Imagine this. You're in the mood, but your partner is sitting across from you on the couch, reading a book, and not seeming interested in the least. What do you do? You could say, "Hey, get over here, let's bang," but let's be real here—is that going to work? For some people, maybe. Some people are totally happy to jump to it and get some without having to work up to anything. There are some that are always DTF. But, that is not always the case by any means. Telling your partner to get over here and fuck you is probably not always going to work, and even if that does work for you right off the bat, there is a chance that just a quick session of wham, bam, thank you ma'am (or sir), is not going to do it.

If your partner is not really in to just being summoned for sex, then doing so will not help you. If your partner is okay with that, you may find that you want to bring your sex life to the next level. Thankfully, you can do both quite simply—all by mastering the art of dirty talk. If you can use dirty talk the right way, you can turn your partner on so much easier than you would probably realize. It is not some crazy, magical act that can only be done in the bedroom either—you can use it to build up that sexual tension to drive your partner wild. All you have to do is know how to use it tactfully.

What Is Dirty Talk?

Dirty talk itself is not inherently dirty in any way. It does not have to be aggressive, violent, disrespectful, or anything else—it is literally just speaking about sex. It is basically just being willing to talk about erotically. Like sex, it is just as personal to the individual receiving it. Not every person is approached in the same way, and you need to be able to tailor what you are saying to the person. It can be offensive to one person or highly erotic to another, and may even vary based on the context

Of course, however, you still have to learn how to do it in the first place. Just as sex requires exploration and learning how to perform and how to create the best time for both you and your partner, you will have to experiment with your partner and talk about what you both like and what you don't, but eventually, you will have it down to an art. You will create the right kind of talk that will drive both of you insane, and you will love it. It supercharges the tension in the air and can really help to elevate the experience.

Dirty talk is surprisingly easy to use—in general; it is as simple as saying what you want and what you like. This essentially allows you to describe what you like at any point in time so that you can drive your partner wild. Men love to watch what they are doing. Women love to hear what is liked. This means that if your partner is a woman, they are already likely to be highly susceptible to the talk in the first place—they will love to hear what you are enjoying.

We will be addressing dirty talk for men and women later on in this book, but ultimately, women are going to take more work to build up to the fullest potential pleasure that they could enjoy. This means that if you want to heat things up quickly, dirty talk is your best bet.

Is It Inherently Disrespectful?

Of course, you may have your own reservations. If the idea of calling your partner crude names and demanding that they do lewd things to you is not your idea of a good time, or if your partner is not receptive to that, you can still talk dirty. There are no rules that say that your words have to be disrespectful or even particularly derogatory. Even saying things like, "Wow, you feel so good," or, "I love it when you move like that," constitutes dirty talk— and that kind of feedback can drive someone insane if you can do it just right.

Of course, it may be that in the moment, you and your partner genuinely do enjoy being more forceful or enjoy being able to call each other names. We all have different interests, and if you and your partner decide that you are into it, that is fine, too. There is nothing wrong with calling your partner a slut if your partner is receptive to it in the moment, and it serves to turn your partner on, and you both consent to it, it is fine. Just as with any other sexual act, all that matters is that both parties are willing.

Bringing Up the Idea of Dirty Talk

When it comes to bringing up the idea of dirty talk, you may be lost. It can be difficult to figure out where to begin, or even if your partner is going to be receptive in the first place. Not everyone is, but you can usually begin to figure out how to understand your partner with some experience. Think about your first time in bed with your partner. Was it great? For most people, first sexual experiences with a new partner rarely are as good as those that happen long after the fiery passion of the honeymoon period is gone, and why is that? Because you learn what turns each other on!

You learn exactly where all of those little physical buttons to press on your partner ar. You learn what he or she likes and what is disliked. You learn what is going to help them get the best orgasm that they can and what is going to ultimately lead to them not finishing at all, unsatisfied and annoyed. It's only natural—you won't know how someone else's body works until you have had the time to experiment with them. It is only then when you learn how their body works, or if you have very explicit instructions on what they like, that you can actually do what they want when they want it the first time.

You need to go through the same learning process with the mind as well. Some keywords may be enough to drive your partner wild, or some words may just be an immediate turn off depending upon their past experiences, and you will need to figure that out with time. If you can go through the struggle of learning what they like, you will be able to really enjoy each other. You can do this by talking about it. Dirty talk really is nothing but asking each other what you like and what you do not. It is talking about what you want to do and what you do not want to do. You can start off incredibly lightly at first, slowly working up to something a bit more intense when you have gotten good responses.

Light dirty talk

To begin with, you want to start with some basic talk. Imagine this; for example—you are at work and really wishing that you could get your hands all over your partner. You could text a quick message saying, "I miss you," or even with a winky emoji added to it or something else suggestive. Or, you could ramp it up a bit. Instead of something not particularly explicit, you would instead send them a message stating, "I miss the feeling of your tits in my hand," or something else similar. NSFW? Sure. But there is nothing particularly demeaning or even shocking in that particular message. You are telling your partner what it is that you miss and what you want. This is one of the unspoken rules of dirty talk; you have to be willing to tell them what you want in the moment so that you can get it, and because you are telling your partner that you want them, you are turning them on too.

Pay attention to how they respond to these light messages of what you want. It is important that you know what it is that your partner will be receptive to. Usually, early dirty talk is much more innocent, so to speak—it is talking about what you like and is usually more affectionate. It involves messages such as:

- I love the way you feel
- I need your body right now

- I'm so turned on by you right now
- I love your hands right there
- You look so sexy right now
- I love what you are doing right this moment
- You feel so good

You usually won't see many protests to most of this dirty talk; in fact, if you tell your partner that he or she is driving you wild, they will probably respond well to you. They will feel that tension building within them, and you will probably have a better time.

Moderate dirty talk

After enough light, dirty talk, it is time to consider some more moderate talk. This is usually a bit more explicit. You may find that at this stage, your partner gets even more excited in the moment, or you may find that you have reached that boundary point, especially if your partner voices that he or she feels taken advantage of, dirty, annoyed, or unhappy with any of this talk. However, if your partner responds well and seems to be turned on, even more, you know that you are on the right track. These are phrases such as:

- I want to dominate you/I want you to dominate me
- You have the perfect pussy/cock
- I love how you ride me
- Fuck me louder
- I'm going to pound you tonight
- I want you to pound me harder with your big dick/cock
- I love sucking your cock/licking your pussy so much

As you can see, at this level, you are getting a bit more explicit. You are starting to use words that, in ordinary circumstances, would be deemed vulgar or inappropriate. They can be offensive to some people, so you will need to make sure that you know where your partner draws that line.

X-rated dirty talk

Here, you are looking at dirty talk that usually is not going to be brought into a relationship that is still new. You are using this kind of talk for a partner that you know is going to be comfortable with it, and usually, you want to slowly build up to this, if your partner is receptive. This is overtly sexual; it is the kind of talk that is going to only be reserved for talking behind closed doors, or possibly through texts in private, but these are not phrases that would, under any means, be appropriate in any context beyond sex with someone.

- Show me how wet my slutty little pussy is
- Fuck me harder
- I want to be your little fuck toy
- I want to ruin your pussy
- I want you to ruin my pussy
- I want you to fuck me harder
- I want to taste myself on you

Some people are into this, but others would balk at such talk at any point in their relationship. It is important to recognize that everyone has their own boundaries that you will need to respect. Dirty talk, even when based in this kind of language, should still be adhering to the boundaries of your partner. Sex is intimate, even amongst strangers or during one night stands. It is a deeply personal act to give your body to someone else, and no matter the context, no matter if you are into BDSM, talking dirty, or anything else, the important part to emphasize is always consent and boundaries. Of course, you only know what those boundaries are if you can talk to the other person to figure out what theirs are in the first place. Communication is key.

Tips for Introducing Dirty Talk

So, you want to add dirty talk into your relationship. It could be great fun for you and your partner, and there is a good chance that you will find something that works for both of you. It may feel intimidating, but the best thing that you can do is get started. Start small and work up to what it is that you want to do. Make sure that you ask your partner during times that are not sexually charged about their own preferences and if anything stood out to them during your last romp.

If you are getting ready and don't know where to start to introduce dirty talk, then pay attention to these tips that are being provided for you. They are great starting points to begin talking about what it is that you and your partner want out of your relationship, how far you are both willing to go, and how you can both get the most potential enjoyment out of it. Try it and start slow—you will probably find that your sex gets even hotter than it ever was.

Talk about what you want

When it comes right down to it, you should make sure that you always talk about what it is that you want. When you are sending messages to your partner, or even just talking to him or her when you are not able to actually get down to business, you can drop little hints to drive the other person crazy. Tell your partner what you want. "I want you right now." "I wish I could feel your hands on me." "I miss the way that your breasts/hips/ass feels." Those are all starting points—you are telling your partner what you ideally want at that point in time, and that will drive them wild.

During sex, tell your partner what you like

During the actual act, make sure that you give feedback to your partner. Tell them what you like. Tell them what is really working for you. Make sure that you tell them what it is that you want if what they are doing is not quite doing it for you. Dirty talk is there to bridge that gap in communication. It is there to get comfortable with the idea of communicating about your own sexual desires and preferences without feeling ashamed or bothered by it, while simultaneously setting the stage for it.

Talk about it before the moment

Make sure that you have some time before you even begin to use it, where you and your partner have a genuine discussion of what you want out of your sex that you are having and what you like to hear or what you dislike hearing. Maybe there are some words that simply drive you insane, and not in a good way—before you begin to add dirty talk to your relationship is the best time to go over that. Make sure that you are communicating effectively.

Learn to be assertive

You have to be assertive in sex. Make sure that you are able to tell your partner exactly what you want or what you do not want. If they ask you if they can cum on your face, but you say that you are not into that, fair enough. You need to be able to say no, or say, "Hey, what you're doing really isn't for me. Let's forget about that." It is okay for you to say no about something that you do not care to do; in fact, you should say no to avoid resentment, which will destroy your relationship far quicker than anything else.

Don't be afraid to ask for something

Similarly, make sure that if there is something that you really want, you need to be willing to communicate about it. Don't hesitate to ask if something that you want is in your mind; you can always ask. Worst case scenario, you are told no, but really, that's better than feeling like you're denying yourself because you are too shy to ask.

Get creative

Make sure that you are using adjectives to describe what you are feeling. Think about the way that you want to describe your partner and see how he or she responds. Are they turned on when you tell them that they are beautiful/handsome, or do they respond better being called dirty or naughty? Everyone has different preferences, and the sooner that you can figure out what your partner's preferences are, the sooner you can begin to use them to entice them.

Don't forget your verbs

Yes, what you are doing is fucking—but use some other words in there too. Make a call to action. Talk about what you want and use verbs that will paint the picture of what you want. After all, "I want to make sweet love to you," has a totally different connotation than, "I want to fuck you so hard that you won't be able to walk tomorrow." Think about what it is that you prefer to talk about and also what appeals to your partner.

Compliment your partner in the moment

In the moment, make sure that you offer your partner compliments. What are they doing that drives you crazy? What makes you hotter? Do you like how they are moving or what they are doing? Compliment it? "God, your hair looks so damn sexy when you're on me," or "Wow, your touch feels so good." When you do this, you let your partner know that you are, in fact, enjoying every moment of what you are doing with them, and that will turn most people on more than anything else.

Narrate what you will do

Another great starting point is to narrate what you are about to do. Make sure that you, in the moment, let your partner know what you are about to do or what you are doing. "I'm gonna fuck you so hard right now," just before you start, or "Fuck, I'm gonna cum" or something along those lines. When you narrate like that, you put your partner in your mind as well. You are showing them the idea that you are enjoying what is happening. You are showing your partner how much you are having fun, and that matters in the moment.

Check in after sex

Dirty talk doesn't end when the fun does—you also need to talk to your partner after the fact. This is a sort of aftercare; it helps to show that your partner matters to you, and that will help to enhance what happened. You can talk to your partner about the actions that you enjoyed or tell your partner what they did so well, and you let them know that you continue to think about them and the fun that you had after the fact.

Take some of your dirty talk outside of the bedroom

When you are standing with your partner while doing something together, don't forget to add in your double entendres here and there to remind them that you are thinking about what you are doing. Even innocent comments can do the job for you. Imagine that your partner wears a deodorant that smells very distinct; perhaps it is a floral one. When you are at the grocery

116

store talking about the candles and trying to choose one out, you can point out one that smells similarly and make a comment about it that lets your partner know that you are thinking about them, their scent, and the passionate fun you had in bed.

Experiment often

If you and your partner are still trying to figure out what it is that you want or like, you can, and should, experiment often. Bring new talk to the bedroom and mention it when you talk. Bring your desires to life all around you. Talk about what you want to do when you get the chance to do so.

Find inspiration

Sometimes, you will see some things that are highly erotic on television, or you'll read a book that has a particularly provocative line in it. Keep in mind that ultimately, television, books, and porn are just fiction—but the words used can still be deeply powerful and can be highly erotic as well. If you are having a hard time coming up with the right words to use, you can make sure that you do talk the right way to the person that you are around.

Get used to talking about sex in all sorts of contexts

A great way to help yourself figure out what you can do to eliminate some of the taboo is to start talking to your friends as well. No, you probably won't be telling your friends that you want to take them, bend them over, and fuck them, but if you can get used to saying so many of those words on your own even in normal conversations, you will be more able to talk to your partner as well. You need to be able to say words that you will need to use in the moment with them.

Expand your vocabulary

Another great starting point is to figure out the words that you are comfortable using. Make sure that you have a list of those that you won't mind making use of regularly. It could be that you are fine calling a penis a dick, but if calling a vagina a pussy or a cunt is a problem, figure out what you do want to call it. There is no right or wrong answer here for you; you can choose the one that is just right for you.

Keep it simple

You don't have to start off talking like you are in the middle of a porno—make sure that you are using words that you are comfortable with, and you can even keep it short. As you walk past your partner, whisper, "I can't wait to have you," for example—that could be enough to drive him or her insane. You don't have to do anything uniquely spectacular or creative or spout off a long ode to your partner's genitalia to constitute dirty talk. Even the occasional comment could be enough for you and your partner to get off better than before.

Channel your senses

When you are thinking of saying something, make sure that you use something that plays on the senses. Sex is intensely sensual, and you want to bring the senses into things as much as you can. "I can't wait for tonight." "I need to taste you." I want to feel you." I love how you smell." Try to hit all of the senses when you are getting started.

Start slowly

You don't have to just rush into things to have good dirty talk. In fact, some of the best, especially early on, involves slowly adding it in. Bring it up, little by little, and tell your partner what you like and what you want. You'll be surprised at the end results.

Be playful

There should not be anything innately hurtful; it should all be in good fun. If you want to enjoy your relationship with your partner, you want to make sure that ultimately, you are using your dirty talk to spice things up and make things more enjoyable. There is no reason to make yourself or your partner feel bad.

Give instructions

It can help to stop and tell your partner exactly what you want in the moment. Instead of asking for it, tell them what you want. This is a great way to really get them in the mood. A lot of people like it when their partner takes charge and tells them what to do; they are happy to comply. If you are interested in something, you should tell your partner what you want.

Try roleplaying

Some people find that the dirty talk, in general, is simpler if they are getting into the mood through roleplay instead. You can ask if you and your partner can try a small roleplay scenario and see if that gets the words flowing.

Try via text or messages if you feel too self-conscious

Now, it may just be that you cannot look at your partner with a straight face and say, "I want you to fuck me. Hard. Right now." Fine, fair enough. It can take time to work up to something like that. But, what you can do is begin to send some suggestive messages. Leave a note in your partner's lunch or in their car to find. Send a text when you know they won't get in trouble.

If something doesn't work, talk about it later

If you find that you have said something to your partner that immediately kills the mood, ask about it later. It might not be something that you can talk about in the moment, but you can usually check in with your partner after the fact. It is important that when you are in a sexual relationship, you are able to check in after the fact, and if you get the idea that you have made a mistake, make sure you ask about it later.

Figure out their sexual triggers

Figure out what it is that your partner really wants. Figure out the language that gets them rearing to go and make sure that you use them regularly. Most people have certain terms that they use, and you should figure those out. What do they say to you when they talk about sex? Do they call it sex? Fucking? Love-making? You want to adopt their language surrounding everything.

Let them know how turned on you are

You should always let your partner know when you want to use dirty talk, when, and how turned on you are. You can let them know what you are feeling, and that brings awareness to it. You are making them feel better because they feel like they can be more confident with you; they feel like fucking you is that much more fun because you are giving them that little ego boost.

One-word dirty talk

Sometimes, all you need is one word. You can say, "Yes,"
or "Harder," or "Deeper." When you add just one word,
your partner knows that they are doing a good job; you
weren't able to say a complete sentence, and they know
that you are enjoying it. Master this, and don't be afraid to
whisper it to them as you go.

Ask them what they want

Sometimes, you can make things sexier in the moment
when you ask your partner what they want you to do.
"How do you want me to finish you off?" or "How do you
want to cum tonight?" are great in the heat of the
moment, and you are letting your partner know that you
will take care of him/her.

Use it when your partner least expects it

One thing that you can do to consistently get others off is
to let them know that you want to do something when
they least expect it. Send a quick message that says, "I
want your pants off when I get home," or something
similar, and you tell your partner that you are thinking
about them.

Use it often

Make sure that you are willing to talk regularly about
what you want. This is a great way to build up that tension
all day long and get your partner's engines revving and
juices flowing. If you want a good fuck, make them want
it.

Do some research

You can learn all about what to say and find new lines pretty easily. You can find online erotica and read over that to get some inspiration. You can get all sorts of new phrases that can be used there, and your partner may even go crazy for them.

Chapter 2: Dirty Talk as Foreplay

Men may be able to go from 0 to ready to go to the bone zone in an instant, but that doesn't mean that they *should*. Why rush to the end? Foreplay is defined as sexual activity of any kind before the actual act of sexual intercourse. Some people prefer foreplay—a lot, and for a good reason. Foreplay is like the appetizer before the main course. It is there to help your partner, and you both enjoy sexual acts more. Your body is not primed to always enjoy sex—there are certain criteria that have to happen. Think about it—have you ever had sex when you were not ready, if you are a woman, or if you are a man, have you ever tried to slide in before your partner was ready? Or before you were yourself? You can't—or if you can, it is not pleasant.

Arousal happens during the foreplay stage. Your body, and your partner's, prepare for sex, and as a result, you and your partner both end up enjoying it that much more as a result. Men get harder. They find that they have more sensation during the act. Women get wetter, making everything that much more enjoyable as well. Blood flows down to the genitalia during arousal, and as a result, everything feels better.

Foreplay is so important—you need it if you want to have good sex. Can you have good sex if you and your partner both happen to be insanely horny at the same time without needing that setup? Sure—but that is the exception more than the rule. If you want good, passionate sex, do not forget the foreplay.

Foreplay doesn't have to be physical, and it doesn't have to happen immediately before you actually have sex. In fact, you can enjoy it all day long, tantalizingly teasing your partner so that you know their blood is rushing, and they are ready for that end of the night finale. It will probably become even more sensual when you have had all day long to drive your partner absolutely crazy with your talk and with your actions. All you have to do is know how to turn your partner on.

Turning Your Partner on With Dirty Talk

During arousal, all sorts of different things happen in the body. Your body literally prepares for the act of sex when it is aroused—it prepares the proper responses that your body will need. Your heart rate increases, along with blood pressure and pulse—this makes sense if blood is being redirected to the genitalia to help with sensation. Likewise, blood vessels will dilate in the genitals so that they can become engorged with blood. The penis swells up as a result, and on women, both the clitoris and labia do as well. For women, the breasts will also swell up, and nipples become erect, and the vagina becomes lubricated naturally.

All of this happens so that the body is ready to have and enjoy sex. It is only when you are actually aroused that sex is actually enjoyable in the first place, and if you are not, you may come to enjoy it in the moment, or you simply dislike it the entire time. Either can happen as a result of what is going on. But really, do you want to enjoy your time? Start with the foreplay. It will put you in the right mood as well. You will be able to build the emotional intimacy that all good sexual relationships need, and you will also be able to lower inhibitions during the foreplay. It is intoxicating and heady, and the more that you play around with each other, physically or verbally, the better your sex will go. Foreplay helps to release the necessary hormones that will lower cortisol—the stress hormone—in preparation for the bonding and affection felt during the act of sex.

Better Sex With Dirty Talk

Foreplay is important—there is no doubt about that. But, if you want to have better sex with dirty talk, you can make it happen. Dirty talk makes sex better just because of the way that it works. We want to be lusted after. We want to feel like we are wanted. We want to believe that our bodies drive our partners insane and that our partners want to get back with us as soon as possible. It's not just about going through the motions; it is about the fiery passion and pleasure. It is about taking someone else's body and making it your own. It is about enjoying yourself more intimately than possible in other ways. Sex is fun, but there is so much more to it than that. It is inherently programmed into us, and it is there to make us bond with our partners. It creates those feelings of euphoria and affection that we associate with our partners. Foreplay and dirty talk will both elevate sex from "meh" to being hot and better than ever before.

Dirty talk makes sex better—we know that for sure. We also know why it does that as well. Let's talk about the ways that dirty talk can create a better sex experience for both you and your partner before we continue on with looking at how to make it happen.

You can tell your partner what you like and dislike

Good sex, the kind that blows your mind, is all about communication—so why not make that communication fun and pleasant? Why not make that communication something enjoyable? Why not make sure that the communication does the work for you as well? You could tell your partner one day that the sex that you have is great when they do that one thing, or you could tell your partner in the moment, "Oh, god, I love it when you do that!" as it is happening. Telling your partner in the moment is going to leave them on fire; it will automatically stoke their inner fire. They know that what they are doing right in that moment is working for you, and that is enough for them.

You are able to connect better

Sex is also about connection. Even with one-night stands, you are still making a connection between yourself and the other person to some degree; you are able to tell your partner what it is that you want or need out of the encounter. Connection matters and dirty talk can help foster it.

You can reignite a lost flame

If you are living with your long-term partner, you may find that your infatuation, that highly passionate, desire-laden feeling is replaced with something that feels less. All too many people will mistake what happens to their feelings with them losing their love for the other person. However, it is normal for infatuation to disappear. However, you can spark that flame of passion again in the bedroom. Dirty talk can help you find those feelings of lust that you thought faded away with the infatuation. With a bit of dirty talk, you can add some variety to the relationship so that you are able to maintain that spark and enjoyment with each other.

It is versatile

Even if you and your partner are not together right at that moment for any reason, whether they have to work or they have traveled or anything else, you can send them pictures that remind them that they are the one for you and that you want them more than they probably realize. You are able to figure out what it will take for you and your partner to keep that spark alight, and you will be able to help create that allure; your partner will be caught up with you and probably spend all day long, thinking about getting back to your bed.

You'll boost your confidence

The act of talking to your partner and seeing the effect that it has on him, or her is a great boost in confidence. If you want to make sure that you are confident, you want to make sure that you can confirm that your partner is attracted to you, and a wonderful way to make that happen is through the way that you talk dirty to him or her. It will make you feel so much better about yourself when you realize that the simple act of talking to your partner is enough to drive him or her wild.

You'll also feel more attractive as a result as well. You'll feel like, in saying those words, you can take control, and you can get exactly what you want when you want it, and that is highly compelling and powerful.

It creates variety

If you can talk dirty to each other, you are able to make sure that your sex life never gets boring. You and your partner are able to figure out everything that you will need to do to maintain your passion for each other. You will be able to try new things and really and truly enjoy them as much as possible to really make sure that your spark never fades.

You can use dirty talk as a segue into talking about new positions, bringing toys into the relationship, and even starting to experiment with new objects. It can help you transition to speaking about, and therefore trying, any of those kinks that you may have had but been afraid to talk about. You will be able to tell your partner about those things that you have kept hidden, not knowing how to bring it up.

It makes you feel better about what you are doing in the moment

When you and your partner can talk to each other about intimate acts like sex, you know that you can talk about just about anything, including aspects of your life. You can alleviate the pressure that comes along with sex—you do not feel like your performance is under complete scrutiny in the moment because you and your partner are both talking about your actions with each other. Your partner is saying what he or she likes and that will give you that boost that you needed to know to help yourself figure out that you do not actually have to worry about the pressure aspect of what is happening. You aren't worrying about if you are doing things right because you can see that ultimately, your partner must be into it if they are dirty talking back.

It makes sex feel better

Sex is not designed to be quiet. Think about it—we groan and moan and grunt sometimes. It is not something that is meant to be prim and proper—it is us giving into our carnal, most feral desires that we have, and that means letting go of needing to be quiet. When you tell your partner how good things feel, you help make it feel even better. You make it real by acknowledging it, elevating it to the next level. This also helps you to create that higher sense of fulfillment that you are looking for as well.

Ultimately, sex is better with dirty talk. We love it—it lets us communicate what matters the most, and it helps us to feel more in tune with our desires. That is highly important to consider, and the sooner that we recognize that, the better. Give it a shot. Let your shame or embarrassment go and talk dirty to your partner. You'll be surprised by how different things can be with it.

Creating Sexual Tension with Dirty Talk

Sexual tension is highly powerful. We see it used in media all of the time because of the effect that it has—it's *hot*. It's so fun to see the ways that people respond to each other when they clearly want to have sex, but are afraid to or they can't, or there is some sort of boundary that cannot be crossed. It typically involves delaying or denying sex. The sex could cause problems, such as at work, or because there is a reason that it would otherwise have social impacts that are wanted to be avoided.

In relationships, however, sexual tension occurs when two people want to have sex and are flirting but can't actually perform for some reason. Maybe you and your partner are both at a big family event, and there is no way to comfortably give in without being caught. Maybe you and your partner are staying in someone else's home, or your children are around, or you're apart for work. No matter the reason, however, you can encourage sexual tension.

While sexual tension between two people that are not sexual partners may be awkward and uncomfortable, in a relationship or with partners, it can help you maintain that hot sex life that keeps both of you going crazy for each other. If you want to be able to build your own sexual tension, you need to know how to make it happen, and usually, it should be happening all day long.

The longer you can stoke that tension, the better it will feel when you release it. After all, what is orgasm other than a sudden release of built-up tension? You can build that tension up higher and higher all day long if you know how to get started. Dirty talk is one of the easiest ways to begin building that tension so that when you get home or when you and your partner are with each other again, you will not be able to keep your hands off of each other.

If you want to create tension, all you have to do is follow some simple ideas, and usually, dirty talk is the easiest

129

way to do so, especially if you and your partner are apart from each other. Your ability to create that tension is going to make your partner completely and utterly addicted to you, and you will be able to guarantee that they will not be able to keep their hands away. If you want that, if you want to know that your partner will be vying to get that release from you any way possible, keep in mind the idea of creating sexual tension.

Start in the morning and keep it going all day

One thing that you need to do if you want to keep that tension going all day long is to start first thing in the morning. We all usually rush through the morning; it is hard to really have time for each other when we have places to go and maybe even kids to shuttle around. But, the morning is the perfect time to start that fire. You can create that spark, leaving the orgasm for later, allowing you to continually stoke the spark until your partner can't stand it any longer.

As you're getting ready to part in the morning, whisper a few dirty phrases to your partner, even if you don't have the time to sit down and make it happen. If you can remind each other of what you are doing and what you think, whispering those phrases of sweet passion to each other, you can get that flame stoked, and in no time, they will be begging for you as soon as you reunite.

Send texts throughout the day

When you have a thought about your partner during the day, let them know. Remind them that you are thinking about them. Tell yourself that you can't wait to get them in bed with you. If you miss them, tell them what you want to do. They will love the little boost in their ego first thing in the morning. You could even slip in a quick picture if you wanted to; they will probably love it.

Get creative with your timing

If you want that tension to build, make sure that you are getting creative. If you are in the theater, you can whisper a comment that will make them blush, and you will probably instantly turn them on. A well-placed hand on a thigh with the right look and the right phrase will build up that tension and make it impossible to forget it. You will be able to make sure that ultimately, they can't stop thinking about you, and that is exactly what you need. If you want to make sure that your partner craves you and will do whatever it is that you want them to, this is one way to drive them insane.

Whisper in their ear or in the crook of their neck

You want to make sure that your partner will be as turned on as possible, and that means that you will want to use all of their senses. Hovering right by their ear and whispering to them when you can to deliver that moment of what you want them to hear is the greatest way to really deliver that double whammy of physical closeness, whispering in an erogenous zone, and then also saying something that you know is going to turn them on.

Tips for Dirty Talk

Now, if you want to start delivering the best possible dirty talk that you can to your partner, it is time to get down to business through all sorts of different tips and tricks that you can use. If you really want to drive your partner insane, you need to be able to use the right words to make sure that they really want you. We are going to go over another 30 tips right now that will help you to bring your dirty talk to the next level during your relationship. You will be able to take your foreplay from average levels to those that are burning with desire that will make that moment of release that much sweeter when you are finally able to satisfy that desire that you have for your partner.

Make it authentic

When you are using dirty talk, make sure that what you say is authentic. If you are really thinking about fucking your partner's brains out, then say that—or if you are thinking about that quiet sensual night that you had the other night, tell them that, too. You should not be afraid of what it is that you are going to say to your partner. Make sure that you are paying attention to the way that your authenticity is being received as well.

Make sure it is mirroring your partner

Watch your partner—pay attention to if they seem to want to engage. If they engage after you have reached out and left a sexual line to grab, then go ahead and continue. If they seem not to be into it for some reason, pushing probably is going to do more harm than good. Make sure that if your partner is the first one to reach out, you reciprocate as well.

Ask simple questions

If you are asking questions at all to be erotic, make sure that the questions that you ask are those that are simple to answer—they should be yes or no questions. Your partner is not looking to be quizzed—rather, he or she probably wants to enjoy the moment and asking too many times how they like something is probably going to kill the moment. Instead of texting your partner saying, "What do you want me to do tonight?" which would put them on the spot and may be difficult for them to answer, you can ask, "Do you want me to fuck you hard tonight?"

Build up to it gradually

If you are building up your foreplay, even for the day, don't just jump straight for the X-rated script that you are thinking about; instead, build up over time, all day long. Start out with a quick whisper of, "I can't wait to get my hands on you tonight," for example, as you are passing by each other to go to work or wherever you go in the morning. Even if it might feel like a good idea to share your passion by saying, "Goodbye, you dirty slut, I'll punish you accordingly when you get home," as you're walking out the door, if your partner isn't feeling it in the moment, you're probably going to do more harm than good. Start out innocently and build up all day long. It's not a race to incinerate everything; slow and steady is always best when you have a whole day of tantalizing messages to share.

Skip the eye contact at first if it is making you uncomfortable

Eye contact can be intense for people, especially if it is not something that they are usually comfortable with. However, you do not have to maintain eye contact for dirty talk. In fact, you can even have dirty talk occurring entirely over digital means without having to see each other in person at all if you wanted to. You can talk to them separately if you wanted to. You don't even have to look at the other person if it is making you nervous. If you find that you lack the confidence that you will need to get to the sexy point that you want to make, find a way to skip out on the eye contact. You can build up to that over time.

Make a promise for later, and follow through with it

If you tell your partner that you plan on bending them over and thrusting with reckless abandon that night during your constant foreplay for the day, you will want to follow through with it. Make that anticipation and reward

133

it later on. Make sure that you always follow through with what you say that you are going to do so that you can make sure that ultimately when you tell your partner something, they know that you will follow through with it.

Inside jokes

Now, jokes may seem like the least sexy thing ever, but think of it this way—when you have inside jokes that are about your sex life, just mentioning the inside joke, or referencing it, can be enough to get your partner going with just a glance and a passing comment and no one else around you will be any wiser to what has just occurred. This is a fantastic way to approach the situation if you are trying to figure out how best to interact in ways that are not overt.

Say something with a double entendre

Imagine that you are eating a popsicle, sensuously sucking on it while making fuck-me eyes at your partner, smirking and saying that, "It tastes so good," or "Mmm..." as you do it. This is going to get your partner desperate for you without ever saying anything that is not really appropriate. The tone is what matters here, and the double entendre is probably enough to help your partner really feel like you want them. This is perfect. You could even lean over and mention something about wishing that you had them in your mouth instead.

Say something subtly possessive

Now, too much possessiveness and jealousy is obviously a problem in a relationship, but if you can play it off the right way and whisper it to your partner as you do, smirking, or flirting with them, you can drive them crazy. We innately like the idea of our partners claiming us as their own, especially when we know that it is not something that is meant from a bad place. It can be kind of sexy to hear our partners stake their claims over us, after all, especially if it is something like, "I want to make you mine."

It's all about the tone

Keep in mind that the tone of what you say is everything. If you want to drive your partner crazy, you have to use the right tone of voice, or you are going to find that he or she is probably going to lose interest. Think about it: would it be sexy for someone to tell you in a flat voice, "I love your cock/pussy."? No enthusiasm. No actual sense of enjoyment in there. Just a flat, robotic, "I love it." Would you believe it? Probably not. Would it stoke that fire within you? Probably not.

You need to master the sexy tone to master the art of foreplay, and that means making sure that your tone is something that you know they will find attractive. Go for something lower, throatier, and softer. Learn the voice. It's your sexy voice. Use it.

Read erotica to each other

If you and your partner are still struggling with being able to talk to each other honestly and from that point of sexual tension, then stop, take some time, and read some erotica that you can read back and forth to each other. This lets you get a feel for the writing and the phrasing. You start to adjust to saying the words in your mouth, and as a result, you get closer to stepping into the zone of being able to use your own dirty talk.

Be bold and take a chance

You never know how your partner will take what you are saying. Try taking some chances and saying some things that ordinarily, you wouldn't say, but that you decided to try out. Be bold. Say things that you think are hot, but that you wouldn't dare to say to your partner normally and see how he or she responds to it. You may be pleasantly surprised.

Make a game out of it

It could be fun to make a game out of trying to make each other blush. The point is to ramp up your sex talk until one of you or the other is blushing. Then, the other person is the winner in the situation. It can be fun trying to think of the sexiest, most blush-worthy comment that you can come up with in hopes of seeing what happens next.

Don't be ashamed as you talk

Don't worry about what you are saying; you are talking with someone that you have had sex with—you don't get much more vulnerable than having someone else's body part in you, or in putting your body part inside of someone else. Allow yourself to really come to terms with the sexual content that you are saying and don't mind it. You're saying things that are typically "inappropriate," but you have a very specific purpose for doing so—you are trying to turn on your partner. Let's face it—the act of sex itself, to someone who is not turned on, may seem a bit strange. It is messy and sweaty, and isn't it a little bit strange how we put our private bits together, and they somehow fit? Sex is strange. Nature is strange. The worlds that you use to try to turn someone on are probably going to seem strange too—but they serve a purpose. Let go of the shame and just do it.

Ask some dirty questions

Sometimes, it can help to ask questions that are dirty. "What do you think I'm wearing? How would you feel if I answered the door and was naked? What should I wear today for you?" Ask questions that start to hint on suggestive but are not all the way there yet. It starts to set the field for what you want to do—which is turn on your partner, and the sooner that you can do that, the sooner that you can get into bed.

Share your fantasies

If you have been dreaming or fantasizing about your partner, now is the time to share it. Talk to your partner about the dreams that you have been having or about what you want to do with your partner more than anything and don't hold back about it—the fantasies should be erotic, and you may find that your partner will even agree to do what you want to do without complaint. You may even find that you both share the same common fantasy!

Ask if your partner wants to take charge

If you want your partner to love fucking you, then you want to ask them if they want to be in control. Even if you are usually the one that takes the lead, ask them what they want. Figure out if they do want to be in the lead, and if they do, let it happen. You may find that you are pleasantly surprised by what happens next.

Tell your partner what you want them to do

If your partner is at home and you are at work, you can send them some sexy texts telling them what you want them to do right at that moment. Make it erotic, but make sure that they don't quite finish up the job without you. Let them know that you want to save the best part for you at home and that you're thinking about them doing it. This builds up that tension for you, and for them, you are both going to be dying to get into each other's arms.

Ask them to play dirty truth or dare

Again, if you want to create foreplay with dirty talk, games can be a great tool to use. You can set up, so you and your partner both play together and see where things take you.

If all of the topics are erotic, you will both probably find that pretty soon, you're both desperate for the other's touch, and that means that your job was very well done.

Message them when you're masturbating

If you're going solo for a session and are apart, consider sending some sexy messages letting them know that you're thinking about them—*really* thinking about them. They will probably go crazy for it, and you can find yourself loving every single moment of it. You will be able to tease them with messages such as, "Oh, it's too bad you're not here, I could use some help ;)" or something similar to that to let them know that even when you're on your own, and even with the entirety of the internet's near-infinite and ever-expanding collection of porn, you chose to think about your partner.

Sexy riddles

You can use sexual riddles that are fun, but still erotic and send them or whisper them to your partner all day long, really building up that foreplay before your grand finale. Riddles can be something silly like, "What's hot and [skin color] and all wrapped up, waiting for you?" or something more erotic as well. Be creative. Be silly about it, but most of all, be erotic and sensual.

Tell them what turns you on

Make sure that you let your partner know exactly what it is that you want to do. Tell them what turns you on more than anything else, and they will probably use that to their advantage later on. Even better, if you are sharing turn ons, just thinking about them will probably get some juices or blood flowing, if you catch my drift.

Tell them what they do to you

If your partner is driving you crazy, let them know. Tell them just how passionate you are for them and just how much knowing that you can't be inside of them, or have them inside of you, right that moment is driving you mad. If you can do this, telling them just how passionate you are, you can boost their egos while also setting up that sexual tension for later on as well.

Tell them what you intend to do when you see each other next/the next time you are in bed

Let them know exactly what you're going to do next—tell them, for example, that you're going to tease them all day long, or that you're going to suck them or lick them or fuck them, or anything else that you're interested in doing. It will get them going crazy for you as well, and you will be able to see just how strong of an effect that you have on your partner when you do it. This is highly erotic and something that many people love to hear as well.

Create a template

If you struggle with dirty talk, it can help to have a sort of template, where you simply follow the lead and fill in the blanks to make it work for you. You could, for example, use some talk about what you love when they do something. Try this format: I love [action] when you [describe the action]. This can help you to begin to get that process down so that you can properly voice your approval or what really matters the most to you when you're getting down to business.

Create IOUs

You can create little sexual IOUs for each other as well. You can whisper to your partner what you want them to do to you that night, as well as whisper to them your promises for what you will do for them when you are able to get down and dirty that evening. The idea here is to create that anticipation for the night—it should be enticing and should drive you both wild. Hearing what you are going to do to each other is a great way for that tension that you need during foreplay to really be built up.

Ask them what they do when they are masturbating

You can also ask your partner what they think about when they are flying solo as well. You can use this information, hearing about what they do with each other so that you can begin to use that when you do have sex. This is a great way to open up conversations and connections about what you both like as well. It is a wonderful influence if you need to make sure that you are both able to talk to each other openly, and even better, it can turn you both on— you get to fantasize about your partner touching him/herself, and your partner gets the added benefit of thinking about you doing what they do.

Let them know about your favorite body part they have

Think about your partner and what attracts you the most to them physically—then compliment them for that body part. Let them know that their stomach or their abs or their breasts drive you insane and tell them all about how much you think about those body parts and what they mean to you. When you do this regularly, you are not only boosting confidence for them; you are also letting them know that you care about them and that you are paying attention to what they look like and how you see them. This is crucial; if you want to have mind-blowing sex, they have to feel confident enough to believe that you are attracted to them.

Talk about your own anticipation

Tell them what you can hardly wait for. Let them know that you are anticipating them. The idea that they are being lusted over is going to be highly erotic for them, and they will likely respond incredibly positively to it, meaning that you'll be able to have all the fun in the world when you can get together. Comments like, "I can't wait to feel you," or "I'm picturing us together naked right now, and I can't wait until we're alone so we can be," are great at stoking those flames and igniting that passion you want.

Chapter 3: Dirty Talk for Men

So. You want to get down with a man, do you? Do you want to make him hard with just a few whispers or a few words typed into your phone? You can make that happen—all you have to do is know what to say, and you'll get his blood pumping in no time at all. As you read through this chapter, you are going to learn all about what it is that will turn on a man with next to no effort at all— all you have to do is be smart about the way that you choose to communicate with him.

Dirty talk can be especially difficult to muster for many women who may feel awkward about what they will be saying. If you're a woman, or even a shy man, hoping to get it on with the man of your dreams, you need to learn one thing: Confidence is sexy. Take control. Take command of the conversation. Make sure that when you talk to him, you are brave about it and that you are willing to go for it. Many men are sex-driven—it is just part of their hardwiring. They are born to fuck, and if they can't, they feel defeated. They may feel emasculated if it is not clear from what you are doing or how you sound that you are enjoying yourself. They want to know what you think of them, especially during sex itself, and they want to hear what you want them to do to you as well.

Whether it is a well-placed moan, a few whispered words of affirmation that he is, in fact, getting you off, or even screaming his name with abandon, head thrown back in sheer ecstasy as you ride him, you have options and dirty talk for men is absolutely not a one size fits all sort of thing. However, one thing is consistent. No matter what, men want to feel validated in knowing that you are satisfied with their sex, either in the moment, leading up to the moment, or even after the fact. All you have to do is figure out how to tell him that.

What Men Want to Hear

Men, when in bed, are simple creatures. They want to know that you are enjoying them, and they want to feel like they are getting you off. If you can give them that, you are already going to escalate the sex to fantastic levels that your partner will most likely thrive on. Think about it—how validating and how much of a turn on is it for you if you are told that your sex is the best, or if you can see that the other person is loving every moment with you?

When you are talking to your partner, then your dirty talk simply has to inform him of one thing: That you want him to fuck you because you think that sex with him is fantastic. If your dirty talk conveys that, you are probably on the right track just like that. How can you do that, then? Simple—you can tell him what you want to do, or you can make use of moans when making out or riding him. You can tell him that he is fucking you so good or that you love it. There are so many options there—you just have to let him know that you are there, present and in the moment and that you would rather be there than anywhere else.

Turning Men On

When it comes to turning your man on, you have no shortage of ways. You could simply take off your own clothes, and he will probably be hard just thinking about the time that he can have with you. You can kiss him or touch him or tell him to fuck you there, or you could do it the long way, building up that sexual tension and making it so that he can't think about anything else. Turning men on is more than just touching some cock and balls or shaking an ass. There are ways to do so without ever laying a finger on him, in fact, and some of those can be even sexier than what you may do to him in bed.

Remember that ultimately, every man is going to be different. Every man is going to have his own preferences that you will need to consider, but if you are able to consider them effectively, you can also usually make it happen in very similar ways through seduction. If you want to turn your man on, consider these options to get that blood pumping and get him ready to go.

Smile seductively

The seductive smile is a great way to get him going, especially if you have just said something that could fall into a double entendre zone. Giving him a quick, sexy smile, especially if you let your eyes undress him within his attention, can drive him wild. You can do this across a room from each other, or you can do it in the middle of a conversation. Make sure that you have an intense gaze as you look at him and try to entice him over.

Be confident

Confidence is sexy, whether you are a man or a woman. If you can speak with confidence, act with confidence, smile with confidence, and more, you will find that he absolutely loves the way that you engage with him. Make sure that, no matter what it is that you are saying to him, you do it with confidence. Even if you tell him something that sounds borderline ridiculous when you first say it, if you can pull it off, you will find that he will go crazy for you in an instant. All you have to do is have that confident attitude.

Compliment him

Men *love* to be complimented. It gives him that ego boost that will help to turn him on even more, and it also shows that you are paying attention to him, meaning that you are getting him ready with two different tactics at once. If you want to make sure that you can get him happy, hot,
144

and in bed, you want to give him the best compliments that you can think of. Tell him how smart he is when he helps you. Let him know that you think he's sexy when he's doing something. When you're in bed together, tell him how you are enjoying it. All of this will help you to turn him on with ease, and the sooner that you turn him on, the sooner that you will find that he will want to stick by you.

Dress sexy

Of course, men also love their eye candy. If you want him to think that you look great, then you have to act the part as well. Make sure that you wear something that you know that he would love. If he is into tight, black dresses, try wearing one. If he is into something else, try wearing that for him. He will greatly appreciate the help and will probably not hesitate to look you over.

Show some skin

Similarly, spending some time showing skin can help a lot as well. Wear shorts, short skirts, or short dresses, and make sure that they are low-cut. In particular, men tend to go crazy for the breasts, thighs, ass, neck, and back. Those are some of the most common parts that can turn a man on almost immediately, especially if he already likes you. You just have to play your part and let him enjoy the moment.

Hold eye contact

Eye contact is sexy. It tells the other person that at that moment, they are the only person on your mind, and that is enough to turn them on, man or woman. When you are able to connect with someone else through maintained eye contact and making sure that he sees that you are interested, you will turn him on.

Whisper what you want with him

When it comes to getting him hard for you, you can tell him exactly what it is that you want. Whisper in his ear that you want to ride him, or that you want his cock in your mouth. If you can tell him what you want to do with him, you will be filling him up with all sorts of anticipation and sexual tension, and he will not be able to get enough of you. You will drive him wild, all through dirty talk.

Dirty Talk Foreplay with Men

Foreplay is great for men and women—it can be incredibly fulfilling to have someone all over your body or even just in your mind. Foreplay, however, does not have to be only physical. You can tease with your voice, with your words, and even over text if you want to. You just have to know what you are doing and let it happen.

If you want to engage in foreplay with your partner, start with your words. Make sure that you tell your partner what you want to do. Don't overthink things—just say what comes to mind. What do you want him to do to you? What do you want to do to him? What are you thinking about right that moment as you are watching and wanting him? Think about those things and then verbalize them. The foreplay follows. As you tell him what it is that you want, you are usually able to ensure that your partner gets turned on quicker and that they are anticipating the sex more so that it is also more enjoyable as a direct result.

You can also talk to him about your secret fantasies—tell him what you're really thinking about and what you really want to try doing, even if you are afraid that he might laugh. Remember, confidence is sexy, and if you want to be confident, the best way to do so is to know what you are saying and how to drive him wild. The more that you drag foreplay out, the more eager he will be to finally get his hands on you for the big event, and you will notice a world of difference.

Dirty Talk During Sex with Men

During sex, dirty talk is easy. Tell him what you like. Tell him what you want him to do. Be as vulgar as you want. There are, of course, some considerations to make. Does he like being called "daddy," or would he prefer that you use his name? Tell him when you are getting close to finishing up and tell him when you are really enjoying yourself. The more that you can communicate how you are doing in the moment, the more turned on he will be as a direct result. If you want him to fuck you, tell him that. If you want him to go quicker or slower, tell him that as well.

Some men may prefer to be the ones in charge, but most of the time, they can respect being told what to do and how to do it. It can be sexy to be commanded about in bed, and men love that. If you really want to turn him on, and you want to do it well, you will be explicitly clear about what you want.

One thing to consider, however, is that you shouldn't try to censor yourself. Keep it vulgar. Keep it derogatory. Tell him that you want his cock inside of you, not that you want his genitals within your own. You want to make sure that it doesn't get awkward and going from sexy small talk to suddenly using anatomically correct terms can be a bit of a mood killer.

Steps to Dirty Talk with Men

Dirty talking with men doesn't actually have to be as intimidating as you may think that it will be. You can follow a few simple steps and figure out how to start talking to your own partner, no pressure involved. All you have to do is know what it is that you want to say, how you will say it, and how to keep it calm and natural. If you can do that, you will find that everything else is simple. You just have to work hard to give your partner that basic level of attention that will help him to feel like he is wanted, and he will be ready to go.

Start Small

Of course, you should always start small. When it comes to dirty talk, it can take a bit of time to get into that learning curve. For some, it is nearly instantaneous, but for others, it is highly difficult to get into the swing of things right away. You need to get to know each other, especially if you are in a new relationship. You need to know that your partner is actually interested in what you are saying or wanting and that your partner is open and receptive to what you are saying. If you can do that, you will find that everything else will follow simply.

Begin in privacy

Likewise, it is usually wise to start in private with your partner rather than being bold enough to get on with it in public. Some people may love whispering those naughty little words into each other's ears, but don't do that without first letting your partner know that they should expect you to do just that by doing it in private before ever attempting it anywhere else. This gives you the chance to make sure that you're both on the same page.

Personalize it

When it comes time to begin, make sure that your dirty talk is personalized. Don't just use random sayings and phrases that are not really tailored to anything. If your partner does not enjoy being called daddy, for example, calling him daddy constantly would be a major problem. Rather than doing that, it is more important for you to figure out what he likes. Does he like being told how good he feels? Does he like being told that he's doing a good job? Does he want you to beg for him to do something or to tell him what you want? Figure out what works for him—you'll know when he seems to get even more eager to fuck than before.

Keep it natural

Finally, don't overthink things. Let things happen naturally and say what comes to mind rather than attempting to come up with the cleverest thing that you can think to say. Rather, you should take the time to just say what comes to mind and see how he responds. It's trial and error, and really, is it that embarrassing to say something to someone that you are sexually intimate with?

Phrases for Dirty Talk with Men

- What do you want me to do?
- How do you want me?
- Your lips feel so good.
- Your [body part here is/are] so sexy
- I want you now.
- I want you to touch me here [guide his hand].
- I want you to fill me up right now.
- Cum in me.
- Fuck me harder.
- I want to do [name what you want] to you.
- I love your kisses.
- Your cock feels so good.

Tips for Dirty Talk for Men

Talk about it before you actually do the deed

This makes it so that you are both currently aroused and therefore are more likely to actually get somewhere with the conversation. Ask about what he wants to hear you say or how far he wants you to go.

Enjoy it in the heat of the moment

Spend time engaging in it whenever you can, and don't be ashamed when it comes to taking the time to enjoy it yourself. It is just as much for you as it is for him; make sure that you are paying attention to what is happening and how much fun you are having.

Pay attention to his reactions

Make sure that in the moment, when you are using dirty talk, you pay attention to what it is that his body language says. Many people do not want to admit when someone has crossed a boundary, especially during sex, but that is more important than ever to stop and point out the problem. If it looks like your partner is uncomfortable with an exchange, remember that.

Check in after the fact

When you are done with the sex itself, it is time for you to spend some time actually talking about what he thought. The act of checking in might serve as extra dirty talk and may turn him on even more. While they don't typically admit it, men are just as emotional as other people.

Take it outside of the bedroom

Your man will probably love a message every now and then telling him just how hot you're getting thinking about what he did the night prior or how much you enjoyed it in the moment. Take that time and capitalize on it.

Don't get discouraged

There is a good chance that sometimes, you will mess it up. Sometimes, you need to practice. It might be awkward at first. It might feel weird to say these things out loud, but it is so important to remember to remain persistent and to keep on trying. If you can have sex with this person, they probably won't judge you for saying something that misses the mark.

Reach out and tell him your current fantasy

Whether you are together or apart, you can tell your partner what it is that you are fantasizing about at that moment. Are you thinking about how much you want his mouth on yours or how much you want to feel his dick in you? Tell him that.

Narrate your enjoyment for him

When you are fucking, men want to hear your interpretation of what is going on. Let him know all about what it is that you are enjoying in the moment.

Invite him somewhere

Especially if you are at an event or something, you can whisper to him that you are going to go into an isolated area and waiting for him. This is a major turn on for most men, and he will love it.

Say things that are meant to be tempting

At random, you can drop something that you know will drive him crazy. Tell him that you're not wearing any underwear or that you've been peeling particularly turned on at that moment. Tell him all about that new wax that you got, or that you have something new in an intimate area that you want to show him.

Mind the voice

If you are talking to him, make sure that you use the best, breathiest voice that you can manage to entice him. Men love that breathy, quiet voice.

Tell him what you appreciate

Tell your man all about what he did last time that was entirely unbelievable to him. When you do this, you will not only turn him on when he realizes that something that he was doing was that great to you, he will also then be thinking all about what he did—further turning him on.

Wake him up with a sexy promise

You can also start by waking your man up in the morning and telling him all about what you will do to him that day at some point. Tell him all about what it is that you want to do to him so that you will be able to drive him wild. You could tell him that you had a sexy dream about him that you're going to reenact that night, for example, as you run your hand up and down his thigh, or you can tell him that you're going to blow him or fuck him or do something else that drives him insane.

Tell him when you're cumming

In the moment, tell him that you're getting close, and as you do finish up, let him know that you are. As annoying as it can seem in porn to some men, they actually find that hearing that they are bringing their partner to orgasm is actually incredibly sexy. So many people say that they are turned on knowing that their partner is turned on, and that is highly impressive for them.

Beg him not to stop in the moment

When you are having sex, make sure that when they are getting the angle or spot just right that you tell him that he is. Tell him how much he is driving you insane and let yourself enjoy it as well. It can seem weird at first to tell someone that you like it right there or like that, but men love the encouragement.

Tell him that you want to do that again

There is nothing more flattering than telling your partner that you want to do exactly that all over again. After all, most people won't bother trying to repeat their sex with people if it is not worth every single moment of it.

Ask for exactly what it is that you want in the moment

You can beg for him to do something else, or you can ask him to, and he will know that you are enjoying yourself and the moment enough to want to keep going and ask for what you want.

Or demand what you want

You can also demand exactly what you want from him as well. Some men are turned on by a take-charge partner, even when they are traditionally dominant, and he may respond well to you telling him that you want him to take you from behind, or to ride him or anything else.

Tell him to take you

When you give him your best fuck me eyes and tell him that you are his for the taking, he is going to be turned on almost immediately. It is sexy to tell someone that you want to be completely taken by them. It is almost like a gift, so to speak, with you offering up your body completely to someone else.

Ask to be used

Sometimes, the best sex is that which is completely without regard to standard expectations. You may not want to be used in your relationship, but there can be something about surrendering in the moment, and men can enjoy that.

Be yourself

Unless you've agreed to roleplay or something else, make sure that, at the heart of your dirty talk, you are still yourself. Don't say things that you don't actually want to say just for him. It is important that you are not forcing things and that you are following your own style. While you may never want to tell your partner to fuck your brains out and choke you (which some people may want), you might find that complimenting him as he fucks you to be your style, and that's okay too. Make it authentic and be yourself.

Ask if you can do something sexy

Sometimes just stopping and asking him for permission to do something for him can be a bigger turn on than just doing it yourself without waiting to hear if he wants to.

Tell him that you can't think about anything but his cock

Men love to know that you have them and their fucking, on the mind, and if you can tell him that all that matters to you in that moment is thinking about fucking them, you will turn them on in an instant.

Tell him that you're touching yourself while thinking about him

What is sexier than knowing that your partner is fantasizing about you while touching themselves? He will love to hear this.

Tell him to cum for you, or even in you

Make sure that you tell him that you want him to cum for you when you are ready, or you could even offer to let him cum in you. Men love being told that, and it can instantly escalate the situation.

Tell him to look at you

Eye contact can absolutely escalate the situation and make your partner go crazy for you, especially during the most intense moments.

Say his name

Men love to hear their names said out loud to them. Yelling, whispering, moaning, it all depends upon the individual man, but they generally love to hear it said. Just make sure that you don't accidentally use the wrong name.

Tell him how good the sex is

Men want to be validated, and you can do that by telling him just how well he's doing. Men love to hear all about how satisfied they are making you, and if you tell him just how much you're enjoying the moment, you will encourage him to go more and harder.

Give him carte blanche to tell you to do whatever he wants

Try spending a session giving your partner the authority to make any decisions that he wants. If he asks you to do something, give it a shot. Let him know that on that day, he is free to do what he wants to enjoy himself.

Pay attention to pacing

When you are speaking to your partner, you should make sure that you get the pacing right. Early on in the encounter, or during the foreplay stage, you will probably speak to each other slowly and breathily. But, as things get heated, you will probably find that your breathing has picked up and that you are likely to speak quicker.

Chapter 4: Dirty Talk for Women

Women are a bit different than men in terms of what they want to hear. While at the heart of things, they want the same thing, to feel wanted, and to feel sexy, they also do not always want to be treated like a sex object. Yes, there are plenty of women who get off on being called a slut or a whore. Yes, there are plenty of women that want you to tell them what to do or rough them up, but there are also women who prefer more subtlety in their bed.

You need to learn to approach women the right way if you want to be able to properly turn them on, and thankfully, you have this chapter. Forego any notion that your woman wants to be called a dirty slut or that she wants you to destroy her sloppy pussy. She might but let her tell you that she wants you to do that before trying to establish it yourself.

The Right Approach

When it comes to fucking and dirty talk, you need to approach it the right way if you hope to turn her on the right way. The way that you approach her or talk to her will determine if she wants to actually get down to business with you or not. If you want to make sure that you are turning her on, you need to take the right approach in the first place. This means that you must remember that really when you're not turned on, dirty talk honestly sounds a bit ridiculous. It does, and that's okay! Think about it—the act of sex itself is honestly a bit ridiculous on its own. How weird is it that sex itself is just the act of rubbing your body against someone else's because you like the feeling? From a practical or logical position, just the act of sex is strange, so is it that hard to believe that narrating out that sex would also be strange?

However, you must make sure that you take the right perspective when you are speaking to women. You should make sure that you are subtle and only as raunchy or dirty as she is comfortable with. After all, dirty talk is meant to be something that everyone is comfortable with. You must make sure that your partner is just as comfortable and happy with what is happening as you are.

There are some words that are off limits as well—don't call her bits a vagina or even a cunt, unless she wants you to. You don't need to be so formal, nor do you need to be so vulgar, especially early on. Rather, make sure that you are making use of words that you know are generally accepted. Pussy, clit, boobs, and tits will do just fine.

Talk and Touch

The most effective dirty talk is able to combine talk and touch to make the most erotic setting possible so that she will enjoy every moment of what is happening to make a sensual, sexy moment that she will love. Mix erogenous zones, the areas on the body that are particularly sensual and create sexual pleasure. Turning someone on is not limited to just being in someone else's pants—all sorts of areas throughout the body are highly sensitive, and they can create that arousal that you are looking for. Women have several different areas in the body that are likely to be delightfully stimulating, including:

- **The clitoris:** This is the most sensitive of the erogenous zones, and if you want to turn someone on and get her off, the best place to focus on is her clit. Women love the pressure and the vibrations that can be used here.
- **The vagina:** The inside of the vagina is full of nerve endings, and deep stimulation is incredibly pleasurable. However, on the outside, lighter touches tend to be preferred.
- **The cervix:** This is the bottom of the uterus and is full of its own nerve pathways that can aid a woman in reaching orgasm.
- **The mouth and lips:** Kissing is essential to a relationship, but it also aids greatly in arousal. If

you want to turn your partner on, you should make sure that you are willing and ready to play with both her mouth and her lips to really get her moving.

- **The neck:** The nape of a woman's neck is highly erotic for most women, especially with a light, gentle touch. If you want to turn her on, gently kiss at or nibble at her neck.
- **The nipples:** Nipples, when stimulated, turn on the same parts of the brain responsible for processing the clitoris and vagina. If you want to turn her on, nipple stimulation, particularly with pressure and vibrations, is a surefire way to do so.
- **The ears:** The ears on women are highly sensitive to touch, thanks to all of the nerve endings. This means that gently brushing over her ears while whispering your dirty talk into them is a fantastic way to turn her on and get her moving.

What She Wants to Hear

Women love to hear their partners making sounds. Silence says that you are not actually enjoying it at all, whether you are or not. Do your partner a favor and actually tell her what you are enjoying in the moment. Women want to hear something—*anything*—during sex, so long as you are not being offensive. Sound like you enjoy yourself, whether you are turning on the dirty talk or even just moaning or sounding like you are enjoying it. Tell her how much you like the sex or how hot she looks. Let her know how much you want to keep going or how you want her to continue. Really, so long as you are giving her positive feedback and you are making sure that you follow her boundaries, you are likely to get some pretty good feedback from her as well. She wants to know that she can feel wanted and desired. She wants to feel like you are having a good time.

Really, just about anything can be sexy if you know what you are doing and how you are talking to her. Follow her cues. Make sure that you are mindful of what she seems comfortable with as well, and don't lose sight that you are talking to her to turn her on, not for yourself. If you can do that, you are likely to have far more luck.

Phrases for Dirty Talk with Women

- You are so fucking gorgeous
- I love what you are doing with your [hand, mouth, pussy, etc.]
- How does that feel?
- I'm going to fill you up
- I want you so bad
- Cum for me
- I'm going to take you
- Your pussy feels so tight right now
- You taste good
- Do you like that?
- I need you right now

Dirty Talk During Foreplay

During foreplay, you have the benefit of being able to talk to her and turn her on. Much like men, she wants to hear you talk about what you want to do or what you *need* to do. Urgency is hot, and women want to hear that from you. If you can make it clear to her that you need her right that moment, you are going to get her wet. You can tell her that you want to do something to her with that urgent, quiet tone, and she will either oblige or ask you to do something else instead.

If you tell her that you are ready to fuck her, or you are able to tell her things that you want to do, you can get her ready in advance. You create that anticipation; you are fostering that sexual tension that will ensure that the big moment will be even better. Remember, women don't want to fuck someone that is disinterested. They want to be wanted, just like men do. They want to feel like they are desired and attractive. They want to feel like their partner is having a good time so that they are able to have a good time, and the sooner that you can make that good time happen, the better. You just have to know what you are doing and how to do it.

During foreplay, try telling her what you intend to do or what you wish that you could do. It will turn her on, and she may even follow through with it if you tell her that you want it enough. If you want to make sure that she's hot for you, you need to make sure that you make her believe that you want her first. There is not much that is hotter than being wanted in the first place.

Dirty Talk During Sex

During sex, things aren't much different—you want to make sure that you are talking to your partner and telling her just how much that you actually want her. Make her believe that you do genuinely want to enjoy her body and let her know how good she feels. Boost her confidence. Tell her that you are so happy with how she is feeling around you as you thrust into her so that she knows that you are enjoying it. Moan a bit. Let her hear just how much you enjoy it.

In the moment, women want to hear that they are good in bed. They want to feel like they are actually bringing you pleasure so that they can enjoy that pleasure as well, and the best way to ensure that that can happen is if you tell them. Of course, you want to tow that line carefully and make sure that what you are doing is something that they are comfortable with. You should always be willing to listen if someone says that something bothers them and make sure that you correct yourself if you continue to try to use that language in the future as well.

Tips for Dirty Talk for Women

Be tactful

Make sure that when you are using dirty talk, you do so tactfully. Make sure that you use it in situations that make sense or that call for it. This means that if you are having a serious conversation about something, you don't tell her that you wish that your hands were on her tits instead of listening to her.

Tell her when you're cumming

Women want to know when you're about to finish. Especially if they are on top, they don't want to continue bouncing away after you're done. Let them know when you're done so that they can accommodate.

Say her name

Just like with men, women want to hear their partners say their name. It is validating, and that acknowledgment brings great pleasure. It can elevate the eroticism of your sex and make it so much better just by dropping her name in there somewhere. Whether you mention her name, or you quietly moan her name to her as she rides you, making sure that you use her name is a great way to make her feel validated.

Sound like you are enjoying it

Make sure that when you are fucking, you sound like you are actually, well, fucking. Your silence is usually taken as being distracted or uninterested. It is far better for everyone involved if you sound like you genuinely enjoy it. Don't be embarrassed by any sounds that you might make—she'll find them attractive and enjoyable.

Tell her she's good in bed

When you tell her that she's good in bed, she'll feel validated and confident enough to want to continue fucking or to want to fuck in the first place. If you tell her how much you're looking forward to having sex and you specify why, you will find that you give her that much-needed confidence boost that will take you far.

Tell her in the moment what she is doing that you like

If she suddenly does something that is particularly enjoyable, such as using her tongue a certain way or touching you or kissing you a specific way, you can tell her that you like it. If you like it, tell her so she can do it again. She will find more enjoyment in the fact that you have complimented her as well.

Check in with her during sex

Ask her if she likes what you are doing, or if she needs you to do something else. See if there are ways that you can change what you are doing to make sure that you are tending to her every need as well. She will also feel more attracted to you when you clearly make it a point to check in with her to make sure that she is enjoying things.

Ask her what she wants you to do to finish her off

When it comes to it, you should make sure that you ask her what she wants, especially to get off with. You want to make sure that you satisfy her completely, and that means that you need communication. When you can feel that she's getting close, you can ask her what she wants you to do to finish her off. Sometimes, it is just that act of caring for her that can make her crave to be with you even more.

Set boundaries

If you are going to be sexual with someone else, make sure that you tell her that she can set a boundary without question. You can tell her that if she is uncomfortable with something, she should tell you. You want to make sure that she is able to tell you when you do cross a boundary. This makes her feel safe, and when she is safe and comfortable, she is going to be willing to unleash the sexual individual within her. If she feels like she is comfortable with you, she will feel like she can continue to be intimate with you and that she can push those boundaries and experiment with you, knowing that she can stop you if she ever feels uncomfortable.

Tell her she smells good

Let's face it—sex is kind of gross if you think about it. There are exchanges of fluids. You are kissing and in each other's faces. You are breathing on each other and getting sweaty as you fuck. She may be feeling a bit self-conscious during the act, but if you tell her that you love the way that she smells, you are letting her know that she is not gross. You are letting her know that she is attractive to you, and that will help her to unwind a bit and enjoy the moment more.

Tell her she's sexy

It can help greatly to tell her just how attractive and sexy that she is. Let her know how much you love to fuck her so that she can feel like she is confident enough to keep moving forward and to keep engaging with you.

Tell her you want to continue all night long

You can also make sure that you tell her that you want to continue your romp all night long to make her feel like she is the most important thing to you. You are effectively convincing her that she is your utmost priority and that above all else, you want her. You tell her that she is not competing against video games, friends, drinking, or anything else—you want her and her alone, and that is erotic.

Tell her to talk dirty to you

If you tell her to dirty talk with you, you will help inspire her further. You can get her to engage more with you when you do this, and that is a major turn on as well. Use this to really get her involved and to make her go crazy. After all, sex is a two-way street—you both have to be involved and engaged if you want the best possible sex.

Follow this pattern

Dirty talk doesn't have to be crass or aggressive—it can be affectionate with a long-term partner or a spouse as well. You can follow this simple strategy to make sure that you are giving the best possible dirty talk that you can: "It feels amazing when you [action] my [body part]" or "Your [body part] is so amazing, I want to [action] them." If you can follow this pattern, you will be able to compliment more than just her sex—you compliment her as a whole, and that is incredibly validating.

Be urgent

Very little is more of a turn on than being needed by someone. If you want to make someone want you, you make it clear that you *need* them. This works with women as well. Urgency is hot. If you want to make her wet, let her know how much you need her. Your voice should be almost a plea—like you need her more than anything else.

Tell her she tastes good

If you are going down on her, let her know that you like how her pussy tastes. It makes her feel like you want to be down in her pussy, pleasing her.

Moan

If you want her, tell her without needing to say a word. As you play with her, let her know just how badly you need her without a single word. Just a well-placed moan can say it all.

Tell her how hard/wet you are

If you have a penis, tell her how hard it is for her. If you have a vagina, tell her how dripping wet it is for her. She will love to hear how your body is working for her and how she is impacting the way that you are able to move and interact. She wants to know that she is ultimately

Comment on how wet she is

As you play with her, you can make mention of just how wet she is and how that makes you feel as well. You can tell her just how hot you think it is that she is as wet as she is so that she can feel a bit more confident about herself as well. Tell her just how enjoyable you find it.

Comment on how tight she is

Whether she is tight around your finger or your cock, let her know. Tell her just how much you like the feeling and how much you want to enjoy it. Comment on the feeling that you have around you and how great it is.

Tell her which position you want her in and what you are about to do to her

When you take charge like this, you will probably set her on fire. Most people enjoy being wanted so desperately that the other person is demanding that they do something. Of course, you must make sure that you are still respecting any boundaries that ought to be respected but let her know what you want.

Tell her how much you want her

Doting on her in the moment, saying just how badly you want her pussy around you, or to taste her on your lips, is going to set her off. It is highly erotic to be the object of someone's sexual attention, especially if there is a mutual attraction there.

Tell her how beautiful she looks in that position

Whether it is from behind, from above, or below, tell her just how great she looks to you in the moment as you are fucking her. She will eat it up.

Experiment until you find what you both like

Take some time to figure out what it is that you both want out of your relationship. Every now and then, in the moment, try something new and see if she responds well to it. She may love what you are doing, or she may wish that you would not do that ever again. Either way, you can get to know each other and what you both want better over time.

Tease her

All day long, tell her how much you want to enjoy her. Make her want you and let that tension build all day long. There is nothing better than making sure that the sexual tension is running high so that you will be able to take advantage of all of that pent up energy later on.

Tell her not to do something because it's turning you on

This goes right back to teasing. If she's walking around the store with you, you can lean over and whisper in her ears that if she keeps walking like that, you're going to have to do something about it at home because she's driving you wild. Of course, she'll then most likely do it more to drive you crazy too.

Tell her that you want to dominate her/have her dominate you

Depending upon the perspective that you take, you can either make her in charge, or you can choose to dominate over her. There is something about being in complete control, or alternatively, to giving someone else complete control, that can be a great turn on, especially when you and your partner are on the same page.

Tell her to scream for you

If you feel like she's getting a bit too lost in the moment, you can escalate by asking her to get loud for you, encouraging her to scream for you. Of course, you should be mindful of neighbors with this method.

Make her think about you by talking about how turned on she makes you

Even if you are not actively having sex in the moment, you can tell her all about how distracted you get when you think about her. She'll then be thinking about you thinking about her.

Tell her just how intoxicating you find her

Women love being doted on, and especially if you are trying to warm her up without just getting everything flowing right that moment, you can try telling her something about how enticing and intoxicating she is. Tell her the smell of her hair is mind-blowing, or that she looks absolutely divine and that you can't keep your eyes off of her. Tell her just how attracted you are to her and that you can't stop looking/smelling/thinking about her.
168

Chapter 5: Digital Dirty Talk

We live in a digital age—there is no way around it. That means that you need to stop and consider that you are no longer stuck talking to each other. You don't just have to talk to each other in person anymore. You have the internet in the pocket of your pants these days—you have an ability to communicate at will if you want it. All you have to do is pull it out of your pocket and use it. That's right, your phone is the greatest facilitator of foreplay and sexing when it comes to turning on your partner with ease. All you need to do is make sure that you know how to write the best sext you can. As you read here, we are going to be looking at how to sext, how to pace things, and how to overcome the initial awkwardness of what you are doing. We will also talk about the importance of being able to take a picture that is enticing but not too revealing, as well as several tips to help you.

How to Sext

Sexting makes one of the greatest forms of foreplay, which you can use just about anywhere at any time. So long as you are mindful of your phone, you can simply send messages back and forth all day long, building up that anticipation and making sure that both you and your partner are driving each other wild. You can tell them all of the fantasies that you have throughout your time. You can tell your partner what you want them to do, or what you want to do to them. You can make sure that you are taking the time to drive them insane as well. When you play your cards right, you can keep that sex desire on their mind all day long, and that means that when you finally are able to come together again, you can enjoy all of that passion again.

Sexting does not have to be difficult or challenging. However, there are a few considerations to keep in mind. You want to make sure that you follow a few rules so that you avoid running into other problems.

Mind the timing

Make sure that you are well aware of what your partner's schedule looks like so you do not send them a message when they are in a place where it would be considered inappropriate. While technically just about any time would be inappropriate, it is important to keep in mind that your partner may be busy at work when you sext them, or they may be with family or other people that should not be exposed to that. Rather than just sending a sexy picture, try coming up with a code word. Ask your partner if they are busy before you do anything at all.

Be slow

Make sure that when you are sexting your partner, you mind the fact that your conversation should move slowly. You don't want to just go from 0 to 60 in an instant—rather, you want to make sure that you start slow and that you want to play. Talk about how much you enjoyed the other night or send a subtly suggestive picture.

Stay within your comfort zone

Make sure that, no matter what, you work within your comfort zone. Your sexting doesn't need to be explicit—you can even just send a message saying that you're ready to have fun with your partner, or you can send pictures of yourself masturbating if you really wanted to. You should start slowly and make sure that you are comfortable with where the sexting is going at any point in time.

Always send a warning before nudes

If you are going to send a picture that's not safe for work, give them that warning. You don't want them to get in trouble at work if your nude popped up on their lock screen, nor do you want them to open the message with others around or within sight of your picture.

170

Have fun

Remember, the whole point of dirty talk and sexting is to have fun and to encourage that sexual tension that will help you to really enjoy the moment. This means that you should enjoy the entire time that you are sexting. You can even draw your inspiration from porn, erotica, and romance novels.

Details matter

When you are sexting, the details are where the bulk of your content is. You need to make sure that you are actively encouraging each other to provide yourselves with the right amount of details. If you can nail that, you will be just fine.

Pacing for Good Digital Dirty Talk

Just like with sex, good digital dirty talk and sexting needs to be just the right pacing, or you are going to run into all sorts of problems. If you want to make sure that you are able to turn your partner on without anything else happening, you want to make sure that you understand the right pacing. You should always start slow at first and build up. When you are just getting started, you should make sure that you lead into it. Talk about how much you miss the other person or that you're thinking of them. Send a few suggestive emojis or a picture that is suggestive, but not revealing.

Think of good digital dirty talk as being quite like sex—you build up to the big moment. You talk about fucking each other and about enjoying it. You go over what it is that you want from each other, enacting fantasies. Think of the following exchange:

I'm thinking of you.

Really? I was thinking about the other night just now. I really liked what you did with your tongue.

Mmm, yeah, I'd like to do that again. I want to kiss and tease you up until you're shaking and begging for more.

Yes, please. I want to feel you tonight.

I can come over and then we can cum over together ;)

Notice how it is not particularly explicit right off the bat. It's teasing, light, and suggestive. It is not meant to be highly explicit at first. It is something that is supposed to build up that tension so that when you are together, you have enough of that tension built up that you can't keep your hands off of each other. Whether you are sexting as your own personal porn as you masturbate or if you are sexting just to build up that tension, you are making sure that you and your partner are ready to go.

Overcoming Awkwardness of Digital Dirty Talk

Sexting can be a bit awkward if you don't know what you are doing, but don't let that deter you. Too many people think, "Wow, I'm not creative enough for this, or I can't think of anything to say." However, that doesn't mean that you can't enjoy it. Sexting can be great. It can be fun and playful while also being erotic. You don't have to start out too explicitly, nor do you ever have to go further than you want to. Start out slowly and work your way up to what you want. If getting a text that says, "This is waiting for you," and a picture of a hard cock is a turn off for you, say something. Make it clear that that is not working for you.

The best way to overcome the awkwardness is honestly just to get started and make it happen. Even if for you it is a compliment or a vague reference to that last time that you and your partner did something highly erotic, that is

172

still something. Even a message as innocent as "I miss your lips on mine," can be erotic. It tells them what you want in that moment and is also an invitation for your partner to take control.

You can also ask questions that can lead to the fantasies and sexually explicit messages that you want. Ask your partner what they are thinking about in the moment to open up the conversation. Ask them what their fantasy is and let them take control. This can eliminate some of the awkwardness for yourself as well.

Consider these different options to start up your conversation with your partner that are able to skip that initial awkwardness:

- I want you to keep me warm
- I'm thinking about you
- What are you up to right now?
- Your lips on my [body part] feel so great
- I miss your hands on my [body part]
- When's the last time you thought about me?
- I'm getting wet/hard thinking about you right now
- Want to try something new tonight?

Taking the Perfect Picture

Taking the perfect picture is important to your sexting life, and the best ways that you can make that happen typically involve having some fun and finding just the right angles. Keep in mind that when you take your pictures, a lot of the time, less is more. When you are trying to choose the right photo, try taking several and looking through them until you can find the right angles for you. Every person has their own angles that make them look amazing—it is just a matter of figuring out where they are.

Start by making sure that you know your angles. This is one time where selfie sticks can be your greatest asset. Make sure that you experiment regularly and that you remember that natural lighting can be a great asset as well. Your pictures do not have to be revealing. They do not have to be anything other than suggestive. You could post a picture of your thighs without taking off your skirt. You could show your cleavage without revealing any nipple. If you are a man, you could show some abs or a toned arm without ever taking off your pants.

You can also work by making your phone your partner. Instead of trying to take a photo just right, you can focus on the image as if your phone itself is your partner, engaging in what is effectively POV pictures that will create that image of your partner being your phone. You will put your picture in the position that you would prefer your partner and then get into the right position, looking right at the camera.

With the right angles and the right attitude, you can usually figure out exactly what it is that you should be doing. Take a whole bunch of pictures and then make sure that the ones that you choose are the right angles and that they make you look great. If you can do that, you will find that you can take the sexiest pictures with ease.

What Not to Do during Sexting

Of course, if you are sexting, there are a few things that you should absolutely avoid at all costs to make sure that ultimately, you are doing the right thing at the right time. Make sure that you keep the following in mind so that you avoid common mistakes that can be problematic.

- **Don't send unwanted photos:** Regardless of whether you are a man or a woman, avoid the unsolicited nudes, especially if you haven't told them that you intend to send any.

- **Don't send photos to someone that you can't trust:** If you have just started dating someone or you can't trust the person that you are dating, don'ts end them any photos.
- **Don't take things too seriously:** Remember, sexting is supposed to be fun. Don't take it too seriously and enjoy the time that you spend teasing your partner.

Tips for Digital Dirty Talk

Offer up something that you want to do

What's sexier than detailing out exactly what you intend to do with your partner? Send them a message with you telling them exactly what you will be doing the next time that you all get together.

Be detailed

Remember that in sexting, all of the details are what do the talking. In engaging with sex, you are able to lead with your body, but in sexting, you must lead with your words instead.

Talk about dreams

Spend some time telling your partner all about a dream that you just had so that your partner can understand just how much you like or are thinking about him or her.

Tell them that you're in the shower

This invites them to text you with all sorts of different things, from what they will do to you when they see you, just imagining you naked and fresh out of the shower.

Be honest

Tell them exactly what you've felt so that they have the opportunity to reciprocate if they want to. This can open up all sorts of fun sexting ideas, and all you have to do is tell them about what it is that you want.

Have your partner turn off image previews

Make sure that your partner is not going to have your sexy picture plastered on his screen in public areas where it could be embarrassing for both of you. If you intend to sext with each other, make sure that your images and messages will not be on display for the world to see at a glance.

Turn on the heat

You can tell them that you are fantasizing about them right there in the moment and ask what they think about what you are saying. This is a great way to turn them on and get them engaging with you.

Express your regret that they're not there with you

This is a great way for you to tell them that you are disappointed that, at the end of the day, they are not present with you. This could take the place of saying something along the lines of, "Man, I wish you were here," to "It's too bad that you're not here right now."

Ask them to guess what you are thinking about

You should also try asking them what they think that is on your mind right at that moment. From being excited about how you are thinking about them, to all of the fun you intend to have encouraged, to guess what is on your mind, and then share whether they are right or not.

Let them know what you are wearing

Or not wearing. Tell them what you have on and ask what they want to do with you. They will probably want to tantalizingly remove each and every item that you are wearing

Ask them to take you

Because you will be in a position where you can say just about anything, try asking them to take you. You would be surprised at the results that you get when they think that all you want is a good, hard fuck, especially if that is you telling them the truth.

Only send messages that you feel comfortable sharing

Unfortunately, a few bad apples tend to ruin things for everyone, and sexting is yet another example of exactly that. Too many people have been burned by trying to sext, only to have their images plastered up online or disbursed among people. This is a major problem, and you want to nip it in the bud so that it cannot be a problem. Don't let anyone pressure you into sending messages that you don't want to send.

Tempt them with previews

Give them a quick sneak peek of everything that you intend to do to them as soon as they get home or to your place. If you intend to drop his pants as soon as he walks in the door and you tell him that, make sure that you are willing to follow through with it.

Play with the senses

Sure, you're apart, but that doesn't mean that you have to ignore the sense of touch, taste, or smell. You can entice each and every sense with the words that you type onto your phone and send off to him or her, and there is a good chance that using those words will drive him insane.

Make a request

These requests can be kind or demanding—you can ask politely for something, or you can tell them that you need them right that moment and that you can't wait any longer to get your hands on them.

Tease them

Tell them vaguely what you are doing or thinking about, only to make them wait a bit before you respond. This will drive them crazy, wondering what they are going to get back from you.

Send a quick video for them

If you are feeling especially brave, send a quick message with a video showing what you are doing to yourself. It could be a quick preview of you masturbating, or even your big O moment to drive the other person wild.

Reminisce about sex that was amazing

Tell them something that they did that you are thinking about at that moment. Talk about how much you miss that moment and what it made you think or feel.

Compliment them

Tell them what they did that you really enjoyed recently and just how much it impressed you. By sending compliments sometimes, you can usually get your partner to start thinking about that time, which of course, is a turn on.

Thank them for something

Sometimes, what they have done is so memorable to you that you need to send them a quick thank you message. Telling them that you appreciate what they have done sexually is a great way to validate them and turn them on quicker.

Come up with your responses for when you're not sure what to say back

Sometimes, you will get a message that you're unsure about how you should respond. When that happens, try saying something like, "wow, that turns me on so much," or "Tell me more." When you encourage them to keep talking, you are engaging even if you don't know what you should be saying back.

Have a roleplay session

You can sext a roleplay. You can write out what you are doing, in your mind, of course, and the other party can reply to you with what they do in response. You might not be able to touch each other, but you can write out your fantasies with each other and imagine it all happening, driving each other insane as you do so.

Be adventurous

Make sure that when you are talking to your partner, you are adventurous. If there was ever a time to pursue and explore your sexuality, it would be during the time in which you are able to engage digitally without any pressure of following through physically. If you discover that you don't like it, then you don't like it, and that's that.

Send pictures

Even if you just send something suggestive, go for it and see what happens, especially if you've talked about doing so in the past. People are visual creatures, and it can be highly erotic to see the impact that you have on someone else's body when they're not expecting it.

Get creative with the language

Make sure that when you are messaging him, you keep in mind that you can only say cock and pussy so much before it is time to change things up. Try to get creative, or even poetic sometimes. You might find that somethings that strikes them the right way and gets them to do what you want more than anything else.

Remember it's a conversation

When you are sexting someone, remember that it is a two-way conversation. You should be paying attention to the way that you engage with the other person and let him or her have some fun getting to talk. Remember that you should both be engaging with each other rather than anything else.

Use sexting as a precursor to dirty talk

Dirty talk in person can be quite awkward, but ultimately, it can be a great way for you to practice talking about what you want and a great exercise in communication that will help to ensure that you are able to talk in the moment as well. You can tell them exactly what you want—tell them that you want them to suck you off or tease you or fuck you via text and, eventually, work up to saying it in person as well.

Be ready to take it live

At some point, be ready to take what is being said live. Your sext session may very quickly turn into wanting to actually video chat or even meet up quickly to see what is going on.

Check in afterward

After sex, you have the ability to cuddle with each other or spoon or enjoy the moment. That is not quite so easy to do when you are engaging in sexting just due to the fact that you aren't close enough. However, you can take the time to check in with the other person and make sure that they recognize that they should be mindful of how they are interacting.

Ask your partner what turns them on

This is a great way to get them thinking about what it is that you can do for them, which not only helps you to know how to address a sexting session but will also ensure that you are able to address those needs in person as well.

Ask what they like you to do or like about you

You want to make sure that you are involving your partner and letting them choose what it is that turns them on. Have them tell you what it is about you that drives them crazy.

Chapter 6: What NOT to Do

Of course, when it comes to dirty talk and sexting, it is important that you pay attention to some pretty important things that should never be done. As you read through this chapter, you are going to be introduced to several things that you should just never do when you are using dirty talk. Make sure that you communicate what it is that you want to do and how you can make it happen as well. You want to make sure that when it comes right down to it, your partner knows what it is that will turn you on more than anything, but you also need to know what not to do.

If you go too far too quickly with dirty talk in general, you can cause some serious problems. You could, for example, completely ruin the sexual relationship entirely. You can destroy any trust that is had or any respect that is necessary for a mutually consensual relationship, and let's be honest here—no one wants to do that. For that reason, it is highly important for you to take the time to communicate what you want, boundaries, and understand what not to do.

This list will provide you with thirty things that you should *never* do in dirty talk. Of course, there will always be the occasional exception to the rule, but if you pay attention to what not to do, you can usually make sure that you and your partner are on the same page enough to ensure that neither of you are hurting the other.

Escalating too quickly

Remember that you can't go from 0 to 60 without first stopping and asking what the other person wants. If it is your first encounter with this person, don't start it off by calling her a dirty little slut with a pussy that needs to be punished for being so sloppy. You could *try* to do that, but there is a very real, very good chance that doing so is going to create a major problem for you and your relationship. Instead, try focusing on what you can do to slowly bring up the heat of what you are saying to what you want it to be. Start slowly and avoid moving too quickly.

Not going far enough

On the other hand, if you are super sterile about what you are saying, you won't turn anyone on at all. You need to be able to follow that bridge between too much and not enough if you want to be able to convince your partner that you really do want him or her. If your voice is flat or you are not talking at all, you may tell the other person that you're just not interested, even if that is not actually the case at all.

Timing it wrong

Make sure that when you are reaching out or using dirty talk, your timing is right. If you are in the middle of a conversation with someone, don't suddenly completely change the mood, especially if the initial communication was there because of the way that you are feeling in the moment. You need to be able to understand that ultimately, there is a time and place for everything.

Not being believable

Make sure that when you talk to your partner, you make it believable. It is not believable to say that you've been jerking it for the last three hours when you are at work, for example, nor is it believable that you would walk around work for three hours pitching a tent. Make sure that whatever you say, you make it believable so that your partner is just as turned on as you are.

Making it seem rehearsed

You also should make sure that you avoid making any attempts to interact with your partner seem too rehearsed. You can't tell your partner the exact same line that you have rehearsed and repeated over and over again and hope that they will listen. If things seem too automatic, you have a very real chance of simply offending the other person rather than actually making any good, clear progress with what you are attempting to do. It is always more important to be honest and realistic than anything else.

Making it too complicated

Dirty talk doesn't have to be complicated, nor should it be. You need to make sure that any dirty talk that you are using is going to be effective and usable without having to worry too much about repercussions. When you are able to talk dirty to someone else, it should not be super complicated, nor should it be full of all sorts of attempts to make you seem smarter or try-hard than you actually would normally be.

Not personalizing it enough

Another common mistake that people make are making their dirty talk too impersonal. Yes, you can say the same thing to just about anyone, but are they all going to respond the same way? Are they all really going to appreciate the way that you have chosen to approach them? Many people find that they are far happier if they are able to have any dirty talk personalized. Instead of just saying, "Fuck me harder," you can figure out how to personalize it—"I love the way you're riding me with that thick cock of yours," for example. Now you are getting specific and personalizing, which allows for more connection and, therefore, more intimacy as well. You need to be able to keep that line just right between not enough and just enough.

Making your partner uncomfortable with it

You should always make sure that you are able to keep your partner comfortable during dirty talk, and this means that you and your partner must have some very serious talks about boundaries to make sure that you are both able to follow along and be comfortable. Of course, this also means that you both will need to be willing to talk about boundaries so that neither of you are unintentionally pushing things too far one way or another.

Repeating back what your partner has said

Even if your partner has just said the sexiest thing imaginable, there is no reason to repeat it back to them. Don't tell them exactly what they just said to you unless you want them to stop and look at you like you completely missed the point. Make sure that you are telling them things that are new and unique to make sure that they are able to understand that you are, in fact, attempting to turn them on, not to make a complete fool out of yourself as you go.

Any mention of pregnancy or making babies

Especially if you and your partner are not exclusive or are not long-term partners, you should leave out any talk of babies. If it is a casual fuck session with your booty call, you should not be telling them that you can't wait to put babies into them. No matter how hot it may seem in the moment, all you are doing is setting your partner up for expectations that are unreasonable and also making it a point to completely avoid the way that you should be interacting. Parenthood is not sexy. While some people revel in it, especially the first year, sex drives can tank,
186

and when that happens, you don't want to be talking about putting a baby into someone else. Likewise, you should not tell your partner that you want them to put a baby in you, either.

Leave food out of it

Unless this is something that the two of you have discussed, don't refer to his or her bits as food objects. Most people don't find calling someone's penis a sausage particularly attractive. It is problematic for most people, in fact, and you can run into all sorts of issues if you are not mindful of the way that you approach the situation. Instead, just leave food where it belongs—in the kitchen and out of your bedroom life.

There is a time and place to be romantic and sweet

Keep in mind that there is absolutely a time for romance and being sweet—and that is rarely during active fucking. Recognize that there is a major difference between fucking, which is usually regarded as almost animalistic in the way that it is used and being willing to sensually make love to someone else. If you are fucking, don't whisper sweet nothings into your partner's ear. If you are making love, don't tell her that her pussy is so tight and wet. Know the difference between romantic sex and passion, no strings or emotions attached sex, and adjust accordingly.

Don't discuss bodily fluids

The only bodily fluids that have a place in your sex life are ejaculate and the lubricant that vaginas make. Don't tell your partner that you want to pee on them, especially if you are just starting out, and you don't know his or her kinks yet. You need to take the time to get to know them and make your actions accordingly. It is only then when you are careful about what you are doing that you can make that appropriate progress. Leave out urine, spit, and any other fluids unless explicitly discussed and agreed to in advance.

Leave the exes out of it

There is nothing worse than enjoying the moment only to suddenly be compared to an ex, whether being better or worse. No matter whether the comment is meant as a compliment or not, you do not want to think that your partner is busy comparing you to see how you stand up against your ex-boyfriend or girlfriend. That's a great way to set up all sorts of resentment and concern that things are going to go wrong if you are not careful. Instead, pay close attention to the ways that you engage with your partner and make sure that you are choosing to give them the respect that they deserve without worrying about the exes that are involved.

Don't make your dirty talk or sexting scenario too impossible

If you are sexting or dirty talking someone else, unless you have both agreed to do some roleplay, don't make your situation suddenly so fantastic that it will take away from the moment. This means don't suddenly be fucking your partner on another planet or something. Make it believable and call it good. This is one of the most important things that you can do to make sure that you are being effective with your small talk. You must make it believable and enjoyable.

Avoid making puns, no matter how tempting

It happens to the best of us at some point in time—that pun comes to mind, and it's really hard to resist saying it. However, keep in mind that when you are using puns with people, you keep those puns out of the bedroom. Most people won't find it attractive if you suddenly drop a pun off of something that you were enjoying just moments prior, and you can completely destroy the moment if you are not careful.

Make sure that you don't say something ridiculous

Similarly, try to avoid anything that is too ridiculous as you are fucking. This is not the time or place for that. Rather, this is the time and place for you to enjoy the moment. Avoid making any jokes at all during this period of time and try to keep your talking as serious as possible in the moment. Say things that are sexy. Don't say things that are going to be annoying, silly, or potentially kill the mood.

Listen to the suggestions that your partner makes

If your partner asks you to do something, you should do it. Make sure that you are regularly doing what your partner has requested of you so that you are able to figure out what it is that you need to do to get the most enjoyment for both of you. After all, if you want him to come back for seconds, or you want her to beg you for it, you are going to want to make sure that your sex is memorable enough for you to want to do it again. The best way to get that memorable nature is to make sure that you are doing whatever your partner has suggested.

Don't be too derogatory (at first)

Unless explicitly told that it is okay to call your partner's vagina a dirty, slutty cunt, you probably shouldn't do it. Especially if your relationship is still new and you are still getting to know each other, you do not want to unintentionally make things worse by saying the wrong things, and the easiest way to push too far is to use derogatory language that is going to turn everyone off from the situation. Rather than giving in to that derogatory language, you should instead consider having a genuine conversation about what it is that you and your partner both want.

Don't tell them to be quiet

If your partner is starting to moan or really enjoy the moment, one of the worst things that you can do is tell him or her to be quiet because they are distracting you. Instead of looking at their moans of pleasure as distractions, consider seeing them for what they are— clear signs that you are doing a good job because the other person literally cannot control the sounds that they are making in that moment. If you were to tell them to quiet down, all you would do is make them feel self-conscious or even make them feel like the relationship not worth continuing.

Don't try to convince the other party to skip the condom

All too often, you will hear men try to get out of wearing a condom during sex. However, that is not only bad practice because you can unintentionally end up pregnant, it is also dangerous if you are not in a committed relationship with someone that you trust. There is no place in dirty talk for risky, potentially dangerous sex, and because of that, do not even try to convince your partner that you do not need a condom. Newsflash—you *do* need a condom, and you *do* need to make sure that you are wearing it the right way.

Don't be too anatomically correct

While it is important to make sure that you are not being too vulgar, you also shouldn't overcorrect—do not tell her that you want to put your penis in between her labia and thrust into her vaginal cavity. That's not sexy. At all. Instead, make sure that you stick to generally acceptable
190

terms. Cock and pussy, for example, are pretty regularly respected and acceptable. However, terms like cunt are debatable for many and should be avoided unless she specifically tells you to call it a cunt.

Don't dwell on something that upsets the other party

If you make a mistake in the moment, it's okay—it happens to the best of us. However, unless you have seriously triggered your partner, you don't have to suddenly stop what you're doing. Rather, you can offer a quick apology and keep on moving forward unless your partner shows signs of wanting to stop. This means that there is no real reason for you to be rejecting everything that you're doing. There is no real reason for you to stop everything to suddenly apologize repeatedly and have a long, drawn out conversation, especially if the other party shows no desire to have one at that moment. You can revisit later if you really want to make sure that you have that conversation.

Don't ask if they are faking things

One of the worst things that you can do in the moment is to accuse your partner of faking something. Your partner should be trustworthy, and you should be able to feel like, if your partner is saying something to you, they mean it. Don't act like your partner is lying to you just because you think that they are being unrealistic. If you are worried about them being truthful, you probably shouldn't be pursuing that relationship in the first place.

Don't criticize your partner's bodies

It should go without saying that during sex or sexual play unless explicitly told otherwise, there is no real room for insulting the body of another person. Unless you have both discussed the idea of playing with degrading each other, there is a high likelihood that you are just going to upset each other and create all sorts of major problems. It is better to leave the degradation out of all dirty talk until you and your partner have had that candid discussion. While some people live by, it is better to ask forgiveness than permission; you can destroy your sexual relationship in this manner relatively simply. Don't even bother risking it—it isn't worth it.

Don't bring up dirty talk during a sensual, romantic sex session

Remember that sometimes, if your session is sensual and romantic, it is best to leave the dirty talk out of it—the aggressive kind, anyway. Rather, focus on the moment, and instead of degrading comments, you should be shifting into talk of how much you are enjoying yourselves, how much you care for each other, and how you enjoy the other person's body. Aggressive dirty talk has no place if you are attempting to woo someone else.

Don't call yourself daddy unless the other party has expressed an interest

Daddy is probably one of the more controversial names that you can call your partner during sex. Some people love it, and others hate it—you kind of have to go with the flow to make it work for you. If you want to be called daddy, then let your partner know and ask how she feels. Likewise, if you want to call him daddy, you should ask in advance. Some people find it a turn on, but others may find that it is a bit weird for them, especially if he already has children that refer to him as daddy. That can be something that is pushing the agenda too far and will get all sorts of backlash. Consider having a discussion about this prior to letting it be used. This is the best interest for everyone involved, and if you don't want to ruin the moment, you will ask first

Don't try to push boundaries when they have been set

While expressing desperation for sex can be hot, begging to do something that your partner has already said that they would not do is a huge turn off. Maybe she doesn't want to have anal sex—that's her right. You can ask her, but if she says no, it is best for you to drop the point altogether. However, if you start to push the point after you have already said no, you are making a big mistake. You will probably turn him or her off quicker than anything else if you continue to push a point that has already been answered. Remember, healthy sex is all about consent, and that consent must not be coerced.

Don't talk about family in bed

Finally, make sure that talks bout real life, such as family, friends, work, or anything else, are left out of the bedroom during sex. Nothing can turn off your dirty talk game quicker than mentioning that your mother is bothering you again. Instead, you should make sure that any interactions that you have with your partner are carefully crafted. Make sure that your interactions are focused on your partner rather than other concerns or problems that may be arising. Are those problems serious? Sure—but they also shouldn't be overwhelming so much so that you are unable or unwilling to have good sex because of them. Be all in or all out, but don't drag your partner down with talks of what your family is doing or why your job is currently driving you crazy.

Chapter 7: Bonus Tips to Spice Up the Bedroom

Congratulations! You've made it through the book and know now how you can begin to implement dirty talk. However, you may be wondering what else you can do to spice up your bedroom life now that you have a pretty solid idea of what to do and what not to do. Thankfully, you are in the right spot, and as you read through this chapter, you will be introduced to all sorts of information that is going to help you really spice up that sex life without much of a hassle at all. All you need to do is make sure that you know what you are doing and how to do it so that you can enjoy your bedroom and your partner. Now, let's take a look at some more tips that you can use to ensure that your bedroom life is never lacking what you are looking for.

Sexy daddy roleplay

Roleplay is a great way that you will be able to spice up your bedroom, and you can do it with dirty talk. You can talk to your partner about a way that you would like to explore. A common one is with daddy roleplay, where one person is the daddy, and the other is the daughter. You can make use of all sorts of dirty talk as you talk to each other, talking in a completely different context. It can really spice things up when you make use of new scenarios in which you and your partner are going to be able to make sure that you and your partner are able to get off together with that dirty talk. Talk to each other about your boundaries and see if that is something that you are interested in trying. It may not be for everyone, but some people love it.

Sexy delivery roleplay

Along a similar vein, a lot of people enjoy spicing things up with other roleplays as well. A common one is pretending to have your partner deliver a pizza. Maybe you have your partner go out to pick up your favorite pizza, and when he comes back home with it, he knocks on your door, and... you don't have any money! You can't find your cash and realize that you have no way to pay for it. However, with dirty talk and the power of being able to seduce your partner, because you happened to be nude with nothing but a robe on when your partner knocked, you are able to seduce him to pay it back.

As you have fun in this way, you can add in all sorts of dirty talk, making a game out of it that you can both get off to. He can call you his little slut for putting out for pizza, and you can rock his world by getting into a role that is completely different than the one that you typically lead. After all, he is not calling you a slut; he is calling the character the slut. You may also consider getting a bit rougher than usual as well, of course respecting any boundaries that have been requested so that you and your partner can both have the best possible time with each other.

Sexy teacher roleplay

Another roleplay idea that is ripe for the dirty talk is the idea of a teacher and a student. One of you can be the newbie virgin that has never had sex before, while the other is responsible for teaching the first one everything that he or she knows about having an awesome sex life. If you want to make sure that you and your partner get the most out of this exercise, introduce all sorts of dirty talk and molding one character to match what the other character is requesting. There can be all sorts of eroticism added in if you have one person pretending to be completely new to sex while the other then gets to do all of the leading. Not only do you set up for dominance there, but you also set up for other situations in which you are able to do so much more as well.

Sexy dirty talk boss and worker roleplay

One last roleplay suggestion is that you make use of a situation in which one of you is the boss, and the other is the secretary worker. You can use this as another position of power dirty talk roleplay. Of course, this is another situation where you can naturally find some ways that you will be able to make use of all sorts of dirty talk. You can have the secretary doing every single thing that the boss wants him or her to do. This is a great way that you are able to spice things up—after all, isn't having that control or power great sometimes?

Sexy storytime

Another way that you can really get each other off in the bedroom is to tell a dirty story as you touch the other person. Maybe one of you is jerking off the other as you tell a story to him. You can tell him all about what you want to do or about a fantasy that you have as you are slowly jerking him as foreplay. Make it full of all sorts of dirty talk as you do, and maybe even get into some rough interactions as well if you need to. It's a great way for you to be able to really get into what is going on. Likewise, you can switch off, so he plays with you while he tells you the dirty, sexy story as well. This is a great little switch off in which you are both able to get that fucking that you want, and you are both able to really turn each other on.

Narrate what the other person needs to do with themselves

You can also try adding in the dirty talk by having one of you tell the other person what you want them to do. You can tell your partner to masturbate your way, using all sorts of dirty talk. You could, for example, tell him that you want him to jerk his cock harder in your face with his balls dangling. You could tell her that you want to see her handle those big tits, pinching her nipples. You get a show out of telling and narrating what you want the other
196

person to do. And because you are able to get that show out of it, you can really spice up that bedroom. It may not be typical to have yourself and your partner masturbating for each other, but it can be enjoyable in the moment. You can even do this over sexting as well to really up the ante and make things hotter.

Sexy narrated blow jobs

If your partner has a cock, this one is for you. You want to make sure that you are giving your partner exactly what he or she wants, and you can do that easily through making use of dirty talk that will blow both of your minds. You will be able to figure out exactly what matters the most in your relationship, and you will figure out how best to ensure that everyone is getting along the right way. All you have to do is make sure that you talk dirty as you suck on his cock.

When you are sucking on him, every now and then, you can moan as if you love every moment. Tell him how much you like to suck on it or how much you like to let your teeth run along it. Tell him to talk dirty to you or to grab your hair and guide you while he talks to you about what he wants.

This can go both ways as well. The woman can get licked and do the talking as well.

Blindfold and dirty talk narration

You can try adding in a blindfold to your relationship too, and if you really wanted to enjoy it, you would have the person who is not blindfolded narrating what he or she is about to do to the other person as it happens. As you do this, you encourage the other person to hear you out and build up sexual tension as well. This is a wonderful way that you will be able to enjoy every moment of that dirty talk as you fuck.

Think about it—what could be sexier than having someone else narrate how they are going to fuck you, just before they do it and when you can't see what they are doing? It can be highly erotic. You can even change things up by blindfolding him first and then taking him somewhere else that he doesn't expect.

Let him/her beg for sex as you deny it—for the time being

Another way to really build up that sexual tension is to tease and tease your partner, through dirty talk, through touch, and any other methods that you may choose to make use of. Perhaps you have a game to it—you are only willing to put out if they do something, but you don't tell them what that something is, and they spend the day trying to convince you what it will take. There are so many options for this—perhaps the magic solution is that you want them to say something in particular—perhaps you want them to literally beg for that sex. You would then use dirty talk to lead them to that particular answer. "How bad does that hot little pussy want me?" or "What will you do to get me to fuck you?" As you lead with all sorts of other dirty talk, you will probably find that your partner is willing to do a lot—and as soon as he or she begs, you then give in because that was what you had decided was going to be the cue.

Dirty talk teasing game

Most people know about the typical drinking games where everyone watches these movies together, and at certain points, there are shots taken. It could be that, for example, you take a shot when the main characters say something that is particularly cringe-worthy. However, have you ever played the dirty talk version? For this game, you and your partner will find some porn that the two of you can enjoy. You will then make a list of different actions that are worth different scores, so to speak. If you hear the woman in the video moan or whine, you may say
198

that you are going to make out for thirty seconds, hands off. If you hear dirty talk in the video, you may have to say something yourself toward the other person and get them involved as well. Set up your scoreboard and let it go.

Dirty talk challenge

Another way that you can spice up the bedroom is by trying the dirty talk challenge. This will serve as foreplay all day long. You will effectively be tasked with messaging your partner all day long as much as is reasonable with your own dirty talk. The goal is that you have to keep his mind on you for most of the day. You want to make sure that he can't think about what he is supposed to be doing so that you can take advantage yourself. Make it as creative as you can and try to make sure that you keep him or her turned on as much as possible all day long.

Write a sexy letter

For partners that you are a bit closer to, you can let your creative juices flow, and hopefully, some erotic juices as well. Take some time to write a letter to your partner with all sorts of dirty talk. The idea is to have your partner turned on without touching him or her once—just by creating the letter and handing it off to them. If you can do this, you will be able to make him, or her want you at will. You will spice up your bedroom by adding in an instant turn on, and you will be able to enjoy everything as well.

If you want to add a different twist to this game, you could write erotica yourself, featuring you and your partner, and then act it out, step by step by step. Make sure that it is plenty steamy—make sure that it is a turn on and that it is also something that you can both enjoy.

Find a porn video that you both like... and reenact it

Now, porn is rarely actually good sex. There is sex that looks good, and there is sex that feels good, and the sex that is able to hit both of those points at the same time is exceedingly rare. However, you might get lucky and find it. Choose out some porn and watch it together, enacting everything that you see so that you can enjoy each and every moment of it as well. If you can do this regularly, you will find that you will totally spice up what you are doing, and you will drive your partner crazy.

Read erotica to each other

Find some erotica online and read it with each other. You can take turns reading it out loud with each other, getting used to the dirty words, and potentially even finding some stuff that you would enjoy trying out yourself if you happen to get lucky. Try out the moves that you read about in the erotica and see if it is actually as sexy to act out as it is to read about. Who knows, you might find your next favorite position this way! There are plenty of different websites online where you can find all sorts of great erotica, free of charge and without any strings attached, meaning you don't have to leave home or buy anything at all to do this.

Mix and match

You can also put several of these different challenges together to really up the ante on it all. If you want to have mind-blowing sex, you need to be willing to experiment and to make sure that ultimately, you enjoy what you are doing. It may be unconventional, but there is nothing wrong with that. It may involve copious amounts of dirty talk, but there is nothing wrong with that, either. It may involve all sorts of things or positions that you never thought you would do, but that's okay too. Sex is one of those things that is not, by any means, one size fits all.

There are so many different options out there for you that you can do, and there are many things that some people swear by that would make other people blanch. So long as you and your partner are finding that it is hot, that is all that matters!

Conclusion

And with that, we have made it to the end of this book. Hopefully, you have read this book with your partner and took the time to really get to know what it is that you and your partner really want. It is important that if you are going to be intimate with someone, whether they are a one night stand, a long-term partner, or even your spouse, you want to make sure that you are communicating.

Dirty talk itself is just another form of communication, but it is one that must be preceded by other concepts as well. If you want to use dirty talk to turn your partner on, you want to make sure that you are always engaging in the right kinds of behaviors. You want to make sure that ultimately, you and your partner are on the right page with everything, and if you can be on the same page as each other, you can usually ensure that the sex that you will have will be mind-blowing. After all, nothing is better than fucking someone that is naturally going to follow your moves, pay attention to your particular desires, and make sure that you are happy. If you can do this, you will have plenty of success.

Before you dive right into dirty talking with your partner, then make sure that you communicate. Is it sexy to talk about boundaries? Not traditionally, but you are conveying your own emotions and that you care about the other person and their boundaries, which is highly erotic itself. Make sure that you and your partner are on the same page with everything that you do so that you will be able to control your enjoyment as well.

From there, all you have to do is get creative. When you know what each other's boundaries are, you can get to work, physically and mentally as well. You can send dirty messages to your partner. You can beg them to fuck you or to let you fuck them. You can encourage them to do things that you may normally have been too afraid to say.

You can make sure that you are in complete and utter control over your sexual relationship, and if you can make that happen, you are going to find that your sex life will be better than ever. You can teach your partner to crave you more than anything else. You can teach your partner to want you constantly, or that you can turn him or her on in an instant just by knowing what they like to hear and how you can really tickle that fancy and get them going. All you need to do is make sure that when you are talking to your partner, you are spending the time to be erotic.

Remember, all you need to do is describe what is happening. Remember that there are three keys here: Say what you are going to do, what you are doing, and what you just did. If you can be descriptive like this, you don't even have to think much about the dirty talk that is happening. All you have to do is just that—narrate what you are doing so that your partner will be even more turned on. Maybe you tell him, "I'm going to ride your hard cock." Then, you say, "Ooh, I love riding your hard cock." Later, when you are done, you can say, "I'm so glad I got to ride your cock." You are essentially just regurgitating out one sentiment in three different ways, but this descriptiveness is a great way to not only turn your partner on because you know that you are already saying things that are narrating actions that happen to turn your partner on.

You should also remember that expressing your desire is crucial as well, especially if you do it with commands. These are all keys to making sure that you can drive your partner wild, and if you can remember these point sand take them into your bedroom with you, you will find that you are highly successful with everything that you are doing. All you need to do is make sure that you are effective in what you are doing.

Thank you for taking the time to read through this book, and remember, dirty talk is a skill. Just like any other skill, it can be natural for some people, but for most, it is something that will take effort and practice. You must commit to what you are doing. You must make sure that you are taking the time to practice and that you are willing to deal with the trial and error. It may not always be the most fun, and it may be embarrassing sometimes, but if you can remember to keep on going, you can learn to say all sorts of things that will turn your partner on instantly so that you can have the time, or the fuck, of your life.

Finally, if you found that this book was beneficial in providing you with tips that will help you to properly master foreplay through dirty talk, or if you feel like the information and activities will help to spice up your sex life, please consider heading over to Amazon and leaving a review with your experience. It could help others find the information that they need to get it going on in bed too, and it would also be greatly appreciated! Your feedback is always well received and helps to ensure that future books are even better than the last ones. Thank you, once more, and good luck, with all your bedroom adventures! May your fucking be fun, and may your orgasms be mind-blowing!

Sex Positions for Couples

Make Your Couple's Sex Life Amazing with The Leading Top Sex Positions and With Techniques and Tips for Awesome Fantasy Time.

of information contained within this document, including, but not limited to, — errors, omissions, or inaccuracies.

Table of Contents

Introduction

First off, I would like to thank you for choosing this book, and I hope that you find it informative and helpful no matter what your needs may be. Congratulations on taking these first steps in improving your sex life. This can be a hard topic for some people, but we are here to strip away all of those awkward feelings about sex. Here, we will celebrate sex as something natural. The goal of the book is to help people improve their sex lives because sex should be something that helps bring couples closer and to improve their overall wellbeing. Sex should not be done only for procreation.

This book will walk you through all of the various aspects of sex and foreplay. The first thing we are going to go over is kama sutra and tantric sex and the benefits of practicing them. These are two common topics that get discussed in the world of sex, but so many people don't actually know what they are or what they even mean. They are not both the same, as you will soon find out, and they will bring something a bit different into your sex life.

Besides that, we are also going to go over how to get your body and mind ready for sex. One of the most common issues people have when it comes to unsatisfactory sex is that they aren't able to get out of their own head enough to really enjoy what is happening. With the right preparation, this doesn't have to be a problem.

Then we will look at some tips that can help out those who may not have all that much experience in sex. Everybody has to begin somewhere, and there is no need to feel ashamed.

After that, the next couple of chapters are going to go over the various ways that can get you and your partner ready for sex. We will go over some tantric massage techniques, preliminary games, dirty talk, and other secrets of a good couples massage. These tend to be things that people like to avoid because they are afraid of messing them up, which makes sense, but you won't have to worry about that anymore after you have read this book.

Next, we will go over the orgasm. This is the main goal that everybody is aiming for when having sex, right? So why shouldn't we discuss it and what it means and how to improve your chances of having multiple orgasms? This will naturally bring us into our next subject, female ejaculation. This has been seen as the lost unicorn in the sex world, but we are going to dispel the myths that you may have heard and explain to you exactly what it is.

Then we will move into specific sex positions for you to try. First, we will go over the best sex positions for him, then the best positions for her, and then the best positions to bring both of your closer.

After that, we will look at some exercises that men can use in order to increase their orgasmic control. This is a common issue that men can run into, and it does not mean that they have anything wrong with them. With these exercises, men can learn how to control their orgasms so that they are able to last long enough to please their partner.

Then we will go over the best sex positions to use when your partner is pregnant. Sex during pregnancy is often seen as impossible or tricky, but there are positions out there that can make sex during pregnancy easy. After that, we will go over the best sex positions for oral. Oral sex is often forgotten about, but it can make things more interesting.

Lastly, we will wrap everything up with talking about things that you can do to improve your sex life. While the goal of the entire book is to improve your sex life, these exercises can be used in addition to everything else that we will talk about.

Making a choice to not be stuck in the same monotonous sex every night is a big decision. Having amazing sex should not be a mystery, and with this book, it no longer will be.

Before we begin, I would like to ask that if you find any part of this book helpful and informative, please rate and leave it a review.

Chapter 1: The Art of Kama Sutra

For many people, when they hear the words "Kama Sutra," they automatically see some contortionist sex positions. They think it requires positions that use acrobatics, yoga, and maybe even some primeval pornography. This is only partly true.

The *Kama Sutra* actually covers much more than what people in the Western world see. To simply say that it is just a book full of spicy sex positions is providing this ancient, sacred Hindu text a disservice.

Kama Sutra isn't something that magically turns everyday sex into sacred lovemaking. That part is only like 20 percent of what it is about. Real, sacred lovemaking is mainly about a deep connection and spirit, which is the reason why the sex positions of the *Kama Sutra* only take up about 20 percent of the text. The rest of it helps to guide you through the art of love. Kama Sutra also helps you with things like:

- Etiquette

- Family life

- Balancing your masculine and feminine energies in yourself and in the partnership

- The philosophy and nature of love

- Proper grooming

- What triggers and sustains desire

- Self-care

- The practice of different arts like poetry, cooking, and mixing

- Many other non-sexual, pleasure-oriented facets of life

It helps you to live a good life and not simply how to have amazing contortionist sex.

Kama Sutra, which is also written as Kamasutra, is a Sanskrit word made of two words, "kama" and "sutra." Both words have different meanings, but when they are combined, the meaning makes up the premise of what Kamasutra is all about.

"Kama" in Sanskrit translates to "desire," and includes both the aesthetic and sensual desires. However, when it comes to Kamasutra, it places emphasis on sensual desire. In the majority of world religions, a person's sexual desire is viewed as taboo.

However, within Hinduism, "kama" is one of the "four goals of Hindu life." Their four goals of life include, "kama," "artha," meaning success and abundance, "dharma," meaning truth and virtue, and "moksha," meaning release.

In Sanskrit, "sutra" means thread or line, but in the sense of Kama Sutra, it is talking about a thread of verses that create a manual.

Where Does it Come From?

Kama Sutra comes from the ancient Hindu book called the *Kama Sutra* that was written by the Indian philosopher Vatsyayana Mallanaga between 400 to 200 BCE. What is interesting is that Vatsyayana said that he was a celibate monk. He also said that bringing together all of this sexual wisdom was the contemplation of deity and a form of meditation.

Vatsyayana wasn't the teacher of this wisdom but simply composed the Kama Sutra from a book that was written much earlier, in the seventh century, called Kamashastra, or *Rules of Love*. This other book is a lot larger, but it also looked at the love-customs and partner compatibility of Northern India.

The *Kama Sutra* was written in a difficult and complex form of Sanskrit. Even when it was translated to English, the ideas still come off as a bit abstract to the modern reader. Thanks to Bhagwan Lal Indraji and Sir Richard Francis Burton, we can look at the complex translation from the Kama Sutra. This excerpt is about the different varieties of moaning that take place during lovemaking:

"The whimper, the groan, the babble, the wail, the sigh, the shriek, the sob, and words with meaning, such as 'mother, 'stop,' 'let go,' or 'enough.' Cries like those of doves, cuckoos, green pigeons, parrots, bees, moorhens, geese, ducks, and quails are important options for use in moaning."

Not exactly what you would think of when it comes to moaning, is it? Luckily, people have studied it more and more translations have been written that make it easier to understand.

Sex and Beyond

As stated above, Kama Sutra isn't just about sex. For example, a large part of Kama Sutra is about flirting and courtship. It states that if a man wants to attract a woman, he should hold a party and ask his guests to recite poetry. When the poetry is read, people should leave out certain parts, and then the guests compete to complete the poem. It also suggests that the man and woman should play together, meaning they should do things together like swimming.

Kama Sutra also focuses a lot on dating with the aim of getting married. Finding your ideal partner involves making sure that you possess the same qualities that you would like your partner to have.

When it does come to sex and intimacy, Kama Sutra also includes the nonsexual aspects. There are eight categories of embrace. The first four are expressive of mutual love, and the other four are to increase pleasure during intimacy and foreplay.

1. Touching Embrace

This helps a man and woman get acquainted, develop the hots for one another, and the man feels passion fire up so that he starts looking for an excuse to get closer with the purpose of brushing his body against her.

2. Piercing Embrace

The piercing embrace happens when a part of the man touches the woman's private parts, such as her breasts, without a known intention, but as an accident. But because of the touch, the man feels an instant sexual urge to grab her breasts when secluded or in the dark.

3. Rubbing Embrace

When a couple passes each other in the dark or down a lonely alley, or even in public, they realize their sexual attraction towards one another, so they make a point or rubbing their bodies against one another because of their desire to feel each other up.

4. Pressing Embrace

The rubbing can move to something else that is guided by intense arousal. This happens when one person pushes the other against a wall and presses their body tightly against the other to bring them closer so that they can feel their partner's intimate parts.

5. Twining of a Creeper (Jataveshtikaka)

This embrace occurs when a woman clings to her man in the way that a creeper twines around a strong plant that stands tall and steady. She then pulls the man's head

216

towards her so that she can kiss him, while intently staring deep into his eyes.

6. Climbing a Tree (Vrikshadhirudhaka)

This embrace occurs when a woman places a hand around his shoulder, reaching to touch the back of his other shoulder. One of her feet is placed on his thighs, and the other foot is on his feet, just like she was getting ready to climb a tree. These moves show that she wants a kiss from him.

7. Mixture of Sesame Seed with Rice (Tila Tandulaka)

You know what it is like to be laying down and to be spooned or to spoon your partner? This is what this embrace is like. Whether you choose to lay face to face or front to back, you both need to be laying next to one another and have your legs and arms entwined.

8. Milk and Water Embrace (Kshiraniraka)

The act of sex is imminent; you become vulnerable to your partner. This is the type of embrace that happens with a sexual union when two bodies are pressed against one another as tightly as you can like you are entering into one another. The woman should be sitting on his lap, facing him, so that they can feel each other up in the best way possible, enjoying whatever sensations happen.

Besides embracing one another, Kama Sutra also covers kissing. The Kama Sutra actually has 26 forms of kisses that range from kisses to showing affection and respect, to those that are used during sex and foreplay. The best kiss for sexual partners is one that based on being aware of the emotional state of your partner when you two are not having sex.

Other aspects of intimacy and foreplay include mutual massages, rubbing, biting, pinching, and using the hands and fingers to stimulate each other, as well as many different forms of cunnilingus and fellatio.

217

Kama Sutra is also inclusive of same-sex relationships, as well as sex "games" like group sex and BDSM.

Chapter 2: Benefits of Kama Sutra

Everybody understands that changing up sex positions and trying new things is good for their sex life. Even still, people choose to stick with what they are used to for one reason or the other. Let's take a moment to look at the benefits of trying new things in bed, specifically Kama Sutra.

- Different Perspective

When you change up your sex positions, you are also changing your perspective in bed. You get to see new areas of your partner's body and experience different types of stimulation.

This is a very important thing for men because their eyes are the second most important zone to his penis. Women love with their ears, but men love with their eyes. Men have visual sex, which is why they are more likely to watch porn. When they get to see something new that is also exciting, it only makes the sex that much better.

For example, in missionary, you only see each other's faces, but if you move to doggy style, he gets a perfect view of her rear end. The same is true if the woman gets on top. They get a nice view of each other's chest.

- Tone The Organism

In Eastern medicine, there is a notion that all parts of the organs and body are connected, and each part can be influenced by another part. Genitals of men and women have many representative areas of every vital organ within the body. During sex, and in various sexual positions, these parts are stimulated. This means that you can be helping other areas of your body when you are having sex.

- Different Sensations

In all the sexual positions that we will talk about in later chapters, the penis will touch a different area of the vagina and enters at varying depths. This changes how sex feels for him and her. For women, they are all different. They feel different things even if they are stimulated in the exact same spot. For men, they feel pretty much the same thing all the time.

- Help Women Reach an Orgasm

The worst thing for a woman is not reaching orgasm during sex. Every woman is unique in what she needs in order to climax, so trying out new things in bed can help her to get exactly what she wants.

Why would you risk your relationship when all you need to do is change up your positions so that she actually has an orgasm? It is important for men to understand exactly how their partner's body works so that they know what she needs.

- Boost In Confidence

Simply following Kama Sutra can help boost a person's self-confidence. The actual *Kamasutra* book provides tips on how to boost a person's confidence and guides you to help make your personality magnetic.

Chapter 3: Trying Tantric Sex

Tantric sex is probably one of the best things to try out if you want to achieve the biggest orgasm of your life. If you don't believe me, then continue reading, If you do believe me and want to learn how, then continue reading.

Tantric sex is a Hindu practice that dates back more than 5,000 years ago. The word tantra is Sanskrit means "woven together." Buddhist and Hindu meditation practitioners often use the union of tantra as a way to help weave together the spiritual and physical, which also weaves women to men, and the Divine to humanity. The main purpose of the practice is to become one with God. The way that the Western achieves this is by teaching people to have slow intercourse without reaching orgasm.

Couples who have chosen to try tantric sex say that they reached more pleasure and have experienced a sense of "becoming one with each other" that is very loving and profound. The main goal of this sexual practice is to be enlightened and not trying to win a gold medal for gymnastics of the carnal type. If this comes off as a bit confusing, this of it this way. If having a quickie is the sexual equivalent of take out, tantric sex is the Michelin-starred meal, lovingly and slowly prepared and more delicious thanks to the wait.

Practice Makes Perfect

You will start things out by facing each other and looking deep within your partner's eyes. Your clothes should remain on while doing this. Remain focused only on the other person's eyes. This is going to help keep the two of you intimate. Some people have said that to keep the tension down during this act is to switch up which eye you are looking at, but some consider this to be cheating the practice. Your eyes are the windows to your soul. The point of this act is that the two of you are gazing into each other's souls.

Check in with your breathing. Yes, you could be breathing wrong during this practice. You should try to get your breathing synchronized with your partners. You both should be breathing in at the same time and then breathing out at the same time. Then you will transition into what is known as breath exchange. You will breathe in as your partner breathes out, and then you will breathe out when they breathe in. This is meant to mimic you breathing into each other. This should be practiced for about ten minutes before moving on.

For Starters

To transition this into tantric sex, you will do the same thing described above but without any clothes on. You are going to sit in your partner's lap, facing them. Next, you will wrap your legs around their waist and start to practice your breath exchange. Now you will start to caress and kiss each other. After some time, penetration can take place, and the two of you can start very slow intercourse. Make sure that you continue to caress and kiss one another. Your eye contact should be maintained through all of this.

Now things get to get a bit more interesting. Once the two of you get more proficient, you could actually build the ability to have longer orgasms. For men and women alike, this is a different way of having multiple orgasms. This will make you remain at the top of your pleasure without actually having an orgasm. You will get to enjoy all of the same feelings as having an orgasm, but it can help you last for several minutes, or even hours, without ever having a regular orgasm. This is able to create an emotional merging, as well as profound sex. There are some women who have been able to have an orgasm while doing specific exercises.

Other Ways to Tantra

What we have gone over is only one way to perform tantric sex. The good news is, tantric sex isn't really goal oriented, so there isn't a right or wrong way to do it. The trick of tantra is to take your mind off of the orgasm and focusing on making foreplay more enjoyable and rewarding until you are both ready to reach its natural end. This is often easier said than done, so in order to delay orgasm, tantric experts offer different methods such as massage, breath control, and meditative techniques.

The first thing you can do is to start by turning down the lights and shutting out the world around you. Loosen up your body. Tantra focuses on moving the energy through your body, so you should shake your limbs vigorously to help energize and unblock your body before you get started.

You may also want to stay off of the bed. Sometimes getting onto the bed will trigger your sleep button, which means that you two will choose to have a quick romp instead of a deep connection and loving sex, which is the goal of tantra.

You can try to lay down with your partner on the floor, with some blankets and pillows to make it more comfortable, and slowly start to touch one another. Take your time to leisurely make your way across their body.

Start experimenting with different types of touches, such as gentle strokes, light feathery touches, and firm massages. The aim of this is to heighten each other's senses in a slow and intense way so that you can build each other to a peak but not taking each other all the way. When done the right way, this is able to prolong the sex and your pleasure for hours.

If you start to find that your mind is wandering, refocus yourself on your breaths. Practice the breath exchange that was discussed earlier. This will help to keep your both focused and bring you closer together.

Above all else, don't give up. The first time you try this, don't be surprised if you don't last more than ten minutes or so. Try again. Tantric sex is going to take some time to get the grip of because we have all become used to our western way of sex. This means that we all expect sex to have an obvious beginning, middle, and end.

Tips and Tricks

Tantra isn't a one-size-fits-all practice. There are different things you can do to improve your practice and to make it more satisfying and unique.

- You don't have to get naked. You can begin things while clothed, and you can remain clothed, or you can choose to remove all of your clothing. The important thing is to do whatever feels comfortable for both of you. This will look very different for everybody.

- Focus on your breathing. Deep breathing is a very important part of tantric sex. When you focus on your breath, it gives you the chance to be present in the moment and to fully immerse yourself in the experience.

- Use all of your senses. Light a few scented candles. Play some sensual, soft music. Slowly touch your partner. Start into one another's eyes. Savor the taste of the kiss. Engage every sense during your tantric practice, and this will help you to feel every ounce of pleasure more fully.

- Go at things slowly. An important part of tantra is to learn how to feel and experience things on a deeper level. The best way to achieve this is to go slowly. You shouldn't rush tantra. Instead, you need to relax your mind and enjoy every second.

- Explore everything area of your partner's body. Stroke you hands slowly over their body. Use your tongue to explore their mouth as you kiss. You can also gently glide your lips up and down their chest. Let them do the same thing to you.

- You can experiment with things as well. For example, kink and BDSM often incorporate tantric ideas. When you are practicing tantra, there is no rule that says you have to stick to traditional practices. You can think outside of the box.

- There is no need to go full tantra. You can add in elements of tantric practices into your bedroom game. This could mean meditation as part of foreplay or focusing more on your deep breathing to help slow things down.

The Importance of Reconnecting

With our lives constantly being over-scheduled, we don't make sure that we take the time to stop and stay focused on our partners. Couples have come to realize that a normal monogamous relationship isn't working for them anymore. There are some couples who decide to have an open relationship for this reason alone. Performing tantric sex is a way to enhance your sexual pleasures and the relationship in several different ways. First, when you emphasize the breath, it helps to connect both of you on a more intimate and deeper level. This alone is able to help open your heart up to being more forgiving, loving, and closer to your sexual partner.

Second, since tantric sex is performed at such a slow pace, this will give you the chance to see how sensual your mind and body can be. Being able to enjoy sex for an hour or more is equivalent to turning a single taco from a fast-food restaurant into a Mexican feast. Either one is going to take care of your hunger, but that feast is going to provide you with more pleasure, satisfaction, and delight.

Last but certainly not least, you may not enjoy the thoughts of not having an orgasm, but his can help both of you create connectedness and ecstasy beyond the normal orgasm.

Chapter 4: Getting Ready for Sex

The secret to an invigorating sex life lies within the mind. Do you remember when sex seemed like a seven-course feast? You didn't know what was coming next, every mouthful made you tingle from head to toe, and once you reached the end of it, you felt content and satisfied. Nowadays, it seems like a bowl of cereal; convenient, quick, and fills a gap, but it's not something you would want to have every single day.

In order to get great sex back, you need to put it on the brain. When you make sure that you turn your brain on before you have sex, it will trigger your libido. Let's take a moment to look at some ways to get your mind ready for sex.

Take It Slow

How come a man can go from watching a slasher film to hopping into bed and instantly feeling horny, but a woman hops into bed and starts to think about everything they have to do the next day? The female brain and the male brain work differently. A woman's brain works by multitasking, but a man's brain typically focuses on one thing at a time.

Studies have found that a woman needs a transition time of 10 to 30 minutes between activities. That means that if you want to have sex before going to sleep at night, turn off the television and take some time before jumping into bed. During this time, you could have a warm aromatherapy bath or a massage to help put one another in the mood. The best scents for arousal are sandalwood, bergamot, chamomile, or lemon.

Just Say Yes

For some, having sex can be like having to go to the gym. Their body and mind start to rebel against is, but once they do it, they feel great. Standard wisdom has said, for a woman, the sexual cycle goes from desire to arousal, to orgasm. There has been new research that has found that women who are in long-term relationships will experience desire after they become aroused. That means, sometimes, you simply have to be receptive to your partner's touch instead of giving in to the voice that's telling you to go to sleep.

When you give into that touch, your brain will start to focus on pleasures that follow and will then increase the blood flow to the right areas. Even if all you have is a quickie and you don't orgasm, the biochemicals released during sex are still released, which will help you to want to have more sex, more often.

There are ways for women to help get themselves aroused instead of waiting on their partners to initiate. You can start by tensing your pelvic floor muscles. All of these muscles support your pelvic floor, as well as your genitals, and helps to stimulate the arousal process.

Morning Person

While most people think about having sex right before bed, mornings are actually the best time for sex. This is the time of day when your body has produced more sex hormones, such as testosterone. If setting aside time in the morning to have sex is out of the question, you should still use those early-morning hormones to help get your mind ready for a night of passion. Simply thinking about sex during the day can often be enough to make you want it.

That means, instead of just giving your partner a peck goodbye, take some time to look deep into their eyes and then give them a long lingering kiss. Wrap things up by whispering, "Our room, 10 pm." This will not just leave your partner anticipating the night to come, but it will also turn you on.

Getting the mind ready is only part of getting ready for sex. You also want to make sure that your body is ready as well.

Fantasy

You can also use your mind to help trigger your desire for your partner. There is a simple exercise you can do for this. You and your partner sit across from one another, hold hands, and then stare into one another's eyes. Don't say a word, but both of you should start to think about the last time that you had sex and really enjoyed it. This helps to create a connection between the mind and body. It works a lot like how you shiver when you recall a scary experience. When focusing on all the little sexy details, it will ignite your body and turn you on. You will also get to see the arousal on your partner's face.

Get Some Sleep

There is nothing worse than falling asleep before sex. One of the main reasons why new parents lose their sex lives is that they are too tired. Sex just doesn't sound good when you haven't had enough sleep. If you have noticed that you are too tired to get intimate, you need to make sure that you make sleep a priority. Make sure that you are getting the recommended seven to nine hours each night. To improve your sleep, you should make sure all devices are turned off.

Ask Questions

One of the most common reasons why you may be turning your partner down is out of boredom. This boredom doesn't have to do with just positions. You also have to rediscover what you both want. You should always ask questions, like: "Do you like it when I do this?" This will help you to feel more comfortable and confident when it comes to asking for what you want. You should also feel comfortable looking outside of your own bedroom for new inspiration.

Talk To Your Doctor

This tends to apply more for women, but men, feel free to talk to your doctor if you haven't been experiencing any sexual desire. For women, you should speak with your gynecologist if you have noticed that you have been having a hard time getting turned on for your partner. There are medical reasons that could cause this. Depression, menopause, hormonal imbalance, and some medications can impact your libido. Fortunately, topical and oral medications, lubricants, and hormone therapy can help get your mojo back. You should never feel embarrassed to talk to your doctor about this, that have heard everything.

Understand Her Cycle

Women are influenced by their cycle. They will find sex more enjoyable at different times of their cycle. From day one to 14, women produce more testosterone, which means it is easier to get turned on and reach climax. Women also experience a surge in libido during days 24 to 28 because of the nerve endings that are stimulated by the thickening of the uterine lining.

Food

We know a healthy diet is important for a long and healthy life, but the foods you eat can also affect your libido. Foods like honey, peanut butter, and bananas contain vitamin B, which naturally boosts your libido. Celery contains androsterone, which can help aid in female attraction. There are a lot of other foods out there that act as natural aphrodisiacs as well.

Kick Those Bad Habits

There are already plenty of reasons to stop smoking, but I've got one more for you. Smoking can actually hurt your sex life. Cigarettes narrow the blood vessels, and this makes it harder for the blood to flow to the genital region, which is very important for both men and women when it comes to sexual stimulation. You should also make sure that you don't drink too much. Too much alcohol will act as a depressant and decrease your libido.

If you make sure that you follow at least some of these tips before you have sex, your mind and body will be ready, and one won't let the other down.

Role Playing

Have you ever felt like you would want to be somebody different behind closed doors? Have you ever felt the need to change up the power dynamics in your relationship? Have you found yourself fantasizing about being a robber, schoolteacher, or police officer? Does it make you feel like you're gross or weird to feel that way?

It shouldn't. Roleplay within a relationship is actually very healthy. In spite of what you might have been told growing up or what might have been said on early morning bad cable shows, sex isn't something that is dirty, and role-play isn't a sinister act that only deviants and sinners indulge in.

Role-play is a healthy practice for couples, married, or otherwise, that can help you to improve and strengthen your connection with your partner. The desire to pretend to be somebody else doesn't have anything to do with dissatisfaction with your partner or sex life. It has to do with safety and trust.

Role-playing is simply the act of acting out your or your partner's fantasies, and this act of playing out fantasies often happens when you feel secure and safe in your relationship. Role-playing is a great indicator of feeling physically and emotionally safe with your partner.

Role-play has the ability to be a healing experience and can help to strengthen the relationship of the individual. It is a great way to express your desires or yourself. While movies and porn may make you think that women and men already have their fantasy roles laid out, that isn't necessarily the case in reality.

For example, if you are the woman in a heterosexual couple and your boyfriend is a high-powered financial analyst, and he wants you to spank him and treat him as a "bad boy," he could be hinting that he doesn't always need to be in control. The two different roles, the submissive and the dominant character in this type of sexual exploration, can change the bonds between people. It can enliven, deepen, and strengthen the relationships, whether you switch between a submissive and dominant role or remain static.

The fantasies you have are a lot more common than you believe. There are three common fantasies:

1. Public or spontaneous sex

2. Bisexual fantasies

3. Dominant and submissive

Chances are, you have had one of these fantasies before.

For the dom and sub fantasies, it gives you the chance to have an unequal power distribution in a controlled and safe situation. It gives you the chance to release your inhibitions and to be taken over by pleasure, and either have a gain or loss of control.

Humans have a subcortical circuit for submission and dominance. The majority of us will display these two sides several times throughout the day. A partner who would like to be dominant might have, or currently, feels weak and helpless during certain points of their life and benefits from getting to feel as if they are in control in a certain area.

With a bisexual fantasy, simply wanting to role play in a bisexual role, doesn't mean that you actually have

232

homosexual tendencies. This, in no way, means that everybody is bisexual, but a lot of people have experienced sexual interest towards a person of the same gender.

With a spontaneous fantasy, it is one of the "just can't wait to have you" type of things. This is something that we have all heard about and thought about, if not, we've given it a try. The thought of having sex in a public setting can be quite invigorating because of the danger behind it.

There is no need to be afraid of the idea of foreplay. It does not mean that you feel unhappy in your relationship, and it doesn't mean that you think your current sex life is boring. Simply wanting to be another person during sex doesn't mean you are going to hurt your relationship and the life that you both have outside of the bedroom.

The key to having a healthy and successful role-play is trust. Without trust, boundaries may end up being crossed, and your lines can be destroyed. It is all about having mutual respect and a good understanding that this is simply an exploration of fantasies, and the most important element of it all is consent.

Through this act of self-expression, there is an opportunity for validation and acceptance from your partner, which can lead to an intimate and emotional connection. The lowered inhibitions and sexual confidence that is needed when you role play can only be reached through safety and trust in your relationship.

If you are able to engage in role-playing with confidence, you aren't being some sexual pariah. Instead, you are proving that you have faith in your lover and partnership with them. If you can comfortably open yourself up to that level of vulnerability, you are reaffirming your connection.

Roleplay equals communication. When you are in tune with your sexual self, you are traveling an enlightened path. You want to feel relaxed enough in your relationship to feel like you can ask your partner for whatever it is that you want without feeling shameful.

In order to have good communication, you have to be in tune with yourself. Having a good understanding of what you desire and being aware of the level of openness and comfort you have to act out that desire is going to help you talk to your partner. If you have a solid relationship, then this communication should be fluid. So what should you do if you think role playing is for you? Here is where you need to start.

1.   Think About What Your Fantasies Are

First, you each need to figure out what you want. In your head, what turns you on? Is it a teacher you had in college? Maybe you have always wanted a massage therapist to take things a step further. You may have even fantasized about being your favorite book character. Your only limit is your imagination. Think about any type of scenario that turns you on, even if it is something as simple as a first date with a person you have lusted over. Your dirty thoughts are the best inspiration for role-playing games.

2.   Talk About It

There are some fantasies that can happen spur of the moment, like pretending to meet them for the first time. Others are going to need some prep work. If it is something really kinky that involves whips, leather, or some type of costume, you are going to have to give your other half a heads-up.

You can start things off by saying, "I can't stop fantasizing about..." Then you can gauge their interest in it. If you notice they perk up a little or get into it, then you can take things to the next level.

3.   Be Kinky or Not

There are some fantasies that are all about power, such as officer and criminal, or student and teacher. One of you is going to have to have power over the other in some way. This is a great way to explore a power exchange dynamic in a playful way. But not every scenario is going to have the power play. Pretending to pick them up in a bar, or acting as if you are on a blind date gives you the chance to be somebody that you don't think you are, such as overtly sexual, aggressive, or bold.

4. Start Slow

For some, role playing is going to feel silly. You may feel uncomfortable or awkward "playing pretend," even if it is something that turns you on. This is why it is best to begin slowly and with something small. You may try sexting about your fantasy at first. This gives you the chance to be imaginative without having to look at the other person or speaking. For some, this is all they want or need. For others, after they get comfortable with typing things, it is going to be easy to say their "lines" as the scene plays out.

5. Dress Up or Not

Imagination is extremely powerful, so costumes aren't always needed. If you aren't interested in buying costumes and the like, then skip it. But if the act of dressing up helps you get into your role, then go for it. If you aren't sure if you need the costume or not, try it with the costume and without to see which way you prefer.

There are a lot of places to buy costumes online. There are adult stores that you can buy things from, and you can also try Halloween stores, especially when they have their sales after Halloween has passed. You may even find some things in your closet that will work.

6. What Do I Say?

The first few things that you say as your character may seem silly or awkward, and that is okay. This is something new, and nobody expects you to be perfect when you first start out. It is okay to fumble and laugh. If the fantasy has a strong connection for you and your partner, then the words will come and you can follow each other's lead.

You might know how you would like things to end. If you do, you need to tell your partner. But you might also want to be surprised; in which case you should imagine what your character would say and go with it. There isn't a critic in your house that is going to tell you what you should and should not do. If the role play ends with both of you naked, sweaty, and satisfied, then you have done well.

Chapter 5: Beginner Sex Tips

If you took the time to compare your sex life to today's dating scene, you might think your sex life is blander than mashed potatoes. That said, you should never get "wild" just because that is what everybody on TV is doing. Research has found that spontaneity and openness are able to lead to a longer-lasting relationship. Don't let other people mess with your mind.

After you have gotten used to talking candidly about sex with your significant other about what you want to try out and what you don't, it will become a lot easier to do in the future. A lot of people prefer to have a partner who feels empowered. This is going to help you to build respect and improve communication between the two of you. So, for those of you who are still new to improving your sex life, or haven't really gotten started with your sex life, let's go over some tips on how you can make some changes.

- Casually Mention It

Every sex expert out there will tell you that if you are having problems talking with your significant other about your sex life, you can let a song, erotic book, or movie provide you with inspiration. The conversation can easily be started with, "I saw this movie," or "I read an article about..." After that, you can let the conversation naturally continue.

- Don't Be Afraid to Be The Initiator

If your partner is normally the one that initiates sex, change things up a bit by showing them how much they excite you and flip the switch so that you can get things started. Everybody loves to feel as if their partner can't resist them.

- Practice Some Non-Sexual Touch

While this may have more to do with putting in some work when you aren't having sex, it can end up leading to an overall better sex life. You shouldn't reserve touching for solely when you are naked. Find a way to add in some hand holding, back rubs, hair stroking, and any other non-sexual touching that will encourage you and your partner to show affection for each other. You will learn more about each others' bodies in a way that is a lot deeper than simply have sex.

- Toys

If you would like to experiment with some toys, begin with simple ones. The easiest one to try is a vibrating ring. They fit over the penis and can be used with a condom. Most guys like these because, well, they vibrate of course. They also provide stimulation for the clitoris, so it really won't matter which position you are in, everybody wins. It isn't just pleasurable for one or the other.

Even if there isn't a penis around, vibrating rings can be used as a massager. You don't have to use them on the genitals.

- No Toys, No Problem

Even though it is exciting when you introduce new things into the relationship, you don't have to have toys to increase the heat.

It isn't always about bringing things into the bedroom. It could be about changing up the location. It might be an erotic book or porn. It might be creating a playlist of songs that turn you on. After two songs, anything might happen.

The most important thing is you don't need to make it complicated. Try to find just a few phrases that you think you can pull off and try them out first. If talking seems too hard, just begin by getting more verbal when you are having sex. Moans and groans can help you get used to

238

being more vocal during sex. This will also help your partner know they are going things that you like.

- Lubes

The easiest thing to add to your sex life is lubricants. Water-based lubes are easier to clean up since the main component is water. These are normally cheaper. There is one drawback to this type of lube. They normally dry up faster than the silicone-based ones. The silicone-based ones last longer and are thicker. If you are having sex underwater, you are going to need a lube that won't wash off. If you are trying anal sex, where lube is very important, silicone-based lubes are your best option.

- Remember to Communicate

This one should be a no brainer, but anytime you begin pushing the boundaries in the bedroom, you have to make sure your partner is consenting to the new things.

If you are into any type of verbalizing or fantasy play that is going to involve your partner saying stop, they need to be able to do that. Everyone needs a safe word. Although you aren't into discipline or bondage, you might need some way to tell your partner it's time to stop.

If your significant other wants to do something you aren't into, say something like: "I appreciate you telling me about your fantasy, and I would like to explore it by talking about it. Right now, it isn't anything that I would be willing to actually try." When you let your partner know that you aren't comfortable with it, you are letting them know that there isn't anything wrong with their fantasy. They don't need to feel ashamed or guilty about asking about it.

Basically, sex is all about what is and isn't pleasurable and comfortable for your partner and yourself. There isn't any way to be an advanced sexual partner. When you have sex with your partner, if it is fulfilling and fun, then it is perfectly fine. Never do anything new just to keep away from a breakup.

Anything you explore needs to be done to enhance your relationship. You need to build on everything you have already created.

Chapter 6: A Massage to Get Ready

Massages are a great way to get rid of any tension you may have, spread healing energies, improve your blood circulation, and when we are talking about tantra, they can help to sexually arouse your partner. Massages are the best way to help sexual partners show one another extra intimacy.

By nature, humans crave touch, and massages are a natural and an easy way to get that much-needed human touch. So how can you achieve this? First, there is no need to head out and get some special certification or training to help you perform your tantric massages. The only thing you really need is to have a yearning and intention to genuinely satisfy your partner through the intricate capacities of your hands.

What Does Tantric Massage Mean?

Before we head into the actual massage techniques, we should go over what a tantric massage is, how it differs from other types of massages and the biggest benefits of it. The tantric massage that we will go over was first created from many different sources, which are mainly a mixture of tantric philosophy and influences from the most important Western thinkers.

The main parts of tantric massage include:

- Experiencing a spiritual awakening is the true and ultimate goal of the practice of tantra and tantric massage.

- You should never wear clothes during the massage, so private parts will, the majority of the time, be exposed.

- It helps to heighten or boost orgasmic or sexual experiences.

- It helps to get rid of blockages in various areas of your spirit, mind, body, and consciousness.

- Tantric massage is focused on using and the potential of your sexual energy so that it will benefit you and won't limit you.

Benefits of Tantric Massage

Just like with any type of massage, a tantric massage comes with many different benefits, as well as some added benefits that make the tantric massage all the more special. The main benefits of having a massage are:

- Increased wellbeing

- Relieves stress, anxiety, and pain

- Improves the mood

- Improves immunity and health

When it comes to tantric massages, you all get these benefits:

- Higher spiritual awareness

- More intense sexual experiences

- Improves sex drive and libido

With all of that out of the way, let's take a look at some techniques and tips to help you get started with your tantric massages.

Getting Things Setup

For those who have never gotten to have a tantric massage, the thought of a tantric massage is often intriguing, if not intimidating. There are some people who think it is taboo, which is an unfortunate byproduct of our society.

Then you have those who have received a tantric massage, and they see it as a unique, irreplaceable, and exciting practice that can do a lot for a person and their significant other's wellbeing. Since most people don't understand what it is and how it works, they don't even view it as an option for them.

In order to have a good tantric massage session, you are going to want you and your partner to take turns massaging each other. This type of massage is going to require the receiver to be completely open and receptive and to be fully willing to surrender themselves to the experience completely.

To help get things underway, the following are some ways to get things prepared before you get started with the massage.

- Get The Space Ready

You are going to want to get the room where the massage will take place ready. This can be any private space you have in your home, like the bedroom or living room. Make sure that you have plenty of comfortable bedding and soft pillows at your disposal. You can also set the mood by adding some candles, and you can use scented candles to help increase the mood. Make sure that you place your candles in safe areas, away from anything flammable, because the last thing you will want to do is set something on fire in the middle of a massage. Turn the lights off or dim them slightly.

You should also make sure you have something drink nearby, like water or wine. You can also have some light snacks close by to help keep your energy up. You can even feed each other. An oil diffuser can be used to give your room a fresh and soothing scent.

- Get Yourself Fully Prepared

Before you get the massage started, make sure that your mind and heart are open. If you have something that is causing you any sort of discomfort, it is a good idea to try to avoid bringing that up right now, but it might be a good idea to take some time to work through your problems in order to relax further. The main discomfort that people will experience is due to self-consciousness and insecurity about different areas of their body. While you massage one another, it is extremely important to keep your attitude playful and show them you are interested in discovering new interactions.

You may also want to take a shower or a bath before you start the massage. It is a good idea to do this together, but make sure that you stay away from any sexual interactions during your shower. Once that is done, stand face to face and stretch to get rid of tension.

You need to also be wearing comfortable clothing. Make sure that whatever you have on is loose enough that you can take it off easily. However, doing all of this fully nude is a very good idea. Since tantra is about the slow accumulation of sexual energy, it is okay to begin things with your clothes on.

- Start by Slowly Building Sexual Energy

After you have taken your shower and you have stretched, sit down so that you are face to face and in a comfortable position. This could mean that you are cross-legged, or you could have your legs draped over one another in order to help the energy from your erogenous zones to be closer.

Simply sit like this and start into each other's eyes for at least five minutes. As we talked about in the tantric sex chapter, the eyes are the most important part. This will likely feel uncomfortable when you first do this but carry on and stare at each other as long as you can. As you begin to feel all of your tension fall away, you have created a real connection. This is what the goal is of this exercise. This is the connection that you have to have so that you

244

can revel in the tantric massage and sex. Do your best to make sure that you don't lose eye contact during this.

Begin the Massage

After you are fully ready, whoever wants to receive the massage first can lay down on the surface that you prepared. There are a couple of simple massage methods that you can use, and all of them are beginner-friendly so that you can use them right away. You will want to have some massage oils to make these massages more enjoyable.

- Start on The Back

Add about two tablespoons of massage oils in your hands. Smear the oil across your hands and then rub them together so that you can get the oil and your palms warmed. This will feel better for your partner. Once you have warmed your hands, place them on their low back and let your hands move up their back, over the neck and shoulders, and then back down the back over the butt.

- The Hand Slide

Now that there is a good layer of oil over your partner's back, you can begin to slide your fingers down the spine and then massage all the way down their low back and over their buttocks. Then make your way back up to their neck, over the should, and down their arms and across their fingertips. Do this around five times. As you are massaging them, communicate with them and ask for some feedback on how all of this feels or what they like about it. If your partner doesn't like to talk a lot, you don't have to push them to talk. You need to remember that this is supposed to give them a sense of relaxation and wellbeing.

- Pull-Ups

To change up the motions, try moving one hand after the other as you move up the sides of your lover's body. Start by placing your hands at their hips with your fingertips pointed towards their spine and then pull your hand up to their spine. Once you do both sides, move your hands to their waist, and make the same motion to bring your hand to their spine. Then move your hands up to the side of their breast and pull your hands up to their spine. Lastly, start at their armpits and pull your hands up to their spine. You want to do both sides with each of these.

- Kneading

This is a crazy easy motion, especially for those who have every baked bread. Even if you haven't made bread, it is still a straight forward movement. All you need to do is squeeze their back and buttocks between your fingers and thumbs in a sinuous motion. Then you will allow your hands to glide to another area of their back and then repeat this action over and over until your kneaded all the way up their back. Then you can move your way back down. When you are working in fleshier areas, such as the butt, you can add a little more pressure, so you shouldn't about squeezing it a bit more and spreading their cheeks as your knead.

- Feather Stroke

Before you move down to their thighs, lightly stroke their shoulders, arms, neck, back, and butt with only your fingertips using an extremely light stroke. You should do this for around five minutes. If you have long fingernails, feel free to lightly scratch their skin. You should do this in circular motions and from side to side. The goal is to have this light and prickly touch to create sensual eagerness for your lover because they don't know what area you are going to touch next.

- Foot Caress

You might need to use a bit more oil for this. Rub your oily hands together and then rub the oil down and across their thighs and calves slowly. Knead the back of their legs as well. Do one leg at a time. The feet, whether you realize it or not, is an erogenous zone, so make sure you give them some considerable attention. Add some extra oil to each foot, rubbing it over the ankles, heels, and between the toes. Using the palms of your hands, slide them along the bottom of your partner's foot a few times. Gently rotate their toes clockwise and counter-clockwise. Then move your forefinger between each toe. Gently pull the toes away from the body.

- Flip Them Over

Your partner is probably feeling pleasured after everything you just did to their back, so now you can bring the attention to their front. Have them flip over as you apply more oil to your hands. Smear the oil over their belly and slowly start to slide up their stomach, over their nipples, and then back down to their belly. Continue to do this a few more times. As you do this, it spreads energy into their bodies. If your partner is a female, make sure that you a gentle with her breasts. Men can handle firmer strokes across their chest. You can also knead a man's chest if you want.

Once you have finished massaging your partner, it's your turn to get massaged. Allow the massages to progress naturally and let what happens next, happens. People who are more experienced in tantra and tantric massages will also use yoga poses during their massages. You don't have to use yoga poses in order to have a successful tantric massage.

Chapter 7: Getting Things Started

The most wonderful thing about playing sex games is that they are all foreplay. Does anybody actually have to justify making sex more intimate, longer-lasting, creative, and playful?

What is foreplay? Foreplay is any type of sexual activity before you have intercourse. With that said, intercourse doesn't even have to be on the menu or the grand finale. Foreplay is hot enough when it is done right. Most women call it "the whole point of having sex." It doesn't matter if it involves a quick text, back rubs, dirty talk, dry humping, spanking, fingering, oral sex, neck kisses, touching each other while spooning, or making out, foreplay is all the sensual things you do before the "huge event," whatever this might mean for you.

Why is foreplay important? There are many reasons why foreplay is so important. It is important for women to feel turned on and excited enough to enjoy sex. Jumping into sex without leading up to it can feel painful, uncomfortable, and boring. Even if you only have time for a quickie, it needs to have some type of lead in so it can be fun for everyone.

You don't go jogging without warming up first, do you? That is all well and good, but it won't get you heated up for sex. All the talking, kissing, touching, and rubbing before sex is just as important as the sex itself. It can help get the blood going to all the right places, boosts the libido, gets you in the mood, and relaxes you. If it is done right, you are going to get your partner primed for an exquisite orgasm.

This definition makes it seem like penetrative intercourse is the only definition of sex. It is best to call it "arousal activities." There are LGBTQ couples who don't actually penetrate each other, and they consider things such as oral sex to be the main event. So, when you call oral sex foreplay, it can be a noninclusive way to look at sex. When you look at foreplay as an appetizer and not the main meal can make it sound like it isn't as important as the man's orgasm.

You should think about foreplay as any activity that can build up arousal, whatever it might be. Sex doesn't need to be a linear experience that begins with a kiss and ends with sex.

As long as all parties involved consent, there isn't a right or wrong way to do foreplay. If oral sex is the main event, then the rubbing and touching that leads to it will give you the arousal you need. Any activity that can get a person "aroused enough to have fun with the other stuff" is considered foreplay.

Here are some classic foreplay activities:

- Spank your partner

- Tell her you enjoy reading her poetry

- Play with your partner's testicles

- Tell him that you love when he plays his guitar (or whatever instrument he might play)

- Nibbling your partner's earlobes

- Fingering your partner's anus

- Biting and kissing your partner's neck

- Fingering her vagina

- Sucking and licking nipples

- Caressing your partner's body all over

- French kissing

- Kissing and licking your partner's anus

249

- Squeezing and caressing your partner's breasts

- Stroking her penis

- Stroking his penis

You can focus on certain body parts like the back of your partner's neck or their pubic bone. The main part is taking the pressure off of yourself and making your partner have an orgasm. If it feels good for everyone involved, then you are on the right track.

Foreplay can trigger physical and physiological responses that make sex possible and enjoyable.

Physical Responses

Foreplay can actually get the juices flowing because it increases your sexual arousal. Don't confuse this with sexual desire, but it can do that, too.

Sexual arousal can cause many responses from your body; these include:

- Increases blood pressure, pulse, and heart rate

- Lubricates the vagina. This makes intercourse enjoyable and prevents pain.

- Dilates the blood vessels in the genitals.

- Makes the nipples hard and causes the breasts to swell.

- Blood will flow to the genitals, which in turn cause the penis, clitoris, and labia to swell.

Physiological Responses

Foreplay does feel good, but it goes a lot deeper than that. When you engage in foreplay, it can help build emotional intimacy that makes you and your significant other feel connected both in and outside the bedroom.

If you aren't in a relationship, no need to worry; foreplay can lower your inhibitions, and this makes sex even hotter between virtual strangers and couples.

If stress halts your libido, foreplay just might take care of this problem. When you kiss, it releases serotonin, dopamine, and oxytocin. This cocktail can lower your cortisol levels while increasing your feelings of euphoria, bonding, and affection.

Foreplay Means Something Different for Everyone

When talking about sex, foreplay has been defined as an erotic stimulation that precedes sex. If you take sex completely out of the equation, then foreplay becomes defined as a behavior or action that precedes these events

Whatever this event is might not look the same to someone else as it does to you, and this is fine.

You don't even have to put intercourse on the menu if you don't want to. Foreplay is its own thing, and it could be all you need to have an orgasm. If fact, research shows that women can't reach an orgasm just by having sex.

As long as all parties are consenting, foreplay could be anything that you want it to be. You can begin before things get heated up. You need to begin somewhere, but why does it have to be during sex. You don't even have to be in the same room to start.

You can use foreplay to prolong your playtime. If you know that you will be getting together in a couple of days or later today, you can use foreplay to start the party and keep going. Below you will find some foreplay tips. You can find one that you really like and try it out on your partner or get adventurous and try them all. The time you spend on your partner's body before penetration increases their pleasure along with yours when the main course happens.

You don't even have to be in a relationship to play sex games that are intended to be used as couples. Anybody who doesn't mind getting closer would be a great candidate for sex games.

When you find yourself needing to break the ice or get closer, take a look at these ideas for sex games.

- Who's More Powerful

This could be a thumb war, wrestling match, pillow fight, or tickle war. The main thing is you have to do it completely naked. The point of this game is competing, getting each other all worked up, and struggling against your significant other. Whatever the case, the person who surrenders first, has to do a sex act on the other. You need to make sure you agree to the act before you begin. Your partner might not like losing, and you might pick something that they don't like doing.

- Leave notes

You don't have to be creative to get your partner going. You can just leave them a note. Put it on their pillow or hide it in their bag. This shows that you can't wait to be with them later.

- Hide and Seek

This is definitely an R-rated version of the children's game. When you know that your significant other is coming home for the day, take your clothes off and leave a trail for them to follow. Make sure the clothes lead to where you are. Once they open the door and see the clothes, give them time to find you. The best part is they get to decide what happens next. You can then switch roles if you would like to.

- Sexting

Foreplay doesn't have to begin in the bedroom. It can begin when you wake up. This is so easy, and you can do it anytime and anywhere. A text telling them what you want to do to them or how hot you get just thinking about them. You can also tell them certain things they can do to get you all hot and bothered. This shows then that you are thinking about them and everyone loves that. Send them a text that says: "Can't wait to get naked with your later" can get your significant other excited before you ever get into the bedroom. If you are careful, you can even send them a nude picture of you to show them what they can expect later.

- Pick Your Tool

Let your partner try to bring you to orgasm by using a toy or object of your choice. This makes for some great foreplay whether you orgasm or not.

- Meeting For Drinks or Dinner

When you meet your partner for drinks or dinner, make out quickly in the parking lot before you go inside. Once you are inside, play footsies under the table, meet in the restroom for another make-out session. You could "accidentally" drop your fork to take a peek at what they might be wearing under their clothes. These are just a few ways to turn drinks and dinner into foreplay.

- Santa's Bag

If you have any sex toys, put them in a bag. Just make sure they are clean. Ask your significant other to reach into the bag without looking and get one. Whatever toy they pick out is the one that gets used for the night. This keeps either partner from feeling self-conscious about adding a toy to sex.

- Kiss Them Like You Mean It

Don't greet them with a chaste kiss on the cheek. Lock eyes with them, press your body against theirs, and kiss them deep and long.

Use your hands and tongue, and be sure to moan enough to make them excited about what is about to happen. Don't forget to end the night with another fabulous kiss.

- Buy an Adult Board Game

There are more of these on the market than you might think. Some will use cards. Others take a pair of dice. Some games are more traditional. There are some games out there that incorporate all three.

You could get a Jenga set if you don't have on already. Take each block and write down a command like "kiss my neck" and keep going from there. When you play with your partner, whoever extracts a block successfully from the tower, their partner has to perform the command. You can also come up with a punishment from when the tower gets knocked down. You can get naughty and creative on the punishment.

- Tell Them It Is Game Time

You don't have to be coy when all you want to do is get them naked and make wild passionate love to them. Tell them as graphically as you can that all you want to do is get them hot and wet or hard and keep them there all night long.

- Red Light, Green Light

This is not the game you remember from your childhood. You are going to lay down on your bed either naked or in something that makes you feel like a goddess. Have your partner stand at the door to the bedroom. You get to see how well they know you by asking them questions about you. The questions can be anything from personal to sexy.

You could ask things like: "Where is my dream vacation?" or "What is my favorite sex position?"

When they get the answer right, they can take a step toward you. If they get the answer wrong, they have to take a step backward. Your significant other is going to learn more about you while going crazy with your teasing. When your partner finally gets to you, let the fun begin.

- Light Candles

There isn't anything like candles to set the mood for all the sexy things you want to do. Tea lights don't cost a lot of money, so stock up and light them when you want to get busy. Plus, candlelight makes your skin look great.

- Timed Penetration

Find some sort of timer. You could use your cell phone, hourglass, or stopwatch. Now choose a time. It could be 30 minutes, ten minutes, or an hour. Now get busy with your partner any way you want. The kicker is there can't be any type of penetration before the time runs out. Once the timer goes off, have all the fun you can handle.

- Turn Music On

Everyone has a song or two that touches them in their special place. You need to find out what your significant other's is and add your to it to create a playlist that will get them all hot and bothered.

Here are a few of my personal favorites:

- o The Weekend – Earned It
- o Nine Inch Nails – Animal
- o Barry White – Let's Get It On
- o Donna Summer – Love to Love You

- Play Truth or Dare

This one is old, but it's still good. You might need to focus on the dares more than the truth. It all depends on your mood. If you think that they might be hiding something, by all means, stick to the truth but be careful, it might blow up in your face and not in a good way. You could dare your partner to try to kiss you without using their hands. Try to pleasure you by only using the tip of your tongue; this is the best time to uncover all your fantasies.

- Dance

There isn't anything hotter than two bodies being pressed against each other. Feeling your partner's hot breath on your cheek while you sway to the rhythm of your sexy playlist can up the heat factor in the room.

- Mirror

You and your partner need to sit down while facing each other. Start by touching, licking, kissing, or lightly touching your partner. Now they have to repeat what you did to them to you as close as possible to what you did to them. This can get very hot. It's a great way to communicate with them about what you like without actually having to talk to them. Then you get to switch roles. This also helps you pay attention to each other better.

- Sexy Underwear

These aren't just for women. If you can find the right one that fits perfectly, you can really turn your partner on. Low rise briefs are always a good choice.

- Make Out Time

You can go old school and make out. Press your partner up against a wall, get them in the back seat of the car, or just fool around on the couch.

- Striptease

I'm not talking about swinging around a pole. You don't even need to have moves. Just dim the lights, put on your playlist, and slowly take your clothes off. Make sure your expression doesn't show any signs of fear or uneasiness. You can totally fake confidence.

- Make An Erotic Picnic

Place a picnic on your bed that is full of sexy goodies that are meant to be shared. Juicy cherries and strawberries along with some chocolate sauce and whipped cream to dip them into can make for a fun night. You can feed each other and then lick each other clean. Chocolate is a natural aphrodisiac, too.

- Slowly Remove Their Clothes

Since foreplay isn't a sprint, it is a marathon. You aren't in a hurry to get finished. Rather than stripping all your clothes off and getting down and dirty, begin by taking off your partner's shirt. Wait a few minutes and then take their pants off, then remove her bra, etc. until they are completely naked. As you remove an article of clothing, focus on the skin that was revealed. After you take their pants off, you can massage their legs. When the shirt is gone, lick and kiss their chest.

- Massage

Human touch is powerful, and a massage can work wonders on the mind and body. Light those candles and get out your massage oils. There are some massage candles that can be used as both.

Begin at their feet and move up their body. Make sure to hit all their sensual points and linger in those special places when you feel like it.

You can begin by massaging your partner's legs from their upper thighs to their ankles. Now, focus on their feet, kneading their heels and all the parts of their feet. Now, work on their toes. Pull on each of them separately. You get bonus points if you suck them.

A bit of warning here, my partner hates having their feet touched, so you might want to ask their permission before you touch their feet.

- Quality not Quantity

If you can improve the quality of foreplay, she won't ever bug you again about quantity. If you just act like you are going through the motions to have sex with your partner, they will notice, and it is going to take longer to get them excited.

Basically, do what you would like to do and enjoy it; if you like her calves, stroke them. If you love how her butt looks in those jeans, kiss it, or give it a smack. When a man loves what he is doing, it will show, and this will turn her on even more.

- Erogenous Zones

A body is full of hot spots that beg to be touched. Nibble, lick, and kiss your way through all their zones.

- Find Out What Turns Them On

If you have any doubts, just ask them what they want. Most women really appreciate it when their partner makes sure that they are satisfied. If they see that you are trying very hard to please them, they will return the favor.

- Skin to Skin

You might remember dry humping from your teen years. Well, it isn't just for teens. The anticipation of two bodies rubbing together in different states of undress is the hottest thing ever.

- Toys

There is a lot more to sex toys than just a dildo shaped like a penis. Vibrators of various sizes and shapes can be used outside the body on any of the erogenous zones.

You can also find nipple and finger vibrators that can take foreplay to a whole new level.

- Sensory Play

All that dry humping and kissing is probably going to get the job done, but you can take it even farther with some props. Put a blindfold on your partner and then tease them with various temperatures and textures by using your tongue, ice cubes, feathers, etc.

- Tell Them What You Want

Talking about what you want during sex isn't just for foreplay. This makes sure you get what you need and want. Tell them what you want them to do to you and what turns you on.

- Soapy Shower

How wet hands and skin sliding across one another's bodies while you are lathering each other up with soap can take showering to a new level. You might not even want to get out of the shower, ever.

It's amazing at all the things you can find at home, or you could buy a seduction kit online.

That's it. Have fun. You might even think of some games on your own. The important thing to remember is that both parties have fun and enjoy each other.

Chapter 8: The Secrets to a Great Massage

We have gone over the art of the tantric massage, but if you don't want to take things to that extreme yet, you can still give your partner a simple massage. These techniques will help to make the simple massage more pleasurable.

In our life, it is very easy to let our emotional distance and stress get in the way of having a healthy relationship with our significant other. An erotic massage can help to create physical closeness and intimacy while helping to relieve stress and letting them get into the mood for sex.

When you add in erotic massage to your relationships, it can help to bring you both closer together emotionally and physically. It does not matter if your partner is always stressed or they aren't feeling inspired; an erotic massage can be exactly what you need to explore brand new levels of sexual bliss.

Three Important Areas of Erotic Massage

For you to get all the benefits of an erotic massage, let's look at the essential elements and how to use them.

- Environment

Setting the scene is very important because the environment could easily break or make the experience. This doesn't have to be time-consuming or expensive. If you incorporate the three things below, you will be doing fine.

First thing, you need to create an environment that doesn't have any distractions. Get any laptops, tablets, or phones out of the room you are going to be in. Unplug the television and cover up any devices that have harsh displays. You will also want something comfortable for them to lay on, and you can use some aromatherapy.

- Mindset

Before the massage, you need to ask yourself:

- How could I make their experience as enjoyable and relaxing as possible?

- How can I stay focused through the whole massage?

- How could I communicate with them to give them the most pleasure?

- What should I look for in their responses or reactions?

How you answer these questions could help you keep the right mindset throughout the entire session. It might take you some time to figure this out; it is going to be worth it to give your partner an erotic and relaxing experience they deserve.

- Technique

Even though the mindset and environment are needed for an erotic massage, it wouldn't be a massage without a technique.

There are some techniques that you can use during the massage:

- Effleurage

At the start of any massage, you should begin with gentle and light touches. These are called effleurage. The reasoning behind this is to get their blood circulating and get them prepared for the massage.

Use the palm of your hand and start with a gentle touch. You can do this in any pattern you want. Circular motions are the most common. They will cover the most area. Make sure you keep the pressure constant and make sure you pay the same attention to all areas of their body.

- Kneading

This is the most common technique that is used during the massage. It is easy to learn how to do.

Use your fingertips and thumb, take the muscle tissue between them, and squeeze at different intervals. This is great for large muscles of the buttocks, upper arms, and thighs.

- Friction

This is normally associated with deep tissue massages. This technique could be used when you need to work out tight kinks. Using your fingertips and thumb, put some gentle pressure on the knot and work it slowly in a circle.

When the knot starts giving away to the pressure, add more pressure while making sure your partner doesn't feel any discomfort.

To lighten the hurts but feels good feelings that are associated with this technique, you can change up the pressure during the session to give your significant other some time to recuperate every once in a while.

- Stretching

If your significant other has some stubborn areas of stress with knots, stretching could give them the best relief. This technique uses manual manipulation on your significant other's joints. You could rotate their ankles and wrists gently, bend and stretch their elbows and knees, and keep working on getting their limbs as loose and free as you possibly can without using force.

- Percussion

The chopping motions that are used with this technique might not seem erotic at all, but this could be a fun way to experiment and see how each other likes it.

There are different ways to do this technique. You could use the side of your hands to make a fast chopping motion to the upper back and things. You could use your fingertips to tap out any knots or kinks your find in their lower back, face, and neck. Percussion is useful to have in your massage arsenal.

The Science of An Erotic Massage

If you have never really entered the world massage, then you may be asking yourself how a simple massage can provide you with the benefits that we went over in the tantric massage chapter. This is a fair question. Humans are sensory-seeking creatures. From a very young age, humans are taught that touch is something we want and is good. We touch people in order to give and receive comfort, show signs of solidarity, and provide warmth.

We touch our partners to show them that we care about them and to provide them with satisfaction and joy. This means that massage can be an easy way to show your significant other that you care about them and their wellbeing. Also, think about the fact that there are certain levels of openness and trust that comes along with a sensual massage.

Very few women are going to be open to receiving an erotic massage from a man if there isn't some level of trust between them, as this contributes to the positive feelings and benefits of an erotic massage.

There are many different processes that the body undergoes when it receives a massage. Some of these processes, like the relaxation of muscles, are local. Others, like the release of endorphins, affects the entire body. But what the exact mechanisms behind the things that are happening?

There are various theories among experts. Some researchers and scientists believe that physical touch through massage session is able to improve circulation.

This will, in turn, increase how much oxygen gets delivered to the muscle and will help to improve the healing process. Others believe that massages engage the lymphatic system.

This will help to remove waste from the knotted area and will improve muscle movement and healing. Still, there are those that believe all of the benefits of massage are based in the nervous system. Touch causes an electric sensation that travels from the original point of touch all the way to the brain, which will release endorphins and other happy chemicals. So which one of these theories is right?

Right now, there aren't any right or wrong answers. It is possible that none of the above are correct, or they all could be. But whatever the exact reason is for those "good" feelings, there is no arguing with the scientific research that backs the benefits that come with a massage.

From lowering depression and anxiety levels to control inflammation following physical activities, massage has certainly shown that it provides many benefits to those who undergo treatment.

Eroticism and Massage

After you have a good understanding of how massage works and all of the benefits it provides, it is easy to see how erotic massage came to be. After all, when you mix two things that help to make you feel, which in this case is sex and massage, it makes sense that those good feelings are going to be amplified.

Erotic massage, though, is not all about sexual pleasure. Instead, there are two ways to pleasure your partner during an erotic massage session. Of course, sexual pleasure is one of these two sources. But, the other pleasure source is from the actual massage.

The orgasm should be seen as a by-product of your massage session, but it should not be the ultimate goal. As you move your hands over their body, your partner is going to feel more relaxed. The tension is going to leave their body, ever so slowly, until all of their muscles are loose and relaxed. This is the reason why climax becomes more likely. As they relax, so will their inhibitions.

With an erotic massage, your partner is going to slowly lose their signs of self-consciousness, anxiety, and fear. This is the magic of an erotic massage.

Targeted Massage Combinations

Knowing the massage techniques outlined above is a great start, but to make sure that your partner receives the satisfaction they deserve, it is important that you know the areas of the body that you should target and in which manner. The techniques can defiantly be used from head to toe, but sometimes a routine that includes targeted combinations of different body parts can provide more satisfaction.

The orgasm is the greatest possible release that a person can experience. While orgasms can vary in intensity and length, with the right massage routine, you can help to increase the strength of the orgasm. That's what this targeted massage routine is going to help you do.

Begin by having your partner lay flat on their back on a comfortable surface, be it bed, table, or floor. You will start with an entire body once over. This is basically a quick rundown of the more thorough routine you will be doing, but it will help to get the blood pumping. With only your fingertips, start at their forehead. Grave the side of the face with both hands and then slowly move your way down to their neck and chest.

Do not touch their nipples, but do lightly touch around the chest or breasts and then down the sides of their torso. Once you get to their hips, you are going to start to

265

branch out with one hand on one leg and the other hand on the other leg.

Simultaneously move your way down their legs. Remember that you should keep your touches light and feathery, and then trace your way back up a little ways and then back down again. Make sure you notice your partner's cues during this once over so that you can be a good idea of where their most sensitive areas are.

Once you have finished the once over, move back up to their neck. You will work your way down their body once more, but this time you will be spending time kneading the tight kinks and knots out of their body, but you should also add in some light touches to excite and arouse them. You can also use some of the other techniques that we discussed early in the chapter, like stretching. Pay attention to how your partner responds to the different methods.

Since this massage is meant to increase the orgasm, you will want to maximize the touches to the pubic region you make to help excite them. If you are massaging a woman, this does not mean you have to spend a bunch of time on her clitoris. Instead, use light pressure just above the pubic bone. Run your fingers over their stomach and stop at the very top of the public bone right above the hips but just below their belly button.

With the palm of your non-dominant hand, press down slightly. Make sure that your partner isn't uncomfortable. With the dominant hand, slowly work across their genitals, gently grazing across the sensitive areas.

When massaging a woman, feel free to insert your middle and ring fingers into her vagina at this point and press the palm of that hand up against the clitoris. As you move your entire hand up and down, the middle and ring fingers will be hitting the g-spot, and the palm will be rubbing the clitoris. When massaging a man, you can start stroking him.

266

As you notice them getting closer to climax, you can press down onto the pubic bone a bit more firmly and increase the intensity of your strokes.

These are only a few of the most common techniques that are used during an erotic massage session. You can experiment with various touches. Just remember to watch your partner and their reactions.

The next time you notice that your partner is feeling stressed out, offer to give them a massage and try out these techniques.

Chapter 9: Trying Dirty Talk

Dirty talk doesn't have to be complicated, weird, awkward, or creepy. Dan Savage, a popular sex columnist, summed up sex talk with this very simple statement, "Tell 'em what you're going to do, tell 'em what you're doing, tell 'em what you did." Simply put, dirty talk should be straightforward and simple.

While it can be and should be simple, most of us end up freezing up in the moment, and we end up saying something we heard once in a porn, and it will come out sound weird, awkward, unnatural, or very unsexy.

Given how easy dirty talk can go wrong, why do we even want to bother with trying it at all? The simplest answer is that when it is done right and is said by a person that you are attracted to, nothing is sexier than vocal sex. The biggest sex organ is the brain, so it only makes sense that we get turned on by what a person says during a moment of passion. This will also work in reverse. When you say your fantasies and desires that normally get kept to yourself to a rapt audience, it can be a big turn-on.

When you will get to the heart of dirty talk, having good dirty talk can take us out of our regular lives and really put us into the act of sex. While you might be physically feeling what is going on, if your mind is not there, the pleasure reward can fall short. This is the reason why people often fantasize when masturbating. Dirty talk helps us get out of our own heads into the body. The simple sounds and tones can help all of our daily worries melt away and remember how amazing our partner feels.

Now that you know why you should try dirty talk, let's look at how you can make it work.

Don't Make It Complicated

You shouldn't try to be a porn start right off the bat. Say the things that feel natural, and definitely don't think you

268

need to have some sort of elaborate narrative before you get things going. This isn't some strange Shakespearean monologue that you have to recite, and there is no need to talk every single time. Dirty talk doesn't have to just happen during sex. Picking the right moment to say something like, "I can't wait to feel you inside me," can do the trick.

Think about your senses, if vulgar or profane language isn't something that you typically use, then don't feel like you have to. Chances are, your partner would be turned off if you all of a sudden started using words you have never used before. Your aim should be to be playful, and you should start early. While your partner is at work or picking up some things from the store, drop a few hints about how you want to play.

This helps to build the anticipation of sex. You can easily send a text that says, "I can't stop thinking about tonight..."

Give Instructions

You have two forms of dirty talk. One form helps to build anticipation for sex, and the other is simply instructional and happens, most of the time, during sex. Giving some direction or instructions can be pretty sexy. You could tell your partner something like, "When you get home, I want you to put on your best lingerie, and then I want you to lay, face down, on the bed, and wait for me to come home and play with you." This combines both forms of dirty talk and can be used to add in some role-playing.

You Don't Have to Go X-Rated

It is very important that you know how to read your partner when it comes to dirty talk. You should not say things that are really vulgar unless all of the signs point to that. You can easily say things that are way too X-rated and then end up turning your partner off. If this happens, it will likely be embarrassing, but you should be able to recover from it.

If Things Don't Work Out, Talk About What Went Wrong

If something you say causes nervous laughter, that is fine, but there could be times when what you say can trigger them. They may not know the best way to verbalize why those words hurt them in the moment, but if you feel as if you took things too far, you should make a point of talking to them about it later on.

It will help to make sure that both of you understand that dirty talk carves out an erotic space and that you don't actually feel the way the person is talking. It is all about play. Think about how some people like to be called "daddy," but they aren't interested in incest. Instead, they like the dominance and authority the word gives them.

If you do take it too far, then do your best to correct it. Honor what your partner is into and what they are comfortable with, and talk with them about the things that they don't like. But, you should never make them feel like that owe you an explanation for the things they don't like. If they want to tell you, they will. This is true for you as well.

Try These Out

So, to make things easier for you, if you really don't know what you should say to your partner, I will provide you with a list of lines that you try using. You will have to fill in the blank on some things, but I think you will get the gist pretty quickly.

1. "Fuck me hard."

2. "I love it when you moan my name."

3. "I want you to use me like a toy."

4. "You taste so good."

5. "I'm going to come for you."

6. "It makes me crazy when you _____."

7. "When I get home, I want you in my favorite skirt with no underwear..."

8. "Yes, please. More."

9. "Right there. Touch my _____."

10. "I've been thinking about what I want to do with you..."

Give some of these a try the next time you want to get your partner in the mood and see how it feels.

Chapter 10: Orgasm

The orgasm has long been viewed as the peak of sexual excitement. It's a very powerful feeling of pleasure, which involves releasing accumulated erotic tension. While everybody's goal with sex is an orgasm, there isn't a lot now about it. During the last few centuries, theories about the orgasm have changed. For example, experts have only recently started talking about the female orgasm. Many doctors in the 1970s claimed it was perfectly normal for a woman not to experience an orgasm.

Orgasms are able to be defined in several ways with different criteria. Medical professionals talk about physiological changes that happen within the body. Mental health professionals and psychologists talk about cognitive and emotional changes. There isn't a single, overarching definition of the orgasm.

Sex researchers have tried to define orgasms in models of sexual response. While the process for orgasm can differ between people, there are several basic physiological changes that often occur in most incidences. Master and Johnson's Four-Phase Model includes:

- Excitement

- Plateau

- Orgasm

- Resolution

Kaplan came up with his own model, but his is different from most sexual response models because it includes desire. The majority of models don't include non-genital changes. It is important to understand, though, that not every sexual act is preceded by desire. Kaplan's three-stage model is:

- Desire

- Excitement

- Orgasm

Benefits of Orgasm

A 1997 cohort suggested that men's mortality risk was lowered when they experienced a high number of orgasms than in men who had fewer orgasms. There is also some research that suggests ejaculation can help to reduce the risk of prostate cancer. Researchers found that a man's prostate cancer risk was 20 percent lower in those who ejaculated at least 21 times a month than those who ejaculated only four to seven times a month.

There are a lot of hormones that are released during orgasm, which includes DHEA and oxytocin. There are some studies that suggest these hormones may help protect against heart disease and certain cancers. Oxytocin, along with other endorphins that get released during the female and male orgasm are also relaxants.

Types of Orgasm

Not surprisingly, since experts haven't come to a consensus in regards to a definition of an orgasm, there are many different types of orgasms. Sigmund Freud stated that immature and young females can only have an orgasm through clitoral stimulation while mature women are able to have an orgasm through vaginal stimulation. We will go over a few of those types.

- Pressure orgasms – this orgasm comes from indirect stimulation of applied pressure. This is a type of self-simulation that is common in young people.

- Tension orgasms – this is a common type of orgasm. It is created through direct stimulation, often when the muscles and body are tense.

- Blended or combination orgasm – these are a variety of orgasmic experiences that blend together.

- Relaxation orgasms – this orgasm comes from deep relaxation through sexual stimulation.

- Multiple orgasms – these are a series of orgasms that happen over a short period of time.

There are actually a few orgasms that both Dodson and Freud discounted, but there are others who believe they are real. For example:

- G-spot orgasms – this is an orgasm that is caused by the stimulation of an erotic zone inside the vagina through penetrative intercourse, which feels very different from orgasms caused by other forms of stimulation.

- Fantasy orgasm – these are orgasms that result from mental stimulation.

The Female Orgasm

Men and women go through similar yet different physiological processes when experiencing an orgasm. Here we will talk about the process of the female orgasm following the Masters and Johnson Four-Phase Model.

1. Excitement

When a woman is psychologically or physically stimulated, the blood vessels in her genitals will dilate. This increased blood flow will make the vulva swell, and fluid will pass through the vaginal walls. This makes the vulva wet and swollen. Internally, the vagina expands at the top. Breathing and heart rate will quicken, and her blood pressure will rise. The blood vessel dilations can cause a woman to look flushed, especially on her chest and neck.

2. Plateau

As the blood flows to the lower vaginal area, it will reach a limit and turn firm. Breasts can also increase in size by 25 percent and increase the blood to the areola, which makes the nipples look less erect. The clitoris will then pull back against the pubic bone, which makes it look like it has disappeared.

3. Orgasm

The genital muscles will experience rhythmic contractions that are about 0.8 seconds apart. For women, their orgasms last longer at about 13 to 51 seconds. Since women don't have a recovery period, they can continue to experience orgasms if they are stimulated again.

4. Resolution

The body will slowly return back to its previous state, with a reduction in breathing, pulse rate, and swelling.

The Male Orgasm

1. Excitement

When a man experiences psychological or physical stimulation, he gets an erection. Blood flow has increased in the corpora, which is the tissue that runs through the penis, which causes the penis to grow and become hard. The testicles will draw up as the scrotum tightens.

2. Plateau

With the increased blood flow, the testicles and glans will increase in size. The buttock and thigh muscles will tense, the pulse quickens, blood pressure rises, and breathing increases.

3. Orgasm

Semen, which is a mixture of 95 percent fluid and 5 percent sperm, is forced through the urethra by contractions in the pelvic floor, vas deferens, seminal vesicles, and prostate gland. These contractions also cause the semen to be forced out of the penis, causing ejaculation. Orgasm for a man tends to last for ten to 30 seconds.

4. Resolution

The man is now in the recovery phase, where he can't have any more orgasms. This is what is called a refractory period, and how long it lasts varies between men. It could be a few minutes to a few days and tends to become longer the older the man becomes. At this point, the testicles and penis return o their original size. Their pulse and breathing will be fast.

Multiple Orgasms

People find the idea of multiple orgasms intriguing and fro good reason. It is perfectly normal to want to experience one right after the other, as well as simply tapping out after the first. Here, we will go over why the female body is designed to experience multiple orgasms, and strategies to make them more likely to happen.

Having multiple orgasms doesn't necessarily mean that you have another orgasm right after your first one without a moment's rest, but you can do that. Multiple orgasms simply mean that you have several orgasms during a single sexual encounter.

In order to experience multiple orgasms, it will require some experimentation on your part. After you have your first, you will need to figure out what can make it happen again. If you find that your clitoris is so sensitive that you can't touch it, use the rest of your body. Try out different forms of stimulation. This could be playing with your breasts or getting your partner to kiss everything except the clitoris. The main point is to continue the arousal in whatever way works for you. Continue this for however long you want, and you can always check back in with the clitoris to see if some of the sensitivity has gone away.

That being said, sometimes stimulating the sensitive clitoris could be the ticket. There are some women who say continuing to run the clitoris gives them the chance to embrace what seems like unbearable overstimulation, which can result in more orgasms. It all depends on what you are able to handle. If you like oversensitivity, then do it. If it hurts or doesn't seem to be creating a pleasurable feeling, stop touching the clitoris to try to have more orgasms.

You can also use Kegal exercises to help extend your orgasms. As you reach your first orgasm, push your hand over your vulva and pulse it between orgasm contractions as you squeeze your thighs. Doing this can intensify and increase the orgasmic contraction and bring you into another orgasm.

You also need to make sure that you breathe during the entire experience. There are some people who will unconsciously hold their breath as the orgasm builds, but concentrating can help. When you reach an orgasm, breathe purposefully, slowly, and deeply while contracting your pelvic floor muscles. This breath work can lead to multiples for some people.

These tips are a great place to start, but don't get upset if they don't work the first time. It takes practice and learning your body.

Chapter 11: Female Ejaculation

Ejaculation has been described as a powerful experience that is only associated with male sexuality and penises. What most people don't realize is that it is possible for a female to ejaculate from the vagina or vulva. This could happen after, during, or even before sex and with or without an orgasm. Since there is a lot more knowledge about women and people, who were assigned the female persona at birth do possess sexuality. We aren't just passive sex objects. We are more aware and open about our sexual appetites, desires, and biology. Squirting is only one small part of it.

What Is It?

While having sex, some people who have vulvas will experience an involuntary release of fluids. This is what is known as female ejaculation or, as some people call it, squirting. Even though everyone who has a vulva identifies themselves as a female, and everybody who identifies as a female won't have a vulva.

"Squirting" has gotten more attention recently because more people are talking about it. There is more accurate information about the sexual reality of people who were assigned the gender of female. Their bodies are still thought of as being a mystery or myth. Squirting is often thought of as something to try to reach or just a part of being completely liberated sexually. This puts a lot of unnecessary pressure on women.

Some people think that squirting is just a party trick that specific people have to perform. But that doesn't make anyone feel empowered. What about people who identify outside the gender norms? How can we talk about female ejaculation?

Squirting History

It seems as if ejaculation has been around for a long time. During 2010, Joanna Korda and her associates looked through numerous ancient literary texts and found many references about sexual fluids being ejaculated.

In the ancient India text the *Kama Sutra*, they talk about "female semen that falls constantly." In a Taoist text written during the 300x called *Secret Instructions Concerning the Jade Chamber*, they talk about the difference between "the genitals transmitting fluid" and a slippery vagina. Joanna Korda and her conspirators concluded that this could easily be considered to be female ejaculation.

Most people wouldn't even consider it to be literature. They see it as pornography. Pornography is a normal way for anyone to learn about sex now. We checked out one popular porn side called Pornhub and found that some of the most popular videos were about squirting. The popularity of squirting increased a lot between the years 2013 and 2015. It still remains as some of their top 20 videos.

According to their data, women search for squirting videos 44 percent more than men do. As people age, the popularity of squirting will decrease.

People from Slovakia, Venezuela, Columbia, Vietnam, and South Africa will search for squirting videos when compared to other countries. In America, people from Wyoming, Montana, Utah, and Nebraska are more interested in squirting videos as compared to people from New Jersey, Maryland, California, and New York.

Most people who are assigned the female gender only experience something like a trickle rather than the large gushes that you see in videos. In fact, most people don't even realize it happened. Just like not squirting or squirting is "better," there isn't a right or wrong way when ejaculating.

What Is the Fluid That Gets Ejaculated?

Just because squirting videos are popular doesn't mean that it is accepted everywhere. During 2014, any pornography depicting female ejaculation was banned in Europe. This ban has been met with a lot of protests because it implies that ejaculating from the vulva or vagina is perverted while ejaculating from a penis is totally normal.

Censors couldn't see the difference between urination and female ejaculation. They consider urination to be and "obscene" act.

Scientists haven't agreed on what exactly is in the fluid of the female ejaculation. Even though it still isn't clear, female ejaculation fluid has shown to contain some urine, and it contains other fluids, too.

Dr. Amy Gilliland, a sex researcher, did a study in 2009 along with Doula and found that studies that have been done on female ejaculation noticed those studies didn't include how the people felt about the account.

Most of the participants reported that large amounts of fluid were released during their orgasm. Some stated there was enough that it sprayed walls, soaked the bed, and scared their partners.

Gilliland saw that some women who felt shameful about their ejaculation learned to feel more positive about their ejaculation later on in life once they heard other people's positive feedback, other's experiences, and learned more about female ejaculation.

Chapter 12: Best Sex Positions for Him

The tantric and kama sutra sex positions that we will talk about in this chapter are great for everyone involved, but it focuses on what will feel the best for him. While this chapter and the next will use the pronouns of he and she, this doesn't mean same-sex couples can't try these positions. They are adaptable to any couple who would like to try them.

Rock-a-Bye Booty

This one can be a bit tricky for people who aren't exactly flexible.

- Begin with the man on his back, and the lady slowly straddles him.

- Once he has penetrated her, he will lift his torso up, and she will position herself so that they are facing each other.

- Both will wrap their legs tightly around each other's buttocks. Both will link their elbows under the other's knees and bring them up so that they are at chest level.

This position will require a rocking motion since thrusting isn't possible in this position. The woman can squeeze her pelvic floor muscles to provide him with a stronger sensation.

Passion Pretzel (Blooming Orchid)

In the scheme of things, this position is fairly simple. If you or your partner have bad knees, then you may want to make sure you have cushions for your knees to rest on.

- To get into this position, start by kneeling face-to-face.

281

- Then you will both place the opposite foot flat on the floor and inch closer until your genitals reach each other.

- You both place your weight on your planted foot, and you both lunge back and forth.

This position places you in equal positions, and you share the reins. Everybody's arms are free to do as they will, as well. This will be a slow grind and not a lot of in-and-out action.

The G-Force

This is a fairly simple move that almost anybody can do. The man will have reins in this one.

- She lays down and pulls her knees as far into her chest as she can.

- He will kneel in front of her and grab hold of her feet and then thrusts into her.

- He can then bring her feet up to his chest. The woman will only have her upper back on the bed or floor.

Baby Got Back

For this one:

- The man will kneel and then sit back on his heels.

- The woman keeps her back to him and lowers herself onto his penis, either in a squat or plie. Her feet should be planted on either side of him.

- She places her hands on her thighs to help her keep her balance. He can also hold her rear to help with support.

- She slowly moves up and down, and she can nest all the way into his lap. She controls the movement with this position.

Tub Tangle

This one will take bath time to a whole new level.

- He will sit reclined in the tub, and she will straddle his lap while facing him.

- Once he is inside of her, he will move his torso up so that they are more face-to-face.

- They will both wrap their legs around one another's backs and link their elbows under the other's knees to pull them up to chest level.

This will require slight rocking instead of thrusting.

Lap Dance

For this one, you are going to need a tall-backed chair that you have padded with some pillows to make things more comfortable.

- He will sit down in the chair.

- She will face him and straddle him, sliding him inside of her, and then lean back a bit. She should rest her hands on his knees.

- One at a time, she will bring her legs up so that her ankles are resting on his shoulders.

- She will then move her buttocks back and forth, and at whatever speed she likes.

This will take some balance power on the woman's part.

The Milk and Water Embrace

This is great for all types of people.

- He sits down on the bed, a short stool, or chair.

- She then sits down on him, with her back to him.

- She then controls the thrusting.

This leaves all hands free to do as they will.

Torrid Tidal Wave

This is great for an intense make-out session.

- He will lay on his back, keeping his legs together.

- She will straddle his penis and then move to lay stretched out on top of him, pelvises aligned.

- She will lift up her torso so that she is resting on her hands.

- The slightest movements will provide pleasing friction.

The Tug of Love

For this position:

- He will lay down first with his legs wide open.

- She will down on top of him and allow him to enter her. Her legs should be on either side of him stretched out in front of her.

- Then she will lean back onto the bed.

- Once both are laying down, he will grab her hands and gently pull them to move her.

This is great for couples who have a foot fetish.

Life Raft

This is designed for sex in the water. You will need a pool and an inflatable pool bed.

- She will position herself on the pool bed on her stomach. Her vagina should be in the middle of the bed.

- He stands behind her with her legs wrapped around his hips. He should not push downwards. He enters and starts thrusting.

The important thing is to make sure the vagina stays out of the water because the water, especially if it is chlorinated, can dry things out.

Brute

This is a very male dominant position.

- She will lay down and pull her knees to her chest.

- He will stand with his back to her, straddling her hips.

- He then squats down and slowly enters her and continues to move slightly up and down.

The man needs to be very careful not to hurt himself.

Piston

This can be quite a tiring position.

- Both are standing and facing each other.

- He will lift her off the ground, placing his arms under her butt and thighs.

- Having a bed or sofa behind him will allow her to let her legs rest on it to help take some weight off of him.

- He will then "piston" himself up and down.

This might be easier to get into if he starts out sitting on a bed or sofa.

Missionary

This is a common one and one you have already performed, but it is a very intimate position.

- She will be on her back with her legs open.

- He will rest on his elbows as he thrusts in and out.

Helicopter

For this, the penis will need to be slightly flexible. Not every man will be able to do this. Basically, if you are standing, you should be able to push your erect penis down towards the ground comfortably before trying this.

- She will begin by laying on her stomach, with her legs straight and wide.

- He will then lay down on his stomach, facing the opposite direction, legs straight and wide.

- He will back into her until his thighs are over hers, and he can push his penis into her. He can then slowly and carefully thrust in and out of her.

Face to Face

This is great when you want to be intimate. Plus, it doesn't take a lot of effort.

- She will need to be sitting on the edge of a sofa, bed, or any other surface that is about 12 to 20 inches off the ground.

- He will kneel in front of her.

- She can drop herself slightly over the edge to help line things up.

- He can grab hold of her legs or waist when he starts to thrust.

Book Ends

Some couples struggle with this one, so you will need to experiment.

- Both will begin on their knees facing each other.

- He will spread his knees so that he can be closer to the bed while she will remain tall.

- Once he has lowered himself so that he is in line with her, he can slip his penis inside.

- If comfortable, he can move his knees back together.

Jellyfish

This can be a difficult position. It requires some strength and balance for both people.

- He starts by kneeling in the bed, his butt resting on his ankles.

- She will straddle him, squatting so he can enter.

- Both will wrap their arms around one another.

You will be doing more of a grinding motion rather than thrusting.

Hang Loose

This is a variation of missionary.

You will do the same thing you did for missionary, except this time, you will be on the edge of the bed so that her head can hang over the edge.

Big Dipper

This is a tiring sex position, so don't plan on being here too long. You will need a sturdy chair that faces your sofa or bed.

- He will position himself so that he isn't quite sitting in the chair, with his hands resting on the chair and his feet on the bed or sofa. He will be completely elevated off the ground. He will look like he is going to do a tricep dip.

- She will then straddle his as she is facing him, but she should not place any weight on him.

- He will then lower himself and push himself back up, moving in and out of her.

Reverse Missionary

This is another one that will require some penis flexibility.

- She will start by laying down with her legs spread apart.

- He will lay down on top of her but facing her feet. His legs should rest on either side of her.

- He will slowly push his penis into her.

Any position that requires him to move his penis backward needs to be done carefully and the partner should never pull on the penis. It is very easy to hurt the suspensory ligaments.

Ballerina Sex Position

This one will require the woman to be flexible to do this comfortably.

- Both will start by standing and facing each other.

- She will raise one leg up until it rests on his shoulder as she balances on the other.

- The raised leg will be pretty much straight so that he can get as close as possible.

- He can wrap his arms around her as he starts thrusting.

Screw

This is a simple position that anybody can do.

- She will start by lying down on her side.

- He will position himself behind her legs and place his hands on either side of her torso.

- She will turn her upper body to face him as he starts penetrating her.

Stand and Carry

This is a standing position that does not use a couch, bed, or wall.

- She starts off lying down, and he will lean over her. She wraps her arms around his neck and her legs around his waist once he enters you.

- He then wraps his arms around her and brings her to a standing position. He can grab her butt to help move her up and down.

Bent Spoon

This isn't one of the most popular sex positions, but it is great if you want to shake things up.

- The man will lay on his back, and she will lay on top of him, back to his chest.

- He will then enter her.

- She will then spread arms out to help keep her steady, and he will spread his legs to keep his balance.

- Once ready, she will bring her knees up to her chest and rest her feet on his knees for support.

X Marks the Spot

This is another variation of the missionary positions.

- She will start by laying in her back with the man on top.

- Hence the name, their bodies will make an X.

This might be a bit tricky at first, and possibly awkward, but once you get into it, it should get easier.

Italian Chandelier

This position is very submissive for the woman and gives the man a lot of power. It is super easy to move from missionary to the Italian Chandelier.

- Begin by getting into a regular missionary sex position.

- He will then come up on his knees, bringing them closer to the woman, which should force her legs apart.

- He then wraps his hands under her hips and butt and then lifts them up.

- She will help out by planting her feet on the bed. The goal is to have her hips and waist pushed into the air.

Down Stroke

There is a lot of stimulation for both people with this move.

- She will lay on her back close to the edge of the sofa or bed and raise her legs into the air so that they are pointed towards the ceiling.

- He will stand in front of her and grab her legs, pulling her toward him so he can enter her.

- Once he has her lifted towards him, he will lift her waist off the bed so that only her shoulders and upper back are touching the bed.

Exposed Eagle

This is one of the hardest Kama sutra positions we will discuss in the book. It requires a lot of strength and flexibility.

- The easiest way to start is to begin in cowgirl position. She will straddle and face him with her knees on either side.

- She will then lay backward until her back in on his knees and thighs. He has the option of raising his knees if she can't bend all the way backward.

- He will then raise his upper body so that he is in a more seated position.

- He can support himself by placing his arms behind him, or he can wrap them around her back.

Bended Knee

This is an easier version of the ballerina.

- Both will start out on their knees facing each other—they need to be close.

- He stays on one knee and lifts the other up and out to plant his foot.

- She will then lift the leg in front of his raised nee and rest her leg over his.

- He can then enter and begin thrusting.

Acrobat

This is a variation of the reverse cowgirl.

- He will begin by lying on his back, and then she will straddle him, facing away from him.

- She will stay on her knees and will then lay back onto him.

Viennese Oyster

This is a more complicated position that will require some flexibility.

- She will start on her back and grab her legs, pulling them apart and back.

- She will want to get her legs so far back that they are touching or almost touching the bed on either side of her. She can then wrap her arms around her legs.

- He can then enter. He could also hold her legs back.

Crab

This is another one that should only be done if he has a great deal of penile flexibility because she will be bending the penis back quite a bit when she sits on him.

- Begin by getting into a cowgirl position.

- She will then move her feet so that they are planted on either side of his shoulders.

- She then bends back, slightly, supporting herself on her hands.

This position should not be used during rough sex because it could damage the penis.

Bouncing Spoons

This is a super simple position that any couple can do.

- He will sit upright in bed with his back supported against the wall or headboard. His legs should be relatively straight out in front of him.

- She will stand over him, back to him, her feet positioned on either side of his legs.

- She will then move down onto her knees and sit back onto him, guiding his penis inside of her.

- She can then lean back so that she is rested against his chest.

Side Ride

This is another variation of the cowgirl position and is super easy to do.

- He will begin by lying down with his knees bent slightly so that his feet are flat on the bed to give him thrusting leverage.

- She will then sit on his lap, letting him enter her. Instead of having her back to him or facing him, she will sit sideways. This means she will face left or right.

Deep Impact

Hence the name, this position will allow for deep penetration. This is great for rough, passionate sex.

- She will lay down and point her legs towards the ceiling.

- He will be position on his knees, facing her.

- She will rest her legs against her shoulders.

- He then grabs her thighs and holds her tight as he thrusts.

Twister

This is definitely an "exotic" sex position.

- She will start by lying down her side. For this example, we will use the right side.

- He will then lay down on his right side. His head will be at her feet and her head at his feet.

- They will both bend their left knees and raise them up to the ceiling.

- She will lean forward and push her body through the newly created gap so that his leg is now over her waist. She should not be lying on his right leg.

- He will be sandwiched between her legs with her left legs over his waist.

- He should now be able to start thrusting.

See Saw

This is fun but can be quickly tiring. This is also a very unique position.

- He will sit down on the bed.

- She will sit in his lap, facing him.

- She should spread her legs wide so that she can get comfortable.

- She can then start to lean back, and either rest her hands on his shoulders or place them behind her.

You can either move up and down or grind on each other.

Intersection

This position will require you to form a cross with your bodies.

- Both will start out lying on their sides. She will have her head at one end and her feet at the other. He will lay across the bed.

- She will open her legs so that he can lay down on top of the lower one and penetrate her.

Doggy Style

This is a position that everybody knows and can do.

- She starts on her hands and knees with her legs spread apart.

- He is positioned behind her on his knees and enters from behind.

Sockets

This is a variation of scissoring.

- She starts by lying on her back with her legs spread wide.

- She will then bend her knees and plant her feet so that she can lift her lower back and waist off of the bed.

- He will then lay on his side at the other end of the bed.

- He should move down towards her in order to enter her. As he does so, he will slide his leg on hers. If he is on his right side, his right leg will move under her left leg and will move his left leg over her left leg. If he is on his left, he will do the opposite.

This is another position where his penis will need to be flexible.

Turtle

This is a variation of doggy and will require a bit more flexibility.

- She will begin by getting into the doggy position by resting on her knees.

- She will lower herself down so that she is resting on her ankles.

- Then she will lean as far forward as she can. She can reach behind and grab hold of her legs to help her lean further forward.

- He will then be on his knees behind her, penetrating her.

296

Lazy Wheelbarrow

While this may have lazy in the name, it still takes a lot of effort.

- He will start by sitting on a sofa with his legs together.

- She then sits down on him, facing away, with her legs together.

- She will start to lean forward as far as she can so that she can place her hands on the floor. Her stomach will be resting on her thighs.

Fire Hydrant

This is another doggy style variation.

- Both will get into a regular doggy style position.

- His knees should be positioned inside of hers.

- He will then start to lift one of his legs up and forwards so that his foot is planted at her side.

- The leg he moved will be under her leg so that her thigh will be resting on his thigh. The goal is to look like a dog peeing on a fire hydrant.

Chapter 13: Best Sex Positions for Her

The goal for these positions isn't to have an earth-shattering orgasm. The journey of lovemaking is about becoming one, being orgasmic, moving, connecting, feeling, and breathing with your partner. When you learn to explore your sexuality while being conscious of everything around you and you learn how to harness its power to experience a profound connection with other humans, you will transcend the need for specific techniques and just get into the flow. This flow will move into every area of your life.

Yab Yum

For this position:

- The guy is going to sit either on a bed or any other flat surface. He will fold his legs in the position of the half lotus. If this is too uncomfortable for him, have him sit on the edge of the bed or a chair and allow his legs to dangle.

- The woman is going to sit on his lap. Her legs will straddle his. She needs to wrap her legs around his waist. If this isn't comfortable for her, she can place a pillow under her bottom. If you are sitting in a chair, her legs could just dangle over his.

- She is going to raise herself up so she can put his penis inside her vagina. It doesn't matter whether it is hard or soft; either one is fine.

- Place your upper bodies against each other to create more skin on skin sensation. You can wrap your arms around one another.

- When you feel the time is right, you can begin to rock back and forth and let your bodies do the rest.

"Fitting On Of the Sock" or "The Rolling Tickle"

These are actually two different positions, but they blend together great and are great if you aren't very flexible.

- The woman will lay down on her back with her head resting on a pillow.

- The man is going to kneel down between her legs. He will sit back on his heels. If he needs to support his knees, he can put a pillow between his heels and butt.

- The woman is going to place her legs across the man's legs.

- The man is going to place his penis along the length of the woman's vulva. He will rock back and forth to stimulate the vulva. He uses his hands to stimulate her other erogenous zones.

- Once the woman is extremely excited and well lubricated, the man can place his penis inside her vagina.

- The woman is going to raise her pelvis up to meet him. Make sure you find your rhythm.

- If the woman is fairly flexible, she can bring her knees up to her chest.

- The man will be able to penetrate her very deeply while she is rolling her things down and up. If she needs help or support, he can place his hands under her bottom.

Congress of a Cow

For this position:

- The woman is going to bend forward at the waist while keeping her feet and hands on the floor

- The man will come up behind her and penetrate her.

- All the woman has to do is keep her balance while he thrusts away.

Yawning

- The woman is going to lay down on her back.

- The man is going to kneel in between her legs.

- The woman will spread her legs as wide as possible on either side of the man's waist. She will lift her legs as high as she possibly can. To alternate the sensations, she can try moving her legs up and down.

- Since you are both supported on the floor or bed, this is a great position to let your hand wander all over each other's bodies.

Tripod

- Both the man and woman will stand facing each other.

- The man is going to put one hand under one of her knees and bring it off the floor. You have now become a tripod.

- The man will now penetrate the woman.

- This works best if both parties are about the same height.

Launch Pad

- The woman is going to lay down on her back.

- The man will penetrate her while staying on his knees and facing her.

- The woman will lift her legs up and bring her knees into her chest. She can rest her feet on his chest if she would like.

- The man can lean over her while she raises her hips so he can penetrate her deeply.

Coital Alignment Technique

- The woman is going to lay down on her back with her legs spread open.

- The man is going to place himself in between her legs and penetrate her. This is just like performing a normal missionary position.

- Rather than him beginning to thrust in and out, he is going to move forward over her body. This changes the angle of his penis. His penis is now going to point down and will be more in contact with her vagina's back wall.

- While the man is in this position, his pubic bone and possibly penis will be in constant contact with the woman's clitoris.

- The woman doesn't need to just lay there. She can move to keep her clitoris in constant contact with his penis and pubic bone.

- The woman can also wrap her legs around his back and pull him farther into her vagina.

- The woman will get more out of this position if she can get a rhythm going with her man.

Swan Sport

- The man is going to lay down on the bed or floor on his back.

- The woman will sit on top of the man while facing his feet. She is going to place her feet on top of his thighs.

- She now has the opportunity to go as fast or slow as she would like.

- She needs to be able to keep her balance while sitting on her man.

- The man can help her keep her balance by holding onto her waist.

Upavitika

- The woman lays down on the floor or bed with her knees bent and feet on the bed.

- The man kneels between her legs and penetrates her.

- Once she has been penetrated, he can straighten his legs out.

- The woman will bring one foot up and place it over his heart.

- She gets to control the situation with her foot over his heart.

The Mastery

- The man is going to sit on the sofa or side of the bed with his feet flat on the floor. He needs to have his butt and thighs on the bed.

- The woman will either kneel down or squat on his lap.

- The woman can then wrap their arms around his neck.

- Help him penetrate you. Once he is firmly inside you, you can lift yourself up and down on top of him, and he can thrust into you.

- You might find it easier to just rock back and forth or grind against him.

- This position puts the woman in power since she is on top. She can find the rhythm she lays to bring both of you to orgasm.

- Since you are facing each other, you get to kiss and fondle each other.

- To change things up, you can place your hands on his knees and lean back a bit. Just be careful.

Pearly Gates

- The man is going to lay down on his back. He needs to bend his knees with his feet on the bed.

- The woman is going to lay down on top of the man. The woman's head will be to the side and above his.

- The man will now penetrate the woman while in this position.

- If you have problems keeping your balance, spread your legs, and keep them bent, so your feet are on the bed. You could also spread out your arms to help you balance, too.

- The man can wrap his arms around the woman's chest or waist to help keep them balance while playing with her breasts.

- When the woman has her balance, she will be able to thrust back and forth on his penis while he thrusts up into her.

- Since his mouth is right by her ear, he can talk dirty to her or nibble on her neck and ear.

Pretzel

- The woman is going to lay down on her side with the leg against the bed straight and the leg on top crooked out just slightly.

- The woman will need to raise her top leg slightly toward her chest and place the arm on top either in front of her or behind her. Just make sure the arms are very comfortable.

- The man is going to come in on his knees and straddle the woman's straight leg while remaining on his knees. Once he has penetrated her, he will keep his torso upright while thrusting into the woman.

- The woman won't be able to do much in this position, so she is at the mercy of her victor.

The Wheel Barrow

- The woman is going to bend forward at the waist with her hands and feet on the floor.

- The man will come up behind the woman and penetrate her from behind. Once he has penetrated her, he can lift one or both feet off the ground. Again this depends on how strong each of you are.

- The woman's hands and arms might become extremely tired while doing this position. If you have to, you can squeeze your legs together a bit to help you keep your balance.

- While the man is thrusting in and out, the woman just needs to keep her balance. That's pretty much it.

The Bodyguard

- You are both going to stand up straight.

- You are going to be facing in the same direction.

- The man is going to come up behind the woman and penetrate her.

- If he is taller, he is going to need to bend his knees a bit.

- Once he is inside, he will just thrust in and out, and you can push yourself back into him.

Asian Cowgirl

- The man is going to lay down on the floor or bed on his back.

- The woman is going to straddle him, but instead of being on her hands and knees like regular cowgirl, she will squat. This means that most of her weight is going to be supported by her feet.

- The woman can use her hands to take the weight off her feet by placing them on the man's chest or beside him on the bed.

Irish Garden

- To start this position, the man will sit on the bed with his back straight. He needs to keep his legs out in front of him and opened wide. He can bed his knees if it is more comfortable.

- The woman will get on her hands and knees, facing away from him and move backward toward him.

- She will lower herself onto the man by straightening her legs out behind the man make sure there is one leg on each side of his waist.

- Now she can lower her shoulders and head to the bed.

- The woman is responsible for all the movement here since she has the man pinned to the bed.

The Amazon

- The man will lay down on his back with his legs raised slightly with his knees bent.

- The woman will come in and squat down on him.

- He is going to need to bring his legs closer to his chest, so they don't get in your way.

- Now, sit on his penis and set your pace.

- The man will automatically push you up with his thighs.

Pump

- The woman is going to stand on a short table, sofa, or bed. Her legs stay bent just a little bit.

- The man will penetrate her from behind while he is standing.

- The woman can place her arms on a wall in front of her if there is one to help her push back against him.

Superwoman

- The woman is going to lay down on the bed on her stomach. Her arms will be stretched in front of her on the bed.

- The woman's legs need to be hanging off the side of the bed. Her waist should be even with the edge of the bed.

- The man will penetrate her from behind while he is standing and will begin thrusting.

Bull Dog

- The woman will get on her hands and knees. Then she is going to bring her legs together.

- This man will penetrate her from behind in a slightly squatting position.

- He will put his feet to the outside of her legs. He can keep himself steady by placing his hands on her shoulders or waist.

Legs on Shoulder

- The woman will lay down on her back and bring her legs up, so they are pointing at the ceiling.

- The man will be positioned on his knees but keeping his back straight. He will penetrate her.

- The woman will rest both her legs on one of his shoulders.

- The man will wrap one arm around her legs while placing the other hand on her stomach.

Prison Style

- Both the man and woman will be standing and facing in the same direction.

- The man will penetrate the woman from behind.

- The woman will bend at the waist until her chest is parallel to the ground, and she is looking at the floor.

- The woman can spread her legs while the man keeps his closed.

- Now the woman needs to put her arms parallel to her body.

- The man will reach forward and grab her wrists and bring her arms behind her back. He gets to control her by keeping her arms behind her back.

Burning Man

- The woman is going to face a table or countertop and will bend forward until her stomach is touching the surface. Her feet will stay on the ground.

- The man will come up behind her and penetrate her.

- The woman's legs are going to act as an anchor that will keep you in place. This allows the man to give some intense, hard penetration without falling.

Praying Mantis

- The woman will lay down on her back with her legs open.

- The man will kneel in front of her pelvis and penetrate her. He will take one of her legs and bring it up slowly so that it points the ceiling. He can then place it on his shoulder or wrap his arm around it.

Betty Rocker

- The man will lay down on his back with his legs slightly apart.

- The woman will straddle him while facing away. While she is sitting straight up, she will place his penis inside of her.

- Once he is firmly inside, she will begin leaning forward while supporting herself with her arms on his legs.

- Now the woman will begin to rock back and forth by using her arms and legs. She could also move up and down on his penis.

Thigh Tide

- The man is going to lay down on his back with his legs straight in front of him.

- He will raise one knee just a bit and put his foot on the bed.

- The woman is going to face away from the man. She is going to place one knee on either side of the man's bent leg while sitting on his penis.

- She will raise herself up and down on him. She can hold on to the man's leg to help keep her balance.

Fast Fuck

- The man will lay down on his back. His knees will be bent slightly and his feet on the bed.

- The woman will straddle him. She can either stay on her feet or knees. She will lean forward while resting on her elbows or hands. She will position herself, so she is raised above the man just slightly.

- She won't be resting on his crotch.

- The man will begin thrusting into her quickly. It isn't going to be a deep penetration, but it will feel wonderful.

Jughead

- The man is going to lay down either beside a couch or bed while keeping his back on the floor.

- The man will put his legs up on the bed or sofa.

- The woman will position herself above the man while being on all fours with an arm and a leg on each side of him.

- The man is going to lift his lower back and crotch off the floor so he can penetrate her.

- The woman will sit on his penis and thrust herself back into him. She can thrust as hard as she wants, or he can just push into her while she takes it easy.

Man Missionary

- The man will lay down on his back with his legs together. He can keep them straight or bend them at the knee.

- The woman will straddle him just like with the cowgirl position.

- The woman will lean forward over the man and rest her hands on his chest or stomach.

- She will then begin rocking back and forth. It is really like the normal Missionary position but reversed.

Chapter 14: Best Sex Positions To Bring Couples Closer

We've covers positions that are more pleasurable for him and for her, so let's look at some positions that will help to increase the intimacy in the relationship. While those sudden and desperate quickies, but nothing is better than sex that is soulful and rich. This can harness the bonding powers of neurochemistry and science.

Lotus Blossom

This is also known as the seated wrap-around and will require you and your partner to embrace one another, which is great for gazing romantically into each other's eyes.

This position can be used even if your goal isn't to have sex or orgasm. You can simply sit in their lap and look at each other or make out. To get into the position, one partner will straddle the other as you both sit in a cross-legged position. The person on top will wrap their legs around the bottom of their partner as you two face one another and embrace. The one on the bottom will enter the person on top with a penis or a toy.

Spooning 69

This position will allow the two of you to give and receive oral play while on your side. You get to have the closeness of spooning while also having the joy of the mouth-to-genital play.

You will both lay on your sides, facing one another but in opposite directions so that your mouth is aligned with your partner's genitals.

Breakfast Spoons

This is the spooning position but with morning sex. While it may not sound special, having sex in this cuddling position before you have both fully woken up brings something romantic to the relationship.

When your partner enters you from behind in the spooning position, they get the joy of being able to kiss your neck, hold your hands, or provide extra stimulation.

The Hound

This is an intimate spin on doggy style. This position allows for slow, deep thrusts, as well as quick, shallow thrusts. It is best to start things slowly and then speed it up. Alternate between deep and shallow. With this position, there is a lot more skin-to-skin contact, and all of her other erogenous zones are easily accessible. They can also nibble on the other's neck or ears, whisper dirty phrases.

How to get into this position. Both will start on their knees. The person doing the penetration will have their legs positioned on the outside of their partner and will curl their body around the other person and enter from behind. The one on the bottom will rest on their forearms and will be able to swivel their hips to get into a comfortable position.

Face-to-Face Standing

Face-to-face sex is great for kissing and intimacy. To get into this position, both partners will stand facing each other. It might be easier if one partner is braced against a wall. The penetrating partner will place themselves between the other's legs. They will penetrate their partner, and if possible, they can lift their partner's legs around their hips.

Drill

Missionary positions can be one of the most erotic positions because it places you in a face-to-face position. This position takes the standard missionary up a notch.

The woman will start by lying down, just like she would with regular missions. She will then raiser her legs up and wrap them around your partner's waist. She can cross her ankles to help keep her legs around him. This will allow you to grip their partner closer and pull them into her.

Teaspooning

This is one of the most intimate positions you can try.

He will start out on his knees, spreading them as wide as he comfortably can. She will then get on her knees in front of him, keeping her knees together. He will move closer to her, keeping his legs on either side of hers. He can then enter her, and his arms should be wrapped around her, holding her breasts, or holding her shoulders.

Sofa Spooning

You will want to make sure you have a comfortable, full-length sofa for this one.

He will lay down on the couch with his back pressed against the back of the couch. She will lay down in front so that they are laying back to chest. He will then enter her and start to slowly thrust with his arms wrapped around her.

This is great for a Netflix and chill moment.

The Mermaid

For this position, she will lay down face-up at the edge of a counter, desk, or bed. A pillow under her butt may be helpful. She will extend her legs into the air, keeping them together. He will stand in front of her, holding her ankles to keep him stable and allow him to thrust deeper.

The Sofa Spread-Eagle

This can be tricky if there is a large height difference.

She will start by standing on the edge of the bed, couch, or on two chairs, with her legs spread wide. He will stand on the floor in front of her. She will need to adjust her stance so that he can easily slide until their pelvises meet.

He'll do all the moving on this one, but she can do whatever she wants with her hands.

Chapter 15: Increasing Male Orgasmic Control

All men are looking to have an intense orgasm and an erection that will last long enough for them to reach orgasm. Reaching an orgasm is simple, but sustaining an erection and enjoying the orgasm will take a little more time and patience. Plus, your partner will thank you for lasting longer. Let's look at how you can control your orgasm and erection.

Muscle Strength

While having a six-pack might get you noticed, those aren't the muscles that help you during sex. To get the most out of your sexual experience, you need to work on your pubococcygeal muscle. These muscles sit on the floor of your pelvis and control your stream of urine and the muscle spasms that happen when you have an orgasm. This is why sex therapists and doctors recommend that you work on strengthening those muscles so that you don't have premature ejaculations and to improve the orgasm.

Kegel exercises aren't something that only women can do. They can also be used to strengthen the man's PC power. When you are urinating, you can squeeze this muscle to stop the flow of urine. Once you have figure out where the muscle is by doing this, you can squeeze that muscle at any time during the day. Hold the muscle for two seconds and then release. Do this 20 times, three times a day. You will start to hold the muscles for longer intervals. You should never stop with these exercises. Kegel exercises have to be performed on a regular basis in order to keep those muscles strong.

Edging

Nothing can help you to strengthen your control and erection better than edging, or holding back right before you orgasm. You stop as soon as you feel like you are about to orgasms, rest until you are in control again, and then continue with sex. This can be done until it becomes second nature. This can be practicing during masturbation, and once you are ready to orgasm, you can stop edging.

The best way to edge is, once you stop yourself, don't start again until your breathing is under control, and then wait 30 seconds before you continue on. If you find this does not work, you can also stop ejaculation by squeezing the top of your penis or gently pulling the testicles right when you are about to have an orgasm. Then you will do this all over again. After edging has been mastered, you will be able to have a dry or contractile orgasm. Basically, you will get the same pleasure sensations of an orgasm, but you won't lose the erection. This means that you can have multiple orgasms before you finally finish.

Stop Masturbating

I understand that I just told you to practice edging while masturbating but hear me out. Masturbating is probably not going to give you and eye-rolling and mind-blowing orgasm for a man at least. The male body releases 400% more prolactin after they have penetrated a vagina than it does after masturbation. Prolactin is the male hormone that makes them feel sexually satisfied. Our evolutionary forces have always rewarded behaviors that are connected with reproduction. Having vaginal-penile sex is something that is passed through our genes.

Deep Breathing

If you ask a sex therapist the best way to have a full-body orgasm, they are going to tell you that controlled breathing will do it for you. If you make sure that your breathing remains regular and deep, this is going to allow for a more intense arousal to build. The orgasm will remain more satisfying. Breathing to quickly is going to increase your excitement and will ultimately push you over the edge.

Breathing can intensify the male orgasm by taking more oxygen into the arousal process. Shallow breaths in through the nose and deep breaths out through the mouth will help to remove muscular and psychological tension that will help to intensify the orgasm.

Use the Brain

Orgasms get started in the brain. Our brains are in control of everything and are active in the genitals. Women have a lot of activity within the brain area that is connected to emotions, whereas men only experience brain activity in their secondary somatosensory cortex that deals with physical sensations. The good thing about this is that in order to have a better orgasm, you have to have your partner focus on the penis while you are focused on the sensation that you are getting from their touch.

Keep Your Feet Warm

This may sound crazy, but scientists have found that men who have cold feet will have a harder time reaching orgasm than those who are wearing socks or have warm feet. When the man is comfortable, he is going to be more relaxed. This relaxation is the key to have better orgasms. If you are afraid of being made fun of for wearing your socks, you can turn the heat up or place them into some warm water before she shows up.

Sex Positions to Sustain an Erection

Maybe you struggle with maintaining an erection, and that is what keeps you from enjoying your orgasm. There are some positions that can help with this.

One way to help things along is by having your partner straddle you. They will sit on your lap, facing you, and will lean back a bit and slide their pelvis up and down along the penis. You will also tease them with your fingers by rubbing their clit. Once you get hard, you can turn this into seated cowgirl, or you can simply stroke yourself while they continue to rub themselves up and down you.

You can also try the wake-up curl. Morning wood is something that shouldn't be taken for granted. This is the time when testosterone is the highest, so have morning sex. Both of you will be on your side, and you will slide up behind her. This means you won't have to worry about morning breath, and she will have a tighter feeling, which will help keep you hard.

Lastly, you can try the pointer dog. This is like doggy-style, but the woman will spread their legs further apart. This will allow you to pull out whenever you need to slow things down or to stroke yourself to keep the erection going. As you do this, you can continue thrusting your fingers into her.

Chapter 16: Pregnancy Sex Positions

Some couples think that they can't have sex once pregnant, especially later on in the pregnancy. The truth is, sex at any point during pregnancy can happen as long as everybody remains comfortable. There is no need to worry about your baby hearing things because they don't understand language, and the sounds are very well muffled.

If both parties are okay with it, then you can try some of the following sex positions. All of these positions help keep him off of the belly and will make things easier for the mom-to-be. That said, there are some women who don't feel like having sex. It is up to the hormones, so you will need to go with the flower.

Some of the best positions for you to try during pregnancy are those that will keep the pressure off of the belly and the woman off her back. When on her back, it can cause blood flow compression, which can cause her to end up becoming lightheaded, and can cause other problems. So the next time you want to have sex while pregnant, try these positions:

- Anal Sex

If this is something that the two of you have already been doing, you can continue to do so. Trying anal for the first time while pregnant would not be a good idea since most women experience heightened sensations, so it might not be enjoyable. For those who are used to it, you can try anal in any position that we are going to discuss.

- Seated

This is a lot like the lap dance kama sutra position, except you won't be facing him. He sits in the chair, or wherever, and you will sit on him. This puts her in control of everything.

- Standing

There are two options with this. You can face each other, or he can be behind her. Which one works best is going to depend on how far along she is. Facing each other isn't going to work late in the pregnancy. After the third trimester, he will probably need to be behind. This will limit his thrusting ability, so it helps for those who are experiencing with heightened sensitivity.

- Doggy Style

This will keep her off her back and doesn't add any pressure to the belly as long as she stays propped up. This places the man in control of the movements, so he needs to check in with her to make sure he isn't too rough.

- Spooning

Both of you will be laying on your said facing the same direction. The man has a little more control in this position, but the depth and speed won't be as much as with doggy style.

- Cowgirl or Reverse Cowgirl

This places the women in charge of the movement and will keep pressure off of her belly. This works well for women experiencing extra sensitivity.

You should also have pillows at the ready to help her get comfortable, and pregnancy pillows are great. You may also want to think about using toys and lube.

While you can do most sex positions while pregnant, there are things that you should never do.

- Missionary is not good with the woman on the bottom because it can compress blood flow, especially after the 20-week mark.

- Any prone position where the woman will have to lay on her stomach.

- And you should never blow air up the woman's vagina. This is something you should never do at any time, whether she is pregnant or not.

Having sex during pregnancy can require the two of you to get creative and figure out what is going to work for both of you. What may be comfortable at one time may not be later on. And you never know how the hormones will affect her.

Chapter 17: Oral Sex Positions

Oral sex can be a great way to get things ready for penetration, or it can be the main event of the night. If you are a woman who is not able to reach an orgasm through penetration alone, oral sex is what you are going to need to get things going. The following positions can give you new ways to perform oral sex so that it doesn't seem like the same old boring oral sex.

Spiderman

Most blow jobs won't allow you to have a good view, but this position will provide your partner with a full view of your body. You lay down on your back on a bed or table. Your head should dangle over the edge. They will come up behind you and lean over so that you are able to swallow their penis. You will be able to use your hands and mouth. They also have the ability to pinch and rub your nipples or clitoris while you are working on their penis.

Sidecar

Both of you will lay down your sides facing one another. Then you slide down until his penis is in your face. This could be called a lazy blow job if you want. Blow jobs don't have to kill your knees.

Leg Up

There are some women who have one side of their vulva that is more sensitive than the other. You will lift up that leg on the side that is more sensitive so that it is exposed. Then you will lick figure eights up and down the vulva to please them.

Deep V

You will start by laying down on your back at the edge of the bed. Grab your thighs and lift your legs up into a V shape. If you aren't this flexible, then you keep your knees bent and let your legs rest on your chest. He will kneel in front of you and start working on you. They can massage your thighs to help bring more blood into your vulva. This can help you to have an amazing orgasm.

Cliff Hanger

You sit on the edge of the bed and keep your legs dangling off the edge. He will kneel between your legs and go to work. They will use their hands to play with whatever they want to help heighten your pleasure.

Sofa So Good

You will start by laying upside down on your couch. Your head and back will be flat on the seat while your legs go over the back. Your partner is going to kneel over your face and facing the back of the couch. You can suck his penis while he licks you.

Doggy Does Oral

This is a very hot position that you will get to control the pressure and angle of. She will be on her hands and knees, just like in doggy, but he will kneel behind you and perform for her. This is also great for a rim job if you want.

Hail the Queen

The point of sitting on a person's face is not to actually sit on their face. You simply straddle their head and work your thighs. You hold yourself a few inches over their face while they work on you. They can still reach up and play with breasts, or anything else that they want to.

Corkscrew

The man will stand for this one as you kneel in front of him. Hold the base of his penis in both hands. Place the penis in your mouth and then tilt your head from side to side as your work up and down.

Fake Deep Throat

You can get the feel of a deep throat without having to gag by putting some lube on your hand and using it on the part of him that won't fit in your mouth. Move your hand as you would move your mouth. To make this more intense, look deep into their eyes.

Peace Out

You are going to be sitting in a chair while your partner kneels between your legs. The will place two fingers on each side of the clitoris and make the same motions you would if you were using scissors as they suck and lick the tip of the click. This will isolate the clit from the rest of the genitals and pinpoints the pleasure.

Swiper

Ask your partner to form some suction on the clit by placing their mouth over the labia and clitoris. Now have them shake their head in circles, side to side, and change the pace up. This is going to mimic how many of us masturbate. You can place some pillows under you to give them better access.

Supersize Me

Once you have your man right at the brink of an orgasm, stop and gently pull a bit on their testicles to stop them from having an orgasm. Give them a bit to recuperate and then go back to it. Once you have them begging, push a finger or vibrator against their penis and watch what happens.

Constellation

If oral sex is uncomfortable for you, you can try it on your side. This is great for people who have spasticity in their hips that makes it harder for them to spread the legs during oral sex. This will provide your partner with access to your genitals without having to be a position that causes pain.

Saddle Straddle

If your partner is more dominant, they will love straddling you as you suck and stroke their penis. You can use your hands and twist up and down their penis, and you lick the tip.

Live Show

If the two of you are into bondage, you can take charge by sitting them down in a chair and then blindfolding them. You can also take a bit further by tying their arms behind the chair. A safeword should be used. Then you will perform oral sex on them and take them to the edge by not allowing them to have an orgasm until you want them to.

Deep-Sea Diver

This is a great position for a rim job. This can be introduced in the shower. The receiver stays standing as the giver squats behind them and performing oral sex.

Butterball

This is another great position for rim jobs. The person receiving needs to be showered and fresh. They will lay down and pull their knees into their chest. This will give the doer the chance to reach the clitoris and breasts of the receive. If the man is the receiver, the woman can play with whatever she wants.

Shark Fin

Since oral sex doesn't work well underwater, the women will lay down with her hips at the edge of the tub. She will open up her legs but keep her feet in the water and enjoy everything her partner does to her.

Chapter 18: How to Have Better Sex

While you may not want to think about exercising when you want to have better sex, exercising has the ability to improve your sex life. Athletes train for years for their athletic endeavors, and sex is no exception. Practicing the following exercises can help to improve your strength and flexibility, which could be the answer that you and your partner have been searching for in order to make your sex life better. All of the exercises are things that can help both men and women.

- High Plank to Forearm Plank

Start by getting into a high plank position with your hands under shoulders. You want your body to create a straight line. From here, engage your core and carefully move your right hand and lower down onto your right forearm. Do the same on the left forearm. With control, move your right arm to bring you back up onto your hand, and repeat on the left side.

This helps to build upper body strength.

- Scissor Kicks

Start by laying flat on your back. Move your hands under your hips. Raise both legs straight in the air with your toes pointed. Try to keep your legs as straight as you can, and then engage your core and slowly lower your right leg to the ground. Don't touch the floor. Bring your leg back up and repeat with the other side. This is one rep.

This helps build up strength in the low back and abs and improves flexibility.

- Hydrants

Start on your hands and knees, keeping your wrists under your shoulders and knees under hips. Engage the butt and core and raise your right knee to bring it straight to the side. With control, bring the leg back down. You will do ten reps on one side and then do the other.

This helps to open up your hips and improves upper body strength.

- Wide Squat

Bring your legs into a wide stance and point your toes out. Keep your shoulders over your hips. As you squat down, make sure that your knees stay behind your toes. Press back up through your heels. This is one rep.

This helps build thigh strength and improves flexibility.

- The Bird

Begin by squatting down with your legs together, arms bent, hands together, and chest high. Keeping this low position, open up your left knee to the side and take a short step to the left. While you step, rotate your chest open to the left and open your arms so that the left arm goes behind you, and the right arm stays straight out in front.

Bring your left foot back to the starting position and bring both arms forward. Do this on the right side and return to the starting position. This is a single rep.

This will help tone up the upper back, calves, glutes, and quads, as well as improving flexibility. This is particularly helpful for women because it can help with woman-on-top positions.

- Squat with Knee Dip

Begin in a play squat position with your legs wider than shoulder-width and your toes turned out. Bring your arms out in from of you and then squat down. As you push back up, you will have all of your weight on your right foot. Allow your left leg to swivel on the ball of your foot so that the knee turns into the center. Bring the left arm back as you do this.

Turn the leg back out and squat back down. Repeat this movement on the right side. This should be one long fluid motion. One on each side counts as a single rep.

This helps to loosen up the hips, strengthen the obliques, abs, and legs, and helps your rhythm.

- Drop It Low

Begin by standing straight with your heels together, and toes pointed out. Clasp your hands together in front of you with your palms facing down. Making sure your shoulders stay over your hips, allow your heels to come, and your knees to point out to the sides slightly as you start to squat down.

As you move down, raise your hands over your head. Engage the core and then push yourself back up through your feet as you bring your hands back down to come to the starting position.

This will help to open up your hips, strengthen the core, butt, and thighs, and improve balance.

- Hip Swivel

To perform this exercise, begin by standing with your legs should width apart and keep your knees soft. Keep your elbows close to your side, bend your arms, and take your arms out to the side.

Rotate your hips to the right and come up on your toes on your right foot, and allow your butt to pop out to the left. From here, drop your right heel and swivel your hips to the left, bringing your left foot up on your toes. You will be drawing a half-circle behind you with your butt and engaging your core. One-half circle to each side is one rep.

This move helps to loosen up your butt and hips and tightens up the core. It also helps to improve your rhythm if you do this to the beat of some music.

Now that you have these exercises, you can turn on your favorite workout playlist and perform three sets of ten reps for each of these exercises.

Conclusion

Thank you for making it through to the end of the book, let's hope it was informative and able to provide you with all of the tools you need to achieve your goals whatever they may be.

The next step is to start trying some of these new positions and games to improve your sex life. One of the easiest places for most couples to start is with the massages. It is a very easy way to bring both of you together and to help get you both into the mood. You could even head out and purchase some massage oils to improve the experience. You can then start to work your way into trying some of the foreplay games and sex positions. If dirty talk is something that you have never done, that could be something that the two of you may want to try out. The possibilities are endless as to what you both can do. The main thing is to make sure that both of you are in agreement with what you want to try.

Finally, if you found this book useful in any way, a review on Amazon is always appreciated!

Description

Do you want to spice up your sex life and improve your relationship? Are you tired of the same old positions night after night? Have you always been a little intrigued by the idea of kama sutra? If you answered yes to any of these questions, then you are going to want to continue reading.

Sex has always been a hush-hush subject because of outdated beliefs and such. This has led to couples getting stuck in a rut when it comes to their sex life. They don't feel that it is "right" to talk to people about their sex life. Times are changing, and more and more people are comfortable talking about their sex life, and that is a good thing. This makes sex less taboo and enables couples to expand their sex repertoire. This new awakening doesn't necessarily mean that couples will find the answer they want or need from people they talk to, though, and that's what this book is here to do.

This book has been brought together to provide information about sex to help couples who are tired of the same old thing every night. Foreplay, that's is the one word most couples dread. For some reason, this is the area where couples end up failing, yet we all know that it is extremely important, especially for women. It helps to place people in the right state of mind and gets things warmed up, so to speak. This isn't the only problem some couples have in their sex life. Sometimes it's simply that things have turned monotonous. This is understandable, especially when you and your partner have been together for a while. It is very easy to stick with the same things because you know what one another likes, or because it is easy. But you both likely feel bored and can easily pass on sex due to the boredom. But things don't have to stay that way, though. You can easily bring the spark back into your life, whether through foreplay or new positions.

This book is here to teach you how you can improve your sex life. In this book, you will learn:

- Why you should bring kama sutra and tantra into your bedroom

- The best sex positions for men and women

- The best sex positions to bring the two of you together

- Sex tips for the beginner

- Foreplay games to get things heated up

- How to practice couples massages

- The best way to start using dirty talk without feeling weird

... And much more.

I get that you might still be skeptical that this book can help improve your sex life. Even if you have tried new things to try and spice up your sex life without success, this book can teach you things that you may not have thought about. The information in this book can be applied to anybody's sex life. You'll even find that within the descriptions of various sex positions, there will be warnings, so you are guided throughout the entire process. I'm certain that if you buy this book today, you won't regret it.

Now is the time to make the decision. If you are serious about changing your sex life, scroll up now, and click "buy now."

Tantric Sex

Ancient Hindu Practice to Expand Your Sexual Energy, Experience Mind-Blowing Sex and Overcome Taboo of Kama Sutra. Level up Your Sex Life and Learn Tantric Massage.

of information contained within this document, including, but not limited to, — errors, omissions, or inaccuracies.

Table of Contents

Introduction

Welcome to tantric sex. If this is your first time with tantra and the power it can bring to your sex life, then you don't know what you have been missing. You are in for a real treat. After reading this book, you will never go back to your old sex life ever again.

This book is about the art of tantric sex and how it can be used to increase your sexual energy to the limit of your capabilities. You will find that true, tantric experience is truly mind-blowing. When you reach the heights of sexual pleasure and ecstasy, you will become a completely different person. In fact, don't be surprised if you discover a whole new way of looking at life.

Now, this book is not a mere collection of sex positions and boring role plays. Those are just games. This book is meant to be your pathway to a life-altering experience that will leave you profoundly changed. It will make you and your partner achieve new levels of sexual connection, unlike you have ever felt.

Be prepared to challenge everything you have seen and heard about tantra. In these pages, you will find everything you need to know about making your sex life everything you have wanted it to be. So, if you thought you knew about tantra, prepared to be blown away... literally.

But don't worry if you haven't experienced tantra before. This book is meant to take you through a gradual process in which you will discover your own sexual energy and combine it with your partner. You'll find that the powerful connection that is created can lead to unbelievable heights of pleasure.

If you have experienced tantra in the past, then you have an idea of just how powerful it can be. However, this book will challenge your current perceptions and take you to the next level. As you go further in this book, you will uncover new levels that never knew were there.

So, the time has come to uncover the wonderful and magical side of tantric sex. The time has come to explore your sexuality and discover your partner's own desires and fantasies. Together, you can take things to the level which you have always wanted to.

However, there is one word of caution: the concepts, ideas, practices, and techniques in this book build on each other gradually. This means that if you, or your partner, are new to tantra, it's best to take it easy at first. It's important to take your time as tantra is not something that you can use right out of the box. It takes some time before you can truly master it. But when you do, you, there will be no turning back. Your partner, or partners, will look to you as "the one."

Let's get started on this journey to a world you have always wanted to explore, but perhaps didn't have the chance to. So, here it is. Here's your chance to make your sex life everything you have wanted it to be.

Chapter 1: The Philosophy of Tantric Sex

Sex is an important part of our lives. Regardless of your preferences and/or orientations, sex is a vital component to making our lives full and complete. Without it, it can be quite difficult to lead a healthy and productive life. In fact, the longer you go without it, the harder it can be to function properly in life.

Now, it should be noted that there is a difference between sex and tantric sex.

Regular, run of the mill sex (which we will be referring to as "traditional sex") is an act which virtually all humans go through at some point in their lives. Unfortunately for some, they go through traumatic experiences with sex. This is something that cannot be disregarded and has an important place in tantra.

How so?

Well, sex is about a physical, emotional, and psychological experience that is meant to take us to heights of pleasure, intimacy, and connection. Sex is about connecting with your partner (or partners, as the case may be) in such a way that you are able to mutually satisfy each other. This mutual satisfaction can lead to a connection that brings out the best in both of you.

Of course, there is a place for love and romance. But as far as this book is concerned, love and romance are a separate topic. The reason for this is that love and romance are not pre-requisites to having a magical experience with tantric sex. In fact, you can conjure up an amazing experience with someone you have barely met. This is possible if you know what you are doing.

Moreover, tantric sex differs from traditional sex in the sense that you are focusing on both yourself and your partner. This is the crux of the matter. If you are selfish and don't pay close attention to your partner's needs, then your sexual encounter won't result quite as good as you might have hoped for.

In fact, if you're plan is to get off and have a merry old time, then tantric sex may not be the most effective philosophy for you. If you're just looking for fun and creative ways to spice up your sex life, then you'll be quite surprised to find that tantric sex goes far beyond that.

When you are committed to making your own sexual experience the best it can be by making your partner's experience as good as it can be, then you know you're in the tantra ballpark. Please bear in mind that this isn't about looks, size, or stamina; this is about knowing what buttons to push and when to push them. Master that, and you will forever go down in history as one of the best.

If that seems like an outrageous claim, don't worry. Once you see what tantric sex can do, especially to someone who hasn't really experienced it before, you'll frame this page up on your wall.

Defining tantric sex

Sadly, most so-called gurus and sexperts pass off tantric sex for a collection of funky positions that don't really anywhere. Sure, it can be fun to try out some new positions, but at the end of the day, if you don't add all of the components that make up a tantric session, then you will be coming up short.

Tantric sex can be viewed as focusing on slow intercourse. This isn't about banging away until everyone comes. In fact, orgasm is not the main focus on tantra.

Does that seem surprising?

If you are unfamiliar with tantric sex, then it surely does seem surprising.

Tantric sex is about synchronizing movements, breathing, eye contact, touching, and even orgasms... it's all about taking your partner and leading the way. As your partner follows along, you can connect with them in such a way that everything moves in concert. Each movement, thrust, breath, touch, and so on, is done with a clear intention in mind.

Of course, there is always room for a quick romp.

But that's not what tantra is about. Tantra is about finding the right place and the right time to get it on. If you are in a hurry, then tantra's not for you. You need to focus and take your time. Otherwise, you won't be able to hit the heights you expect.

Tantric sex and love

If you are planning to engage in tantric sex with a loving and committed partner, you will find that your sexual encounters will become unforgettable. Tantra becomes easier when you have a history with your partner in such a way that you are both comfortable with each other and have a high degree of trust.

However, this doesn't mean that you have to be in love with them.

As a matter of fact, it is quite common to find tantra practitioners who hook up just because they know they are going to be in for a real treat. When two experienced practitioners get together, fireworks light up. As such, you don't need to be in love with your partner, though it certainly helps if you are.

It should also be said that tantric sex isn't really a one-night stand type of thing. If you believe that you can hook up with someone on a random night and have a mind-blowing tantra session, then you might be disappointed.

344

Ideally, tantra works with someone you know, someone you trust and with whom you can build a connection. That is something which you can't really do with someone you meet at a club or a bar. Often, it takes some time to get to know someone before you can really go through the roof in a tantra session.

Tantric sex is a mindset

When you really get into tantric sex, you'll find that it's mostly a question of mindset. When your head is not in the game, tantra doesn't work. You see, tantra is about making your energy flow. When this energy flows, it's like an electric charge that pulsates through your body. As this charge courses through your entire being, your partner will pick up on that. As your partner's energy flows as well, then a circuit is complete. This circuit enables the energy to flow through both of you.

That is why tantra isn't about orgasm; it's about prolonging the experience as much as possible. But that doesn't mean that you have to go for hours. In fact, those who master tantra are quite efficient at achieving orgasm (we'll be defining that in a bit).

That being said, tantric sex isn't about spending hours in bed. It can be something as short as 10 or 15 minutes. But even if it's just 15 minutes, if your mind is really into it, you can achieve pleasure that will literally blow you away.

Please keep in mind that focus is key. You can't expect to have a full tantric experience while you are concerned about this thing or that thing. Most experienced tantra practitioners find that disconnecting while in a tantra session is a means of release. So, turn off your phone and forget about emails. When you are ready for a tantric session, the world around you goes away. All you need to focus on is you and your partner.

In a manner of speaking, tantra is like mindfulness. Mindfulness is about focusing on the "here" and the "now." This is why you will hear tantra experts say that tantra is like meditating. And when you truly think about, that's what it is. Tantric sex is like meditating on your sexual energy.

The slower, the better

One of the worst things modern culture has taught people is that fast and hard are the "hottest" ways to have sex. You often see that in movies, TV shows, and books. Perhaps the worst of all is pornography. Most porn films feature fast and aggressive movements that don't really foster any kind of connection. After all, porn is just acting.

This is the main reason why porn is so damaging to those who believe that real sex is like porn films. When you break it down, going as hard as you can, while exciting to a certain degree, does not foster the connection and intimacy that is needed to achieve real tantric ecstasy.

Consequently, the phrase, "the slower, the better" ought to become your new mantra. If you get it in your head that taking your time is the way to go, then you will find that opening the door to tantra is quite easy.

Of course, going slow can be hard for some, especially men. For guys, it can be hard to go slow, and controlling arousal and orgasm can be a real challenge. This is why tantra is not something you can just read through and put it to use. Tantra is the type of practice that needs time and dedication.

But there is some good news. The practices we will outline throughout this book will help those who have trouble controlling their arousal find the means of settling down and allowing their energies to really flow. This is why the mantra, "the slower, the better" will make all the difference in the world.

Taking the leap

Now that we have defined what tantric sex is all about, you are ready to take the leap into the world of pleasure. So, to kick things off, make a concerted effort to put your current way of looking at sex behind you. Now, make a conscious decision to embrace a new way of looking at sex. This new way is based on being open-minded. When you are truly open-minded, you are open to the new experiences you are about to encounter.

Please don't think we're talking about bondage or that sort of thing (well, if you're into it...) We're talking about being open-minded in such a way that you are focused on experiencing everything that sex has to offer you, everything from a wonderful physical experience to a deep, emotional connection. With that mindset, you can't go wrong.

If you are in a committed relationship, then please take the time to talk about this with your partner. Talk about what you expect from your sex life. By talking about it, you can both be on the same page. This will allow your tantric sessions to be focused on what fulfills you.

For instance, some couples value touching and kissing a lot more than penetration. Other couples place a higher emphasis on rhythmic movements as if they were dancing. Other couples value the sensory perception of their encounters above everything else. A good example of sensory perception can be scents or sounds that are arousing or soothing.

As you can see, there really is no "standard" way of enjoying tantra. There isn't some formula that you need to follow. Sure, there is a path you must go down, but at the end of the day, this path leads to different outcomes. In fact, don't be surprised to find that practicing tantra with different partners leads to completely different results. Naturally, everyone is different, so it's logical to assume experiences will be different, too.

So, here is your first exercise: the next time you have intercourse with your partner, try to set the stage so that you have no interruptions or distractions. This means no phones, no gadgets, no nothing. If you must get away somewhere, then do it. It could even be just booking a hotel room in your city. The point is to devote your entire time and attention to your partner, even if it's just a couple of hours. The secret here is to give your undivided attention to what you want and what you want to give your partner. That alone is enough to make your next sexual encounter a great one. So, please get into the habit of blocking out the world around you and focusing your energies and attention on your partner and nothing else. It's totally worth it!

Chapter 2: The Difference Between Sex and Tantric Sex

At the beginning of our sex lives, we don't really know what to do or what to expect. Even when your parents give you "the talk," you really don't know what's happening until you actually do it. Then, depending on the amount of sex education you get, you learn more and more about sexuality and how it actually works.

However, most people don't really take the time to learn as much as they can about sex. It's funny that we should act in this manner, especially since sex is such a significant part of human life. In fact, most of what we learn is generally on the fly. For example, you hook up with someone who's older and more experienced, they show you what to do, and that's that.

For some guys and gals, teaching a virgin about sex is a thrill they relish. Then, there are some who are caring and strive the show a younger partner how to really enjoy. Sadly, these people and experiences are hard to come by.

That is why your interest in this book is a testament to your desire to learn about the best ways in which you can unleash your sexual potential. Through the art of tantric sex, you can unlock all of the repressed energy within you.

Yes, that's right, repressed energy.

Even if you have intercourse ten times a day, the energy is stuck there within you. Your sexual energy is never released unless you give it the time it needs to fully unfold and envelope you. When you are open to such experiences, you allow your core to absorb every minute detail of intercourse.

In this chapter, we are going to explore five important differences between traditional sex and tantric sex. These differences will enable you to have a crystal-clear understanding of what tantric sex and what it can do to improve your sexual life exponentially.

So, let's get right into it.

Difference #1: It's not about orgasm

When most folks think about sex, they see orgasm as the ultimate goal. This is particularly true for most men. Most guys tend to believe sex begins with arousal and ends with orgasm. In between, there is intercourse. However, intercourse is just a means to an end, so to speak.

This mentality is detrimental to a healthy and fulfilling sex life as sex, itself, is much more than the mere act of intercourse. In a manner of speaking, it's like reducing a meal to just dessert. So, instead of enjoying every bit of food in your meal, you simply rush through the first course just to get to dessert. Once dessert is served, you wolf it down and be done with it.

When you look at sex in this manner, you won't ever truly enjoy everything it has to offer you. In fact, it even seems transactional to a certain degree. That is why sex is much more than just reaching orgasm. It's about the entire experience surrounding the encounter.

For a lot of women, reaching orgasm can be a challenging endeavor. Often, this is due to the lack of synchronicity with their partner. There are times when it seems that there is no communication whatsoever. When this happens, one partner gets off, and the other... may not.

That is why the entire scene that surrounds tantra begins well before actual coitus. It begins with both partners fostering intimacy. It begins with being in touch with each other's needs and desires. From there, the overall experience of the encounter makes sex much more enjoyable. At that point, orgasm is a natural consequence. For women, this can lead to multiple orgasms. And, believe it or not, it can also lead to multiple orgasms for men (yes, that's right!)

Difference #2: It's a sensory experience

Sex goes beyond the mere act of intercourse, be it through penetration, touching, or oral. It involves all of the senses in such a manner that everything works in sync. When all senses are involved in a single encounter, the sensory experience is much broader.

This is what leads to the mind-blowing experience.

When you are committed to a full sensory experience, you begin sex with visuals such as dressing up (whatever you fancy is perfectly fine), sounds such as music or any other auditory stimulus, smell such as your favorite scents, touch such as massaging, and of course, taste (food and drink can also be part of the experience).

To put this into perspective, think of all the mating rituals that humans go through prior to hitting the sack. For example, dance is a powerful mating ritual. The most sensual dances mimic sexual movements in such a manner that they foster intimacy among the couple. When a couple is able to hit it off on the dance floor, they can be confident they can hit it off in bed. While this doesn't necessarily constitute a guarantee, it's a heck of a place to start.

Another powerful mating ritual is food. This is the reason why most dates (especially first dates) involve food in one way or another. Also, drink plays a vital role in mating rituals. Just look at films and TV shows. Most dates begin with dinner and drink, and then end up in the sack. The sensory perception that is built with food and drink carries over into coitus.

So, if you are keen on really getting a full, tantric experience, don't skimp on the entire event leading up to sex. While it is not necessary for you to put together an elaborate evening, it is certainly helpful if you set the stage in this manner. This can be especially helpful while you learn the ways of tantric sex. Eventually, you won't need such an elaborate setup.

Difference #3: There is no domination or control

One of the most interesting dynamics of traditional sex is the need for domination and/or control. Sure, most couples have one partner who leads, and the other tends to follow along. But in the world of tantra, this isn't about having one partner dominate the other such as in the world of BDSM. The fact of the matter is that tantra practitioners don't seek power, domination, or control. What they seek is to please their partner, and as a result, themselves.

Now, that happens if you are naturally dominant? Does that mean that there is no place for you in the world of tantra?

That's hardly the case!

In fact, dominant individuals take great pleasure in guiding their partner through the road that leads to pleasure and ecstasy. This is the ultimate rush that a dominant individual can derive from tantra.

Think about that...

What could be better than blowing your partner's mind? Imagine how incredibly satisfying it can be to give your partner the best sex of their lives... this is a feeling you can't get from "dominating" your partner.

You see, in traditional dom-sub relationships, the dom derives pleasure from the power rush that comes from having their sub at their mercy. This is a one-way relationship in which the sub doesn't always derive pleasure from their position. In fact, there are many cases that subs go along with the game simply because they want to feel "loved" in some way. As such, subs comply with their dom's bidding with the hope of gaining the dom's favor.

While this type of dynamic works perfectly well for some couples, it's not the type of relationship that is built for mutual pleasure and fulfillment. This is one of the reasons why dom-sub relationships tend to run their course; that is, they aren't meant to be long-term relationships.

With tantric sex, the focus is on mutual satisfaction and fulfillment. This implies that all parties have the chance to get what they want out of the relationship. Now, it should be noted that "relationship" doesn't mean a romantic partnership. If anything, a tantric relationship can be strictly sex with no strings attached. But the relationship and the dynamic that evolves from the practice of tantra can lead to a relationship that is far more fulfilling than your run-of-the-mill romantic partnership.

Difference #4: Nothing else matters

This is one of the biggest mistakes that couples make: they let other things get in the way during their encounters. Please bear in mind that tantric sex is about the here and the now. So, when you are getting it on, nothing else matters.

This concept doesn't apply just to phones and email. It also applies to anything else that might be creeping up in your mind.

For example, if you are concerned about your physical appearance, say, you're concerned about being overweight, then you will find that you won't be able to get as much out of your encounters as you'd like. Based on this concept, you really, truly, need to let go.

So what if you're not physically perfect?

So what if you're not the biggest?

So what if you're not the most attractive?

If you are attractive and desirable to someone who is willing to engage in tantric sex with you, then it's just a matter of going with it. In the end, you'll enjoy the relationship far more simply because you are able to let go of your hang-ups.

The fact of the matter is that we get in our own way. Most of the time, there is genuine attraction and chemistry. But when you don't give yourself a chance to really enjoy intercourse, then you find your mind more concerned about a million other things. Needless to say, this isn't the most exciting mindset.

The overwhelming majority of tantra practitioners would much rather get with someone who shares their same mindset rather than someone who's merely good-looking. This means that tantric sex is much more than just looking good; it's about being able to translate your passion and desire into a tangible force that can open up the floodgates to amazing experiences of pleasure and ecstasy.

Difference #5: Surrender at all times

By "surrender," we're not talking about some kind of domination thing. We're talking about letting yourself go and giving yourself to your partner. This is the core tenet of tantric sex. You must be willing to give all of yourself, even for a brief moment, before you are truly able to channel your energy into the powerful force that tantric sex can unleash. If you are holding back, then you won't be able to fully harness your sexual energy.

If you are a more submissive person by nature, this might be easier to achieve. By nature, you don't need to be in control. So, it's far easier to simply go with it. But for naturally dominant individuals, surrendering may represent a monumental challenge.

Surrender happens at various levels. Firstly, anyone who engages in sexual intercourse (unless it is against their will) surrenders physically. Often, folks think this is the last thing you surrender.

That could not be farther from the truth!

Surrendering your body in the act of passion is one of the easiest things you can do. It's surrendering everything else that becomes the hardest part.

As such, the next level, the emotional level, is paramount to tantric sex. Again, we are not talking about "love" here. Love has nothing to do with tantric sex. While it certainly helps to love your partner (it certainly facilitates the process), what you really need is to be emotionally invested in what you are doing. This implies that you need to be ready to give this person all of the care and attention they need during your encounter.

This is what fosters intimacy.

Then, the third level becomes a deep, spiritual level. When you are able to achieve this level, you are able to really hit it out of the park. Your connection is so profound that mind-blowing sex becomes a regular occurrence. Again, love is not a pre-requisite. But a deep understanding of each other's wants and needs is.

So, take it upon yourself to be ready to give all of yourself to your partner, even if it is for the brief moment you are together.

Chapter 3: The Need for Tantric Sex

Throughout this book, we have talked about how important sex is in the life of humans. After all, if sex wasn't important, then there wouldn't be so much attention paid to it. It would go practically unnoticed. If anything, it would serve for reproductive purposes, and that would be the end of it.

The fact that sex is so important in our lives forces us to make sex as enjoyable as possible. That's where tantra really shines. Tantra is all about situating sex in its rightful place. By giving sex the importance it deserves, you can lead a much more satisfying and fulfilling life.

In this chapter, we are going to be taking a closer look at the need for tantric sex. Now, we're not just talking about sex in general; we're talking about tantric sex. And yes, there is a clear need for it. There is a clear need for having the best possible sexual experience of your life. If you believe that tantric sex is just about massages and playing soft music, then do read on.

Sex is meant to be enjoyable

In popular culture, sex is objectified to a degree in which it is seen as a transactional occurrence. For instance, sex is used as a currency in order to obtain benefits from people. In addition, sex is reduced to a mere physical act in which one, or hopefully both, of the parties involved, get a physical rush out of it. If you are more adventurous, group sessions (or sex with multiple partners) is seen as some type of thrill that doesn't really lead anywhere.

This is where people end up feeling shallow and empty. Sure, they may be sleeping with very attractive people, but at the end of the day, they don't get as much fulfillment out of it as they would expect. In fact, this is where you see extremely attractive people debase themselves simply because they don't enjoy intercourse.

Then, you have committed and/or monogamous relationships. There are folks who view sex as a chore in such relationships. So, sex isn't about having a great time with their partner. Rather, sex is viewed as a necessary evil in the relationship. Under these circumstances, you can't expect sex to be fulfilling. At best, it would be able to provide physical release. But the reality is that sex under those terms would only prove to be a monotonous event.

So, what can be done about it?

If you find yourself not enjoying your current sex life, then you really need to ask yourself: what do I want to get out of my sex life?

This question will lead you down a path in which you must explore what you really want to get out it. If you view sex as a currency that will get you everything you want, then tantric sex might not be right for you. However, if you view sex as something pleasurable that you would love to share with your partner (whoever that might be), then tantric sex is a must in your life.

Additionally, a healthy sex life is part of a well-rounded lifestyle. When you have a satisfying sex life, you can be sure that this will rub off on other areas of your life as well. So, there is no reason why you shouldn't strive to incorporate tantric sex into your life right away.

Traditional sex gets old... fast

Traditional sex is fun and exciting whenever you have a new partner in your life. Even the same old positions and routines become hot and steamy when you are in lust for someone. During this phase, a quick romp is enough to get your blood boiling. However, if there is no substance to your encounters, that passion can quickly fizzle out, leaving you with mundane encounters. This is why many relationships don't survive for too long.

Of course, it's true that relationships aren't solely about sex. There are other components surrounding sex which make relationships more or less enjoyable. For instance, if you and your partner share the same pursuits, then you can be sure that your relationship outside the bedroom will be fun, too. But if things aren't working as well as they could in the bedroom, then there will always be something missing.

When you look at traditional sex for what it is, physical enjoyment and attraction are the only things that can keep you coming back for more. When attraction wears off, then there had better be something else to your relationship.

This is where tantric sex makes all the difference.

When you engage in tantra, you are moving beyond physical attraction. You are moving into a realm of emotional and even spiritual enjoyment. While you could theoretically achieve this with anyone you meet, the truth is that it doesn't happen with just anyone. It takes two people (or perhaps more...) who are willing to surrender to each other during the time they are together.

Please keep this in mind at all times!

Surrendering yourself to your partner will allow you to open the floodgates of your sexual energy. Sure, there is heightened physical pleasure that comes from tantric encounters. But the fact is that the physical response is expanded by the non-physical components that are involved. In the end, the physical enjoyment you are able to get out of a tantric session will leave you feeling full. It's kind of like taking your time to savor your favorite food. In the end, you have not only enjoyed your meal but also satisfied your hunger. Ultimately, this leaves you with an amazing feeling.

Good sex is key to a healthy life

Multiple studies have shown the importance that sex has in our day to day lives. For example, sex can boost mood and improve cognitive performance. This is due to the release of chemicals by the brain after a satisfying sexual encounter.

Those studies are based on traditional sex, that is, people who engage in a "regular" sexual relationship. Now, if traditional sex can do that, imagine what tantric sex can do for you. In essence, what tantric sex does is help you circulate your sexual energy. When this occurs, it's like a wave of electricity that begins to power various aspects of your mind and body.

When you don't have sex, or you simply "get off," you don't allow your sexual energy to circulate through your body. This is why tantra calls for you to take your time. The more you rush a sexual encounter, the less chance you give your energy to flow.

According to ancient beliefs, sexual energy is located at the base of the spine. From there, it moves up your spine and circulates throughout your body. And while this is an automatic process, it doesn't happen automatically.

Wait a minute...

You see, when you don't take the time to release your energy, you exert physical energy through the mechanical act of coitus, but you don't give your sexual energy the chance to get moving and flow upward. As such, the mere act of reaching orgasm doesn't necessarily imply that your sexual energy is flowing to the maximum of its capabilities.

Here's how this works:

For men, sexual pleasure is equated with ejaculation. If a man ejaculates, this implies orgasm, and all is good. However, this belief is hardly ironclad. Any guy will tell you that ejaculation does not necessarily mean orgasm. While it may feel good, it doesn't necessarily mean that a man has reached the climax of sexual pleasure.

The reason for this is that an orgasm is a chemical process that goes on in the brain. When a person reaches sexual climax, the brain floods the body with pleasure-causing chemicals. When these chemicals are released, they flow through the bloodstream and feed all of the organs and body systems. In fact, orgasm causes the penis to get harder and not softer.

Think about that for a moment...

For a man to reach orgasm, he needs to focus more on the action that is happening, on his partner's pleasure and, of course, his own. This means that he cannot be focused on how good it feels and that he can't finish too soon.

This is where he needs to let go!

He needs to forget that he is feeling pleasure and focus on the here and now. That can open the door to the chemical reactions that are produced as a result of pure sexual pleasure. In the end, a man who can master this mindset may find himself having multiple orgasms well before ejaculating once.

As for women, orgasm is a mix of emotions, physical sensations, and a sense of security. When you combine all of these elements, it's possible to reach unbelievable heights of sexual pleasure. However, women can be betrayed by their emotions. For example, if a woman feels uncomfortable about anything surrounding the encounter (such as feeling guilty about it), reaching orgasm can be quite difficult. By the same token, if she feels insecure about her physical appearance, this can also lead her to have difficulty reaching orgasm.

Again, this is why tantra is about the here and the now. When a woman is able to focus on the "task at hand," so to speak, she can let herself go. This is an emotional response in which she isn't focused on what is happening in the world around her; she is only focused on what's happening between her and her partner. That's all that matters.

Making orgasms count

One of the most common misconceptions about tantric sex is that orgasms keep coming and coming. While that may be true for some people, the fact is that it doesn't quite work that way. For many couples, having one orgasm is more than enough to make the session memorable. This is why we say you should "make orgasms count." When you really make orgasms count, the overall sensation that comes with them is incredible.

Now, it may seem paradoxical, but if you aim to reach orgasm, then it will be harder for you to get there. So, your aim in a tantric session is not to reach orgasm. Your aim should be to just enjoy it. The orgasm will come when it comes.

Do you see the difference?

When your pursuit of a sexual encounter is orgasm, you will find that it's nearly impossible to get it. It's like when you're unemployed and in need of a job. If you get desperate, you will project that in job interviews. Plus, each day that passes without a job seems like an eternity. After just a few days of job hunting, you are so stressed out and anxious that you might even get sick.

The same goes for orgasms.

If you are fixated on reaching orgasm, you'll find it nearly impossible to focus on what you are actually doing. You won't be able to focus on enjoying your partner. If anything, it'll feel good up to a certain point, but nothing else.

On the flip side, if you choose to enjoy coitus for what it is, you'll find it's a lot easier to relax and let your energy flow. When you are able to do this, reaching orgasm comes naturally. As a man, you're not worried about finished too fast. That's why you're going slow. In the case of a woman, you're not concerned that it takes you forever to reach orgasm. All you're concerned about is enjoy each passing moment with your partner.

This is the core essence of tantric sex. All of the components that make up tantric sessions are building blocks to a wonderful experience. Consequently, everything you do, from dancing to massages, is a precursor to the big "O." That way, when the big "O" does arrive, you'll be ready to literally burst at the seams.

So, make every orgasm count by letting yourself go and surrendering to your partner.

Chapter 4: Setting the Scene

In tantric sex, setting the scene just right is as important as anything you do with your partner. Often, setting the scene is about setting up a comfortable atmosphere in which both of you can just be yourselves.

This is the main point here.

The right stage can make your tantric sessions that much more enjoyable. The proper atmosphere can turbocharge your senses, thereby making the overall experience memorable. In fact, having the right atmosphere alone is enough to take traditional sex into tantric territory.

But first, let's talk about what we don't mean by "setting the scene."

If you are picturing an elaborate situation in which your bedroom is flooded by candles and rose petals, then you might be taking things a bit too far. Sure, if that's the type of thing you are into, then so be it. However, you don't have to remodel your bedroom to set the right scene. If anything, you'll find that trying to hard to set the right stage will end up killing the mood altogether.

Here is a quick example:

Let's say that you want to surprise your partner with a truly special evening. So, you go pull all the stops to make your bedroom look like a scene out of a movie. You have soft music playing in the background, champagne on ice, and even some visual stimulus on the television. While this scene may seem perfect, it could backfire as it creates pressure on your partner to deliver. After all, how would you feel if your partner surprised you in this way? You'd feel pressured to make it worth their while. Of course, we're not talking about a transactional relationship, here. But, you would still feel pressured not to disappoint your partner.

Based on this example, it's plain to see that taking things too far can create unnecessary pressure on your partner. The higher you set your expectations, the harder it will be for you to enjoy yourselves.

So, let's take a look at what you can do to set the scene just right.

Talk with your partner about what they want

First and foremost, talk with your partner about what you both want in the perfect setting. It could be that you both have very simple tastes. Perhaps the décor isn't as important as privacy. Moreover, you and your partner may value quiet and darkness more than a fancy setup.

Most couples who engage in tantric sex often set their ambiance to that of peace, quiet, and privacy. The main idea here is that whatever happens in the bedroom stays in the bedroom. The last thing tantra practitioners want to worry about is the neighbors overhearing them. If they have kids, they don't want to worry about what their kids are doing while they are getting it on.

As you can see, for most folks, setting the right scene isn't so much about the visuals of a room that looks right out of a magazine. For them, it's the peace and quiet that makes all the difference. This is why it is vital that you and your partner communicate your preferences to one another.

Setting up the right visuals

Visual stimulation is essential to fulfilling tantric sex. By "visuals," we mean everything that your eyes can possibly take in. This can range from the décor and ambiance to the actual physical appearance of you and your partner.

Regarding physical appearance, anything goes!

For instance, wearing sexy lingerie, costumes, or just wearing a birthday suit can provide you with the visual stimulation you seek. Some couples enjoy dressing up with a theme in mind. Others enjoy role plays. Some prefer watching racy films to set the mood. The fact of the matter is that anything goes so long as you are both on board.

This is important to keep in mind, especially because anything that makes you or your partner uncomfortable can become a mood killer. This is the last thing you want to see happen. As such, setting any and all visuals, as long as you are both comfortable, will go a long way toward making your tantric session memorable and enjoyable.

Taking in the sounds

This is a tricky one. The traditional playbook (such as what you generally see in films) calls for soft music or smooth jazz playing in the background. However, some folks find music, or any other sound, for that matter, to be distracting. So, this doesn't mean that they don't enjoy it; it's just that background sounds may lead them to become distracted from the actual encounter itself.

To put this into perspective, imagine this situation:

Suppose you are studying for a big exam. This is an important mid-term that you need to focus all of your mental energies on. So, do you study in silence or have music blasting in the background?

Your answer to this question should give you a clear indication of how you would react to music (or any other sound) during our tantric session. In fact, it could be that you enjoy having smooth jazz playing in the background. But your partner may not. So, this is where you need to strike a balance.

One common practice is to play music while things are heating up. This could be during a massage, kissing, touching, or just cuddling. But when it comes down to intercourse, the music is off. While this doesn't mean that you are going to be in absolute silence, it does mean that there aren't any other sounds that could potentially distract you from what's going on at the moment.

In fact, turning the music off is quite useful when you are syncing your breathing. You see, when there are other noises around, it can be hard to hear your breathing. As such, you might have a hard time syncing up. But when you don't have any distracting sounds around you, it's far easier to sync your breathing. This is especially true if you close your eyes and let your other senses take over.

One other thing about sounds: don't feel compelled to make a huge ruckus during sex. One very persistent misconception is that yelling your head off is a sign of enjoyment. While that might be true for some, there are plenty of folks (women, especially) who have a mind-blowing orgasm without feeling the need to scream their head off. So, if you, or your partner, aren't the screaming type, then that's perfectly fine. Everyone is different, and it's something we need to embrace.

Lighting to set the mood

This is another one of those tricky areas. Lighting can really set the mood for you and your partner, or it can throw a monkey wrench into your session.

The rule of thumb here is that there is no rule of thumb.

Some couples feel perfectly comfortable in a well-lit area, while others prefer darkness. Again, this is all about what makes you feel comfortable. As such, it's a question of being on the same page.

In this regard, some folks like to "see what they are doing." So, a well-lit area for them works perfectly fine. They don't mind having the lights or getting it on during the daytime. For other couples, they prefer the anonymity of darkness. Thus, you'll see them drawing blackout curtains during the daytime while perhaps leaving their environment pitch black at night.

As a matter of fact, you'll find that experience tantra practitioners prefer the dark as it cancels the visuals out and forces them to feel and hear everything they are doing. For some, it's hard to concentrate when there is a large amount of visual stimulation around them. For others who are a bit more self-conscious about their physical appearance, darkness gives them the opportunity to forget about the imperfections they perceive in their body.

Once again, this is a call that you ought to make as a couple. That way, you can both feel comfortable. In the end, it's one less thing to worry about.

Using scents to your advantage

Scents are paramount in tantra. The right scents can give you the chance to focus on a different kind of sensory perception. Scents are very useful when it comes to triggering positive emotions. This is why scents are practically a cliché during massages. Everything from scented candles to essential oils is highly recommended.

When selecting scents, it's important to choose ones that trigger positive emotions. For instance, your partner is nuts for chocolate ice cream. So, using chocolate-scented oils can work wonders during a massage. In other cases, essential oils such as lavender can provide you with the olfactory stimulation you seek, that is, entering a state of relaxation.

Now, here's one naughty trick you can use to get things started in a very discreet way. Pick a scent that you both find pleasing. It could be a perfume, cologne, essential oil, scented candle, even some kind of food. Then, set a rule that this scent is only used during sexual encounters. This is a type of code that indicates that you are ready to go over the moon.

Here's the trick: use the scent well before you actually get it on. This will signal your partner what you intend to do. Even if you are nowhere near the bedroom (or your chosen place), the scent is enough to begin triggering the emotions that you associate with intercourse. By the time you actually get "down to business," your mind and body will already be in a state of readiness. In a manner of speaking, you have gotten a head start on your pleasure.

Things don't always happen in the bedroom

If you believe that an amazing tantric session only takes place in your bedroom, then you might be surprised to find that tantric sex can happen anywhere! Yes, practically any place is good for a tantric session.

To choose a place for your sessions, it must meet your criteria. Otherwise, it wouldn't work at all. Now, when we say "criteria," it's a question of meeting your requirements in terms of lighting, mood, privacy, and so on.

This means that if your garage fits the bill, then your garage would be the place to be.

It's also important to keep in mind that lifestyles are quite varied. Some couples have very busy lifestyles and so on. That's why they seek to get away from it all to be together. So, some couples find hotel rooms or go on a trip somewhere to really get it on.

Ultimately, the actual location of where you do it doesn't really matter so long as it's a place that works for you. When you find this place, then you have a huge head start. Having the right place and the right atmosphere is just as important as any of the practices you can do. In fact, you could be a master practitioner of tantra, but if the mood and ambiance aren't right, you'll find that your experience just won't be the same.

At the end of the day, tantra is a combination of factors. If any factor is off, for any reason, then you might find it hard to make the most of your sessions. That's why communication is key. If you and your partner are on the same page, you will find it much easier to make the most of your time together. Even if you are naturally dominant and your partner is naturally submissive, being able to communicate what you both want is an essential part of tantra.

A healthy and rewarding sex life is all about being able to connect with your partner at a profound level. This is where tantra can lead both of you to levels you may have only dreamed about. Perhaps it might seem far away at this point. But with some careful planning and an open mind, you'll find that anything is possible in the world of tantra!

Chapter 5: Fostering Intimacy and Touching

Not everything in sex is about intercourse. Sadly, in our culture, sex is reduced to some kind of penetration, that's all there is to it. As a matter of fact, a harmful myth that persists is the belief that sex isn't really "sex" unless there is some kind of penetration.

While this is certainly an important part of sex, it isn't the only part. There are so many things that can happen during an encounter. This is why you need to be aware of the various options at your disposal. Truth be told, some of the most exciting and steamy parts happen outside of traditional penetrative sex.

That's why this chapter is centered on intimacy and touching. The main point is to focus on foreplay, or perhaps post-coitus activity. This is very important to keep in mind as there are so many things that can happen before and after intercourse.

Fostering intimacy

Intimacy isn't just the act of sex itself. Intimacy is an emotional connection that is felt between two individuals (or more as the case may be). You can potentially develop an intimate emotional connection with anyone without being in a committed relationship or being "in love." In fact, our lives are filled with intimate connections, such as those we cherish with family and friends. These types of intimate relationships have nothing to do with sex. It's the emotional connection that counts.

As such, it should be noted that the cornerstone of tantric sex is intimacy. Without it, achieving the truly uplifting heights of ecstasy can be hard to come by. While it is not impossible, it will take some additional effort to get there.

Fostering intimacy is not nearly as hard as you might think. The biggest step you can take with your partner(s) is to be honest about what you want, your expectations, and what you bring to the table. By being transparent in your intentions, you will find an unmatchable sense of liberation. It is so much more fulfilling to have an intimate relationship with some who you really connect with as opposed to someone with whom you have a superficial interaction.

This is the reason why mind-blowing tantric sex with a stranger is not quite that easy. It is possible if both parties are experienced in the ways of tantra. In that case, it might be quite easy for both parties to let go and surrender to the moment they find themselves in.

If you are in a committed relationship, intimacy is something that you ought to work on all the time. There are a plethora of activities that you can do to foster intimacy without even coming close to intercourse. When you make a concerted effort to foster intimacy in your day to day interactions, you will find that sex is just an extension of this usual interaction.

Building intimacy every day

Intimacy can be built every day through a clear and concerted effort to do so. For example, hugging, kissing, and meaningful touching (in a non-sexual way), is a great means of fostering intimacy.

Think about it for a minute.

If you don't even touch each other during the day, then how can you suddenly turn it on in the bedroom?

When you take the time to foster these kinds of interactions with your partner, you will find that playful touching, constant touching and kissing can easily transition into the bedroom. What you will find is that this type of behavior simply translates into sex without much effort. In a manner of speaking, you are ready for sex all the time.

Now, what happens if you are in a long-distance relationship?

In such cases, it's hard to build intimacy since you aren't physically present. This is where you need to get a bit more creative.

But before we get into it, a word of caution: if you plan to use photos and videos, please make sure that you are both on the same page about it. Unfortunately, photos and videos can fall into the wrong hands or can be misused, particularly when a relationship ends. So, it's important that all parties involved be on the same page.

That being said, the use of photos, videos, racy messages, or sexy calls over a webcam can really foster intimacy when physically separated. Please bear in mind that intimacy is more of an emotional and psychological phenomenon rather than a physical one. If anything, these types of exchanges tend to build up so much pressure that, by the time you are physically together, the fireworks are truly memorable.

In addition, building intimacy doesn't always involve racy content. Something as simple as being aware of your partner's needs on a regular basis can be enough to light a fire... and keep it burning.

The role of trust in building intimacy

When building intimacy, trust plays a key role. You have to trust your partner to some degree in order for you to be able to truly surrender yourself. This is something which can be hard when you don't really know someone.

By the same token, if there is an issue getting in between you and your partner, building trust can be quite complex. Without trust, achieving true tantric form can be more challenging. Given the fact that tantra is built on emotion and even spiritual connection, trust needs to be present at all times.

Now, it's important to note that we're not talking about trusting your partner with life and death decisions. This isn't about given them power of attorney. This is about trusting them enough to know that no harm will come to you while you are with them. This type of trust is so powerful that you know you won't have to worry about being hurt in any way. So, that leaves the door entirely open for you to relax and enjoy your encounter.

One of the biggest issues that pops up in committed relationships is infidelity. When one partner, or even both partners, are unfaithful, trust can be shot down. This drives a wedge between both partners in such a way that it may be nearly impossible to truly trust one another. As a result, this could make building your tantric experience somewhat more challenging.

If there is anything on your mind, it's best to talk about it with your partner. Get it out in the open. That way, you can clear the air and move on. That alone is enough to open the floodgates for most partners. It is incredible how unresolved issues can fester to the point where sex is no longer an enjoyable activity. In fact, sex may even become non-existent.

One other thing: it's important to discuss each other's limits. This is especially true if you are planning on engaging in some kind of BDSM activity. Trust needs to be put at the forefront of your mind. That way, you can be certain that your experience will be as pleasurable as you wish it to be. Please keep in mind that having sex with someone puts you in a vulnerable position regardless of whether you are a man or woman. So, the last thing that you want to have in mind is feeling insecure about anything that's going on during your encounter.

The power of touch

Touch is an incredibly powerful force. There is immaterial energy that is transmitted through touch. When you think about it, we can communicate so much more with a simply touching gesture than we could with words.

This is why handshakes are so important in business communication. When you go to business seminars, trainers often tell you that a handshake says much more about your character than your resume could ever say.

When it comes to sexual relationships, touch is a foundational element. You cannot expect to have the best sex of your life without incorporating touch in one way or another. However, not all touch is the same in the world of tantra.

Thus far, we have talked about the kind of touch you can do outside of the bedroom. This type of touch is great at fostering intimacy while keeping you "on your toes," so to speak. It's the type of silent communication between you and your partner that says you are always ready for action, even when you really aren't.

Now, most tantra books limit touching to sensual massages. And while we will be covering massages extensively, it's important to note that touch is so much more than that. Many times, light, sensual touching can produce unbelievable effects.

Using touch effectively

To heighten the sensation of touch, you really need to set the stage. This can be done through the atmosphere that we described earlier. In addition, hugging and cuddling can give you the opportunity to use touch effectively before you engage in actual intercourse.

Many couples enjoy genital touch, such as mutual masturbation, while cuddling and kissing. This is by no means meant to replace the entire act of coitus. However, it can be a power foreplay technique. All you need to do to make this technique effective is to relax and let go. In fact, many couples who have sex for the first time would rather spend a good deal of time touching well before engaging in intercourse.

Another important benefit of touching as part of foreplay is that it eases any anxiety prior to the main part of the show. This is important as genital stimulation allows you to become aroused at your own pace. Naturally, not everyone gets aroused in the same manner. For some, it takes longer than others. As such, touching can allow you to take all the time you need to get aroused at your own pace. That not only takes the pressure off, but it also allows you for variety.

Some tantra practitioners like to mix things up. For instance, they engage in intercourse and then separate in order to spend some time cuddling and kissing. This can be a good way of resting, particularly when you are planning to spend a good deal of time together.

Touching is incredibly useful, particularly for me. After ejaculation, there is a period in which the penis needs to recover before becoming erect again. This is a perfect time for touching. It's a way of keeping the party going without having to put additional pressure on having another erection right away. Furthermore, touching is incredibly powerful when one partner is essentially done while the other would like to keep going. As a matter of fact, some women report that they have more powerful orgasms following oral and manual genital stimulation (particularly stimulation of the clitoris) as compared to penetrative sex. While this may seem paradoxical, it actually makes sense. You see, when you are engaged in coitus with your partner, you are more focused on pleasing them rather than yourself. But when it's you that receives all the attention, it's far easier to just let go and enjoy the moment. This is when ecstasy can be taken to powerful heights.

As for post-coitus touching, please bear in mind that true tantric intercourse is a powerful event. This implies that simply shaking hands and being on your merry way doesn't really work. There needs to be some kind of touching, kissing, or just plain cuddling to bring your encounter to a natural conclusion. While cuddling after sex may not be your thing, at least acknowledging the fact that you had an amazing time is a great way of fostering intimacy. After all, you just had a great experience with some you enjoy being with.

So, do take the time to use touching as a cool down, so to speak. This will help you bring your encounter to a natural ending while leaving you connected with your partner even if you won't see them for a while. Please keep in mind that touch makes the experience all that more powerful while ensuring that you are building an intimate bond with this amazing person.

Chapter 6: Breathing and Relaxation

When it comes to tantric sex, being in sync is absolutely paramount to an effective session. When you and your partner move as one, each movement becomes that much more enjoyable. However, being in sync isn't something that happens automatically. It's something that takes some time and effort to develop.

In this regard, breathing is of vital importance. Breathing is not only useful when it comes to regulating physical exertion, but it's also the best tool that you can use to stay on the same track. You see, tantra looks for both partners to be going down the same path together. This implies that you are focused on where you and your partner are heading as opposed to focusing on your own path toward pleasure.

In this chapter, we are going to look at the role that relaxation plays in tantra and how you can achieve this through breathing. Plus, we're going to be focusing on how breathing is the ultimate road map which can lead you and your partner down the same path toward mutual pleasure and intimate connection.

The role of relaxation in tantra

There is no question that relaxation is essential in any good tantric session. Stress, anxiety, and distractions are the most common culprits of poor sex. These factors wreak havoc on libido and desire.

Just think about that for a moment.

You are trying to get your groove on, but you can't stop thinking about a problem you had at the office. Naturally, it's an important issue that's occupying your mind. And yes, you are eager to get with your partner and have a good time. However, your head is simply not in the game.

In the case of men, this leads to added pressure, which can result in trouble getting an erection. So, on top of the anxiety and stress at the start of the session, tension mounts, even more, when the pressure is on to perform. This can be a real mojo killer.

As for women, stress and overall anxiety can lead to trouble reaching orgasm. Sure, the session might be fun and enjoyable, but things just don't feel right. So, no matter how hard she tries, she just can't seem to get there.

If you have ever been in any of these situations, you can appreciate how tough it is to not only satisfy your partner but yourself. Needless to say, this does not make for an enjoyable romp in the bedroom.

So, what can you do about it?

The first thing to consider is being honest with your partner. If you let your partner know how you feel, they can help you settle down and relax. This is crucial as your partner is there to support you. They can help you calm down and enjoy your time together.

Nevertheless, that is easier said than done.

This is where breathing comes into play.

In addition to massaging, breathing is effective in relaxation. To use breathing as a relaxation technique, there isn't much that you need to do. One great exercise involves hugging and cuddling. You can sit on a sofa, lie in bed, or even stand. All you need to do is hold your partner (or be held) and simply breathe in unison. As you breathe, close your eyes and use your hands to "see" your partner's body. Don't be afraid to let your hands wander. If they should go to intimate places, then so be it! That's the whole point of the exercise.

One great way of incorporating structure into the exercise is to use rhythmic movements as if you were dancing. This could mean swaying from side to side or rubbing body parts such as the back, buttocks, genitals, breasts, or face. Each caress, each movement, each touch is intended to move in concert with each breath, that is, as you inhale and then exhale. Before you know it, you'll be moving in sync. This will eventually lead to arousal, which then leads to showtime.

Calming your mind

To say that your mind plays tricks on you is an understatement. When you are stressed out, anxious, or simply distracted, your mind gets the best of you. Consequently, you don't have the freedom to enjoy sex as much as you would like.

In fact, it's quite easy to get caught up in any number of thoughts.

For instance, you can get caught up in your physical appearance. You might end up being too overly concerned about your body to the point where you can't really enjoy what you are doing. In fact, being insecure about your body (both and men and women) can lead you to feel bad, or even guilty, about sleeping with someone.

Your mind can also have a detrimental effect on your sex life when you let it run the show. This means that you can't let your mind get the best of you during sex. For example, you can't expect to have a mind-blowing session while you are analyzing what your partner is doing, what you should do next, or why things are happening the way they are.

Even though sex does call for careful thought and consideration, once you're in the bedroom, there is no need for sex to become a mathematical equation. Yes, you need to focus on what you are doing, but this doesn't mean you should be knit-picking everything that's happening.

As a matter of fact, if things aren't going right, you can always slow things down, spend some time touching, kissing, hugging or cuddling and regroup. If you can't trust your partner enough to take a time out and regroup, then perhaps you might be better off finding someone in whom you can confide.

So, here is a great exercise which you can do to calm your mind.

Now, whether you are actually having intercourse, or just getting warmed up, you can use your mind's eye to project what you want to happen. To do this, imagine that you're feeling a bright-colored light pulsating through your body. This light is coursing through every part of your being. It can start at the base of your spine and radiate onward. As you feel this energy flowing, imagine it is passing through to your partner at whatever point of contact you have. This could be through the hands, mouth, genitals, or any other point in which your bodies are in contact.

Next, imagine the light enveloping the both of you. Don't pay too much attention to the pleasure you are feeling. That will be there. It's something that you can't ignore. Just imagine the light connecting both of you. This light is the energy that you are sharing during your time together. Please keep in mind that there is no need for penetration to actually take place in order for this light to pass through the both of you. All energy needs is a channel which it can run through.

Now, here is the real kicker: as this energy, in the form of light, returns to you, what you are receiving is a recycled form of energy that isn't yours anymore. It belongs to the both of you. As this energy gets stronger and stronger, the pressure builds up in such a manner that when the big "O" comes, it's explosive. However, the big "O" does just end there. It's just a means of feeding the system in a closed-loop so that the pleasure keeps building and building, thereby leading to a stronger and stronger orgasm.

380

Syncing your breathing

In most tantra literature, you read about the importance of syncing your breathing. It should be noted that it isn't breathing per se that leads to connection. What leads to connecting with your partner is the fact that you are both moving in unison. The role breathing plays is to enable all parties involved to progress at the same rate or at the same pace.

To sync up your breathing, especially during intercourse, here is an effective exercise:

When you are in the midst of intercourse, you might find the action getting hot and heavy. As such, it's quite common for one partner to speed up while the other is moving along at a slower rate. It's important to remember that tantric sex is about taking things slow. This means that if your partner is racing along, you can slow the pace of the game down talking to them. Tell them to breathe in and breath out with you. You can help them by modeling the way they ought to be breathing. That way, you can slow things down and sync up your breathing.

As you get into the same rhythm, the actual speed of intercourse can move from a faster and more superficial tempo to a slower and deeper one. In fact, one highly effective practice is to mix things up. You see, when the rhythm of intercourse is fast and furious, it can't possibly last very long. It's just a matter of time before one, or both, simply explode and end up unable to recover. By the time they're ready again, the moment might have already passed.

So, when you mix things up, going fast and then slowing down, you will find that it gives you the chance to better manage your pleasure (and that of your partner's) while taking the time to savor the sights and feelings. If you are looking to take in the visuals, you will have enough time to feed your sight. If you are more inclined to the sensations of it all, you will have the time to savor the moment.

Now, if things appear to be getting out of control, don't be afraid to stop and regroup. Often, all it takes is a momentary pause to regain your breathing and then resume. Please keep in mind that experienced tantra practitioners are not afraid to take a breather even when the action is hot and heavy. In doing so, you can ensure that you are making the most of the time you are spending with your partner.

Don't forget to breathe!

For a lot of folks, breathing becomes an issue at the height of pleasure simply because they forget to breathe. Yes, as silly as that may sound, there are times when you might simply forget to breathe. This occurs because your entire nervous system is fixated on the pleasure you are feeling. However, when you stop breathing, you stop supplying oxygen to your body. Now, it's not like you are going to suffocate or anything. It's just that if you are looking to really enjoy your session, it's a good idea to be cognizant of your breathing.

Breathing is a great way to keep track of yourself. You see, when things are going really well, it's easy to get so caught up that you might end up losing yourself completely. While that is not a bad thing, it might cause you to neglect your partner. This is important, especially if you are very keen on pleasing your partner.

Consider this example:

As a man, it's easy to get caught up in the moment and lose control. When you lose control, you might feel compelled to finish. While this is not the issue, there might be an issue when your partner doesn't feel that they have gotten their fair share. For instance, the other partner hasn't reached their orgasm yet.

382

This situation exemplifies how breathing can help you stay in the moment. By focusing on breathing, both men and women can quell their mind, manage their emotions, and heighten their sensations. A simple way of using your breathing to your advantage is to simply focus on inhaling and exhaling. That's all. You don't need to count to ten, nor do you need to repeat some mantra in your mind. All you need to do is feel in the air entering your lungs and leaving your body. This alone is enough to get your body the oxygen it needs to perform up to the level you expect it to.

Chapter 7: Using Toys

One of the most common questions that surface with regard to tantric sex is the use of foreign objects, that is, "toys." Now, it should be noted that we're not talking about anything that could potentially cause harm such as artifacts used in BDSM. Also, we're not talking about any items that don't typically fall under the "sex toy" designation, such as sharp objects, machines, or even torture devices. In this discussion, we're talking about the types of things you would find in a regular sex shop such as dildos, vibrators, rings, plugs, beads, or even clamps.

Now, tantra purists will point out that textbook tantra doesn't call for the use of toys. If anything, toys can be considered as a distraction that can hinder reaching full tantric ecstasy. However, the use of toys can actually enhance pleasure particularly during a "warm-up," and especially during intercourse itself.

So, in this chapter, we are going to be discussing how you can incorporate the use of toys, should you choose to do so, under the scope of tantric sex. Moreover, we'll go over some recommended ways in which you can get the most out of the toys you bring into the bedroom.

Talking it over

Like anything in sex, the use of toys should be a mutual decision. These types of objects should not just be thrown into the mix. Sure, it might be a nice surprise, but if you haven't used toys before with a specific partner, it's always best to talk about it first.

For most women, the use of sex toys is not unheard of. In fact, you might be surprised to find most women are comfortable with the idea of using sex toys. After all, what's wrong with mixing things up a bit? The truth is that sex toys, like any other aspect of sex, are there to enhance enjoyment and pleasure.

For some men, the use of sex toys can actually be intimidating, especially if they have never used them before. This is due to the fact that the male ego may view the use of toys as a sign of dissatisfaction on the part of their partner.

This could not be farther from the truth.

A sex toy, no matter how good or pleasurable it may be, can never replace the type of interaction that comes with having sex with another person. As such, there is nothing to be worried about, or threatened by, when it comes to using sex toys.

That being said, it's important to discuss what types of toys you are both comfortable with. If you are new to the sex toy scene, perhaps you can start off with one and see how it goes. If you have had prior experience, you can talk about what you like and take it from there. By having an honest talk about what you like and what you would like to incorporate, you can ensure that your experience will be that much better.

Another important issue to talk about is boundaries. It is crucial to set your limits clearly. While you might be up for anything, there might be a certain thing you're not comfortable with, at least not yet. So, it's important to bring up these boundaries as this would avoid any potentially uncomfortable situations. The last thing you want to do is shut things down because you don't feel comfortable with anything. Please keep in mind that trust is an essential part of tantric sex.

Toys during warm-up

Prior to actual intercourse, you may choose to have a "warm-up" phase. This warmup portion of the program can be devoted to taking turns in giving and receiving pleasure.

This is where toys can really spice things up.

Consider this situation:

You are holding your partner while allowing your hands to touch all over your bodies. This touching is a great way of leading the way to arousal. Now, at this point, you might be inclined to focus on your partner's genital area. For the sake of this example, let's assume that it's a man who is stimulating a woman. The man's touch on his partner's genital area is soft and slow. The intent is to arouse his partner so that she can be receptive to intercourse.

At this point, rather than jumping straight into intercourse, why not try out a toy? For instance, a vibrator can be a perfect complement to the manual stimulation in the woman's genital area. This stimulation can go as far as you want it to go.

In fact, you can even try syncing your breathing while your partner is progressively becoming more and more aroused. While the man isn't necessarily receiving any direct stimulation, the emotional and psychological stimulation, that is, the sensory perception is a great way of boosting arousal. If you like, you can take your partner all the way to orgasm. In doing so, the woman can feel satisfied and fulfilled and... ready for more!

This example is a great way of aiding arousal. As such, toys can be used as precursors to the main event. Once in the main event, both partners can feel satisfied that they are thoroughly enjoying the situation.

Now, it should be noted that most sex toys are geared toward women. However, this doesn't mean that there aren't toys for men. It's worth taking the time to do research in order to find suitable toys based on a man's preferences. There are varying degrees of openness with regard to male sex toys, so if you're a man reading this, take some time to go through what toys are out there. If you're a woman reading this, you can peruse online catalogs with your man. That way, the experience of searching for sex toys can be a mutually bonding experience.

Toys during intercourse

The use of toys during intercourse is often debated. There are some who love the additional stimulation, while some dislike them completely. So, let's take a look at both sides of the argument.

For those who love toys during intercourse, these can provide additional stimulation. For instance, the use of clitoral vibrators during intercourse can provide another layer of arousal and stimulation. In fact, the combination of penetrative sex and clitoral stimulation can produce mind-bending orgasms. In a manner of speaking, it's like combining two foods that you love into one dish without them tasting weird.

Another facet of toys during intercourse is anal play. Some couples love using toys to stimulate the backside. This can also offer another layer of pleasure to the receiving partner. For women, anal stimulation during vaginal intercourse can produce an incredible sensation. And of course, there are men who also enjoy anal play during coitus even if they are heterosexual. Ultimately, the use of toys during intercourse is a question of finding the best way to get the most out of your experience.

On the flip side, there are those who dislike toys during intercourse altogether. The most common objection is that it becomes a distraction. For some, the use of toys during intercourse might mean fumbling in the dark for it. When looking at it from that perspective, it can certainly be seen as a distraction.

Additionally, some couples would rather not use toys during intercourse as they seek a unique experience in which it is them, and only them, who are involved in the action. While this is perfectly valid, it should also be noted that it ought to be a mutual decision. This implies that both parties should be on the same page. If one of the partners is reticent about using toys, they should at least give it a try. If they find that it's definitely not for them, then at least they gave it a try. However, it could be that once they try it, they can see just how good using toys can be.

How to determine if toys are right for you

There really is only one way to find out: try it!

If you don't try, at least once, to use toys during a tantric session, then you may never know if you are really missing out or not. It could be that you are missing out on a great experience without even knowing it. It might very well be that your hesitation about the use of toys is based on preconceptions that aren't really founded on anything.

Naturally, this argument is not intended to coerce you into trying out toys. Still, it's worth giving anything a shot at least once. In many cases, folks are reluctant to try toys out because they are afraid of being judged or seen negatively. The truth is that there is nothing wrong with the use of toys. It's just a natural part of human nature. If anything, denying yourself this opportunity can end up causing more harm than good.

Furthermore, if you commonly use toys during solo sessions (yes, both guys and gals use toys during solo sessions), then it only makes sense to carry that over into tantric sessions with your partner. As we have stated earlier, the use of toys is not about replacing your partner, or any other person for that matter, it's about enhancing the experience that you share with your partner.

Consequently, trying out toys is definitely worth a shot. If, after trying it, you feel it's not for you, then that's fair game. After all, tantric sex looks to push your boundaries. If you find yourself comfortably ensconced in your comfort zone, then you may be missing out on what could be one of the best experiences of your life.

Not all toys are created equal

It's also important to do your homework on the toys you plan to use. This is important as there is any number of toys out there. Some are rather straightforward, while others come in a variety of shapes, sizes, colors, textures, and functions. You can't really know what works for you until you try them out. So, it's always best to start off with the basics and move on from there. This is especially true when you haven't experimented with toys before.

When you go about purchasing your first sex toys, you might be tempted to make a big splash. However, you might not want to spend any big bucks until you are sure what's best for you. In fact, for most folks, simple works best. So, dishing out a pretty penny for the fanciest toys may not be the best choice, at least not at first.

Getting over the mental hang up

If you have no qualms about bringing toys into the bedroom, along with your partner, then make the most of your opportunity to enjoy a pleasurable experience with your partner... and some added stimulation.

However, if you are on the fence about bringing in toys, then it's worth going over the worst-case scenario. When you really think about it, what's the worst that can happen? If you really trust your partner, then there should be no reason why toys would get in the way. For instance, if you choose to try something out, but realize that it's not for you, or it didn't work the way you expected it to, then you can simply chalk it up to experience. If anything, it could be that you haven't chosen the right one.

Please keep in mind that this chapter isn't meant to convince you to use toys. It's meant to convince you to try new things. When you are truly committed to exploring the depths of tantra, you need to be prepared to open yourself up to new experiences. Otherwise, you will never get out of your comfort zone. As such, you may never be able to truly surrender yourself to your partner and the depths of pleasure that can emerge from liberating your hang-ups. When you let go of your hang-ups, you are truly free to be yourself!

Chapter 8: Exercises During Tantric Sex

Thus far, we have focused on the various factors that make tantric sex the best sexual experience of your life. It may seem like a big claim to make. But when you really think about it, all the time and effort you have put into learning about tantra makes it truly possible.

That is why this section is devoted to specific exercises that you can use to help you achieve the heights of sexual pleasure and ecstasy you seek to achieve. As we have mentioned throughout this book, ecstasy isn't something that happens automatically. There is a certain number of elements that go into sex before you can truly hit the heights you seek.

In this chapter, we are going to focus on exercises that you can both do solo and with your partner. Ultimately, these exercises are meant to help you stimulate your own sexual energy and that of your partner. In the end, you will find these exercises to be quite simple and very enjoyable.

Going solo

First of all, let's take a look at exercises you can do solo. These exercises are great when you don't have a partner. They are also very effective when you do have a partner. The key thing about solo exercises is that you are on your own meaning that there is no pressure to perform for anyone else. These are exercises which are yours and yours alone. So, there is no going wrong. If you find that you're not quite getting what you want out of it, then keep trying. In fact, you may find these exercises worth trying on your partner later on. It could even make for a nice surprise.

When going solo, the end game isn't always masturbation. Most people have the false assumption that anything that involves touching yourself, in any way, is about masturbation. However, this could not be farther from the truth. The exercises we are going to reveal are about self-exploration. They are about getting yourself in the right condition so that you can channel your sexual energy in a positive and meaningful manner.

Solo exercise #1: Meditation

Yes, meditation. While this isn't traditionally considered to be a "sexual" exercise, it is a must if you are really focused on mastering tantra.

In this exercise, you are focusing your mind on your energy, your sensations, and the overall arousal you feel. This will help you to explore the emotions and sensations you feel during arousal. Moreover, you can use your mind's eye to help you picture the outcome you want in a sexual relationship.

Here is a great exercise you can put into practice right away:

Find a comfortable position. This could be lying on your back in your bed or perhaps on a comfy sofa—the more comfortable the position, the better. Now, begin the exercise by breathing slowly. Inhale and exhale to the full capacity of your lungs. As you fill your lungs, picture the air entering your body. Once your lungs are full, hold your breath for about 3 seconds and then exhale. Repeat this breathing exercise as many times as you like. Don't keep count as that will only serve to distract you.

Next, picture your energy flowing through your body. Picture your sexual energy building up and coursing through every fiber of your body. If you feel slightly aroused, that's perfectly normal. Try to focus on your breathing and your energy. As you feel the energy flowing, imagine how it feeds your body. Picture how it is nourishing your cells.

Try to hold this state for as long as you can. At first, this state may only last a few minutes. As you gain more

392

practice, you might find yourself in this position for quite a long time. Don't worry if you happen to fall asleep. Sometimes, you might be tired and stressed out. So, this type of exercise gives you a profound state of relaxation, thereby causing you to fall asleep.

Solo exercise #2: Self-massaging

Self-massaging is about exploring your own body. It's about understanding every part of your body, and in particular, the areas of your body that are most susceptible to arousal. While everyone can be aroused by touching the same areas (such as the genitals), it is also true that different folks find different parts of their bodies susceptible to pleasure. That is why this exercise is about exploring your own body. After all, if you don't know what feels good, how can you expect your partner to figure it out? Sure, they will eventually, but you can shorten the learning curve by guiding your partner.

In this exercise, start out by relaxing in a comfortable position. You can undress if you like, wear a bathrobe, or perhaps stay in your underwear. The idea is to find whatever makes your most comfortable. Then, begin by breathing just like in the previous exercise. As you relax, start by touching yourself slowly and softly. Try to get a feeling for every part of your body. Don't hold back.

As you make your way around your body, try to take in the sensations produced. You may be surprised to find that some parts are more sensitive to others. Make a note of which areas are more sensitive. Try to focus on how everything feels. If you find yourself having erotic thoughts, try your best to steer your mind back to what you are actually feeling.

One great addition to this exercise is the use of oils and lotions. These can help make your touching smoother while adding a pleasant scent. Play music if you like or use other scents such as essential oils, incense, and so on. However, try to refrain from any visual stimulation as the idea is to help you see with your other senses and not just your eyes.

Solo exercise #3: Masturbation

The intention of this exercise is not to just get off. It's about exploring pleasure and what makes you feel truly satisfied. As such, rushing orgasm is not the best way to go about it. In this exercise, the main focus is to take your time to explore your genitals and all those sensitive areas of your body.

Don't hold back!

Remember, you are alone. So, there is no one judging what you are doing. This can give you the freedom to explore all areas of your body. The worst that can happen is you find something you don't really like. Nevertheless, it's worth exploring every inch of your body.

You can set the mood just like the previous two exercises. In fact, you can do these exercises in sequence. First, start off with some meditation, then some self-massaging before masturbation. Please bear in mind that the ultimate goal is not orgasm. The ultimate goal is to manage your sensations so that you can control your arousal.

This is especially important in men. By going slow and managing your arousal, men can get more control over ejaculation, thereby prolonging the time of intercourse. As for women, this is a perfect opportunity to find what type of stimulation works best in pursuit of the big "O." Oh, and by the way, use toys if you wish!

Working with a partner

These exercises are intended to help you and your partner find the right combination of stimulation, intimacy, pleasure, and arousal. While that may sound like a great deal of things in one package, the truth is that all of these elements interact together in a single cycle. So, when you hit one target, that activates the next and so on.

So, here are three great exercises you can try with your partner:

Team exercise #1: Foreplay

There is a lot about foreplay in sexual literature. In fact, we have talked extensively about foreplay in this book. However, we haven't honed in on a couple of aspects that are essential to tantric sex.

Please bear in mind that foreplay is essential. It can be as long or as short as you like. There might be times when both of you are ready to go, while there may be others when a little more warming up is needed.

For this exercise, you can choose to undress, dress, wear costumes, lingerie, whatever hits the spot for you. Also, you can lie in bed, sit on a sofa, stand in the kitchen, be in the car (somewhere that isn't too public), or anywhere you can find the privacy and intimacy that you seek.

First, by syncing your breathing. You can use the same breathing technique we presented in solo exercise one. Now, take the time to look at each other. Explore each other's bodies with your eyes. Try to take in every aspect of your partner's body. Then, begin by touching. You can use lotion or oil if you wish. This isn't just a massage; it's touching that's meant to arouse you. As the energy builds, you can take turns touching each other, especially in those areas where you feel most sensitive. Don't forget to kiss your partner as much as you like.

At this point, you can take things to the next level. Here, you can make use of toys, or perhaps oral stimulation. If you choose, you can take turns stimulating one another. Or, you might choose to stimulate each other at the same time. Anything goes!

Please bear in mind that the point of this exercise is not sex per se. The point is to build arousal and intimacy in such a way that both of you learn what truly turns you on. In fact, you may choose to avoid sexual intercourse and perhaps bring about orgasm through the use of toys, fingers, oral, and manual stimulation. The fact is that there is nothing carved in stone. If you wish, you can have sex and make it the full package.

Team exercise #2: Snuggling or cuddling

Earlier, we described this exercise as a means of fostering intimacy. In this variation, we are going to spice things up so that it can be used as foreplay, or just as a means of stimulating arousal.

To carry out this position, we are going to be "spooning." This is a position in which both partners lie on their sides. Then, the partner that is behind the other holds the other. This creates a "giver" and "receiver."

With this exercise, you can take it as far as you like. You can lie there breathing in sync or take it up a notch. For instance, you can undress and touch. The giver takes the time to explore the receiver thereby arousing and stimulating them. If this leads to sex, then the "spoon" position is there for your enjoyment. Or, you may choose to engage in or oral or manual stimulation. Please bear in mind that this exercise isn't intended to lead to sex. It's about getting you to feel comfortable with each other's bodies so that sex becomes that much more potent.

Team exercise #3: Sex

Traditional sex is defined as intercourse, that is, penetration of some kind. Well, this isn't traditional sex. In this exercise, "sex" is anything you want it to be. In fact, you can even mix things up. Some couples feel the need for penetration every time they have sex. Other couples use penetration as the final act following the exercises outlined in this chapter. Other couples use penetration as a lead into other events such as oral or manual stimulation. And then, there are toys...

After you have truly become comfortable with your partner, sex becomes a natural occurrence that stems from stimulation and arousal. In fact, you don't really think about "sex" when you are with your partner. All you think about is enjoying your time with them. Then, things can go any way you want them, too. The main thing is to be on the same page and enjoy your encounter.

That is the bottom line. Whatever you choose to do at this point, please bear in mind that giving is just as good as receiving. So, if you feel compelled to take turns, then so be it. If you feel compelled to reach the big "O" together, then you can take your time to work yourselves up to that point.

Chapter 9: Positions During Tantric Sex

Much is written about positions in tantric sex. However, most of what you will find is a collection of various positions that don't really espouse the philosophy of tantric sex. Sure, it might be fun to try a different configuration. But at the end of the day, if your head is not into the tantric frame of mind, then the positions you try will not lead you to the ultimate ecstasy you are seeking.

With that in mind, this chapter is about taking sex positions that are a staple of tantric sex so that you can incorporate them into your own sex life right away. Sure, you may have tried them before, it's a guarantee that you haven't tried them like this before.

So, try to keep an open mind in this chapter. Now, you may not be surprised by these positions, but when you see the spin that we have put on them, you will regret no having tried this sooner!

Going on the power play

This might sound like you're playing hockey, but the power play is all about that, "power."

In this position, we're not really talking about intertwining your bodies in one manner or the other. It's about giving your partner free rein to do what they like with you. By surrendering your power, you allow your partner to take you to places you may not have been to before.

But first a disclaimer: when trying out the power play, it's important to talk about boundaries. For instance, you might say that anything in the backdoor is off-limits. Also, make a point of telling your partner what you like best. By the same token, pay attention to what drives your partner crazy. It could be that you already know how to push all of the right buttons.

That being said, the power play isn't anything like BDSM (unless you're actually into it). This is more about letting go. For instance, the use of blindfolds or masks is highly useful. The idea is that when you cancel out senses, you force the others to make up for it. Thus, your heightened sensitivity makes you feel pleasure in a whole new level.

Here is a simple yet effective angle on the powerplay.

Let's assume you are giving pleasure. Lay your partner down on their back. Use a blindfold, sleeping mask, or any other means of blocking their sight. Now, slowly undress your partner. Do it in such a way that they can anticipate your movements. The only rule is that they can't move or push you away. If you feel inclined to use handcuffs or any other type of restraint, then by all means. Now, as you approach the genital area, slowly caress their inner thigh.

At this point, you have two options. One, you can continue the caressing and proceed to masturbate your partner. In the case of a man, slowly stroking the penis will not only cause a great deal of pleasure but will allow him to control his need to ejaculate. Use lubrication if you like. In the case of a woman, stimulating the clitoris can be a great way to get things rolling. You can then choose to take your partner all the way to orgasm, or perhaps use this exercise as a warm-up.

The second option is to perform oral pleasure on your partner. The same rules apply here. You can work your way slowly so that the sensation is that much stronger. You can take your partner all the way to orgasm, or just use it as a means of setting the stage.

One of the great things about this technique is that you can use it as a means of controlling orgasm. For men, it's a great way to help control the urge to ejaculate. The trick is to get close to the "point of no return" before settling back down again. In the case of women, building up "pressure" so to speak, can lead to a massive "O." Other women may feel inclined to just have multiple orgasms as a result of oral or manual stimulation, or both.

Also, the use of toys is perfectly fine here. Just make sure that you are on the same page about the toys to be used and how they are meant to be used.

Take things slow

Throughout this book, we have talked about the importance of going slow. This is very important when you are starting out with tantra. Please bear in mind that this isn't about how hard and fast you can go. If anything, tantra is about taking things slow and relishing every moment with your partner.

At first, it's a great idea to start out with traditional positions such as the missionary and the cowgirl (or reverse if you like). With the missionary, the male is on top of the female. Now, it's important to resist the urge to go fast. Rather, the goal here is to go slow. Ideally, slow, deep penetration works really well.

Here's a simple way of ensuring this position works wonders.

Count to 4. Yes, that's right. Start out with three shorter, shallower thrusts and one deep, hard thrust. The fourth thrust should last just a little bit longer than the first three. This technique will allow you to get into a rhythm. Please bear in mind that tantra is all about finding a rhythm. When you get into that rhythm, then the female can experience a rather predictable outcome: a big "O."

In the case of the cowgirl (or reverse cowgirl), the female is on top. As such, the female is in control of the movement. So, it's a great idea to play the same 4-count: three shallow thrusts and one deep, prolonged thrust.

400

This will allow the female to control the sensation thereby enabling a rhythmic movement.

You will find that even though these are very traditional positions, they really work very well when you are able to build a rhythm. Eventually, both of you will be able to sync everything, movement, breathing, and eye contact. If you choose to cancel sight, then breathing becomes highly important in order to ensure you are on the same page.

The final lap

This is the classic tantric sex position. In this one, the man sits upright, preferably with his back up against something firm for support, legs stretched out (not crossed). Then, the woman sits on his lap. The woman's legs should wrap around the man's buttocks. Kneeling is not recommended as it can get quite tiring very quickly. She can then wrap her arms around the man's neck or use her hands to caress him. The man can also wrap his arms around the woman or use his hands to caress her.

This is a very intimate position as it always for a number of things. First, kissing is the go-to option here. Also, it's great for breathing exercises. You can simply hold each other and attempt to sync your breathing. In addition, you can caress each other in unison. For instance, massaging each other's backs, buttocks and chest are all good exercises.

The other great thing about this position is that you can achieve penetration with it. So, if you want to take it up a notch, then it's certainly an option. One interesting thing about this position is that due to its nature, you can't move very fast. So, it's ideal for tantra. Plus, the level of intimacy you can achieve with this position is excellent.

The reverse lap

This position is essentially the same as the previous with a twist: one of the partners sits with their back to the wall while the other sits on their lap but with their back facing their partner. As such, the first partner only sees the back of the second. The second partner is essentially the recipient of the former's attention.

When engaging in this position, the first partner essentially has access to the second partner. They can caress just about every part of their partner's body while having the option of kissing the back of their neck, shoulders, and upper back.

One of the great things about this position is that you can switch things up. So, the man can hold the female, or the female can hold the male. So, it's great for taking turns and pampering each other. If you choose to penetrate, the female can sit on the man's lap and do so. At this point, the position works pretty much like a reverse cowgirl. And just like the previous position, there's not much room to move fast. So, you really don't have much choice but to take it slow.

One very nice variation of this position is that it can be done in a bathtub, jacuzzi, or a swimming pool. If you're in public, well, you have to keep it civil. But in private, you can take it up as far as you want to. A bubble bath is one of the go-to moves for this position.

Spooning

Earlier, we talked about how spooning can be a great tool for fostering intimacy. In this case, it's also a great position for having intercourse. Additionally, it works really well because you can't move very fast even if you wanted to. Spooning can work both ways as the female can hold the male and vice-versa. If you are intent on penetration, then it works very well, especially because it favors syncing your movements. Plus, it's one of the most intimate positions you will find in the tantric sex toolkit.

The other great thing about spooning is that it can be quite erotic without necessarily leading to sex. It's good for syncing breathing and it's also good for post-sex cuddling. In fact, lots of couples love sleeping like this. So, that's an added bonus.

One other twist to spooning is the ability to masturbate your partner. This works well if you're keen on pleasuring your partner. In fact, you can practice syncing up your breathing while masturbating your partner. As you can see, it's the position that keeps on giving!

Mutual masturbation

On the subject of touching, mutual masturbation is a great way of syncing everything up. This technique works well to sync breathing, practice eye contact, and also kissing passionately. So, let's take a look at a couple of ways in which you could make this work.

The first is by both partners lying on their backs. Then touching ensues. But the key here is that the touching needs to be at the same speed. If one goes faster than the other, you might get a big "O" ahead of time. Also, it might be a bit hard to focus when your partner is going at a different rate than you are.

Another position is lying on your side, facing one another. This position allows you to make eye contact, kiss, and basically have access to the entire front part of your partner's body. This variation is great if you are just looking to lie in bed, spend some time together, and throw in a fun ending.

The third variation to sit, facing each other. For this one, both partners sit upright on the same surface. So, one does not sit on the lap of the other. This variation is great for eye contact and breathing. It also allows you both to touch each other slowly. Given the nature of the position, you can't go very fast. That is a great thing in the world of tantra, of course.

So, there you have some great position which you can practice today. Please keep in mind that anything goes in tantra. You can do any of the positions you enjoy. However, the ones we have presented in this chapter are intended to help you get into the rhythm of tantra. Eventually, you'll be able to mix things up as suits your mood.

Chapter 10: Massages During Tantric Sex

Massaging has to be the most recognizable part of tantric sex. All experts on the topic recommend the use of massaging as a means of engaging in tantra. However, not too many experts take the time to explain while massaging is such a useful tactic when it comes to tantric sex.

The main reason behind massaging's effectiveness is that it promotes a sensory response that other techniques don't really provide. This is important as tantra is based, first and foremost, on sensory perception. After all, traditional sex is "traditional" because it's just about finding the quickest way to orgasm.

When you take the time to practice massage, you will discover a two-way street that you had no idea already existed. First, the incredible sensation that comes with receiving a tantric massage. The second, the unbelievable satisfaction that comes with giving your partner a tremendous experience. Both of these situations can leave you feeling both satisfied and nurtured.

Massaging roles

Basically, there are two roles in tantric massaging, the giver and receiver. The giver is the person performing the massage while the receiver is the one who is the recipient of the massage. Both roles are important in tantra as each partner connects to the other, thus producing the tantric experience.

If you are more inclined to a dominant or submissive role, massaging provides a great opportunity to feed this side. For example, more dominant individuals can take their partners into their hands, literally, and give them an extraordinary experience. If you are a more submissive person, then you can fully surrender yourself in your partner's touch.

However, massaging is also great at inverting the power dynamic. More predominantly submissive individuals can take the opportunity to be in the lead. They can give their dominant partner some much-deserved attention and pampering. The dominant partner has the chance to relinquish power for a short while. This can be a refreshing change that can help a dominant individual get away from their comfort zone to find a different role in the relationship.

Massaging also allows each partner to take turns. It's a bit hard to massage each other at the same time. So, the best way to go about it is to just take turns. Now, it can be hard to receive a massage, pop up, and then give one. As such, you might work out a deal in which one receives a massage on one occasion and then the other on the next occasion.

Still, taking turns can work well if you plan on simpler things like a shoulder rub or foot massage (this is awesome if you have a foot fetish). So, do make time for massaging as part of your love life. If you haven't given it a try, you'll regret not having done it sooner.

Setting the stage

Setting the stage for a massage is highly important. If you are keen on pulling out all the stops, a massage table is the best way to go. Alternatively, just lying in bed is great. Lying on a couch also works, but because of the design of couches, it can be a bit tough to access all of your partner's body.

Scented candles, essential oils, or incense are great ways of providing a pleasant smell. Soft music, nature sounds, or some smooth jazz can also enhance the mood. Visuals are important too, such as dim lighting or perhaps candlelight.

One very important aspect of setting the stage is to minimize distractions. This means blocking out the world around you. Please keep in mind that both the giver and receiver ought to focus on the events as they are happening. So, eliminating distractions is a must.

An interesting twist could be to massage your partner in a tub or jacuzzi. You can make use of bath salts to create a pleasant atmosphere. This works exceptionally well when you are looking to alleviate stress. Water has a great way of making aches and pains go away. Plus, massages in water tend to be a lot more intimate than say in bed or massage table.

Using equipment

This largely depends on what you are going for. You can keep things very simple by just using your hands and some oil. There are various types of oil that you can use on your partner. The most common type of oil is regular baby oil. It serves as a very nice lubricant while also stimulating the skin. There is also a wide range of massage oils. Some are scented while others vary in texture. So, it's up to you to experiment with whatever you feel would work best for you.

Additionally, if you are inclined to use any sex toys, feel free to bring them into the mix (more on that in a minute). Any other props such as mallets, rubber balls, or vibrators could enhance the experience. In a way, massaging is about trial and error. This means that you can try out various things and see what works best for you. If you find that one thing doesn't work, then you can just move on from it.

A good piece of advice here is to avoid rushing out to buy a bunch of massage gear. Start out with your hands and move on from there. The best equipment which you can use is your hands!

The proper technique

When using tantric massage, the question of the "proper technique" comes to mind. Often, folks are unsure about whether to rub, or stroke, or do karate chops. The fact of the matter is that you don't need to be a professional massage therapist to give your partner a pleasurable experience. In fact, you can just start out by running your hands down your partner's limbs, back, and shoulder. In addition, the use of oils can greatly reduce the amount of friction when rubbing your partner down. So, that creates the warm sensation of being touched while also allowing yourself to control the movements you are doing.

One interesting spin is to take a couple's massage class. In this type of class, a trained professional shows you how to rub down your partner. So, it's not them doing the rubbing; it's you, but with the guidance of a pro. For couples looking to build an intimate experience, this class actually works really well despite having a third person in the room with you.

Alternatively, online tutorials can help you get a good sense of what to do and how to handle your partner. In fact, watching such tutorials can even create arousal. In a manner of speaking, it provides a great visual.

With that in mind, here is a great four-step plan you can put into practice right away.

First, let's start with relaxation. To get ready for a massage, you can practice breathing with your partner. The receiver lies down on their back while the giver sets the pace for breathing. The giver can begin by providing light caresses on the legs, arms, or just simply being there.

Next, as relaxation sets in, work your way up. To do this, begin by providing a foot rub, working your way up on the calves, shins, and thighs. You don't need any particular technique here. Basically, all you need is light rubbing with your hands or the oil of your choice. Lotion works well, too.

After, try to avoid the genital area at this point. While you might be tempted to go for it, it's best to wait until you have completed the entire body massage. While you might have a happy ending for your partner in mind, the main point of the tantric massage is to foster intimacy and give your partner the best experience. As such, you can caress their inner thigh, eventually working your way up their stomach, chest, and down their arms.

Once you have reached the shoulders, ask your partner to flip over on to their belly. Now, you can work your way down their back to their buttocks and the back of their legs. At this point, you can focus on their thighs. Here, you can decide to stimulate the genital area if you wish. You can ask your partner to flip back on to their back to focus on their genital area.

Lastly, it's important to be aware of what the point of the massage is. If you want to use the massage as a means of foreplay prior to sexual intercourse, then certainly stimulating your partner's genital area serves the purpose. You can use your hands or even perform oral pleasure. The use of toys can also work here.

If the point of the massage is not sexual per se, then you can leave it at that. Please bear in mind that if you are not planning on any sexual activity as it relates to the massage, then make this clear to your partner, so there are no expectations. However, the chances are that you may not resist and choose to take it further.

Happy ending?

This question always comes up when discussing tantric massages. In general, you can provide your partner with a happy ending if you are both comfortable with it. This is important to note, as you may not be comfortable with this idea at first. Generally speaking, the giver may feel left out if the receiver orgasms while they don't receive any reciprocal pleasure.

One of the deals you can make it to take turns. You can choose to pamper your partner one day while you are in line for the next round. Otherwise, you could take turns massaging one another before sexual activity.

The fact of the matter is that massages provide you with the opportunity to foster both intimacy and to pamper your partner. Please bear in mind that one of the core tenets is to provide your partner with the attention they seek. By the same token, you should also be on the receiving end. This is why we have stated throughout this book that tantra is a two-way street. Of course, communication is the key in this regard.

What to watch out for

While tantric massages are more about providing your partner with an experience that goes beyond the actual massage technique you are using, it's worth mentioning that you and your partner should communicate on what feels good and what you enjoy most. For instance, you might have highly sensitive areas. As such, your partner needs to be aware of this. Likewise, you need to be aware of which areas are sensitive to your partner.

Also, setting a time and place for massages is key. While that may sound mechanical (like having to set an appointment) the fact is that improvising a massage session may not provide you with the results you seek. This is why many tantra practitioners make time for themselves and their partners. Since you want to dedicate as much time and attention as you can to the occasion, making time for your partner is a must.

On the whole, tantric massage is a technique that evolves among partners. Over time, you will find what works for both of you. Then, you can take that knowledge and translate it into an experience which makes sense for both you. That way, your massage sessions will become as pleasurable as they can become. If this leads to sex, then so be it. If it doesn't lead to sex, then it's still a wonderful experience that can set the stage for further sessions.

Please keep in mind that tantra isn't necessarily about sex. This misconception tends to permeate the minds of folks all over. When you see that tantra is just the overarching theme that also happens to include sex, you will find that your overall feelings about your sex life and your relationship with your partner change drastically.

So, make the time for yourself and your partner. You won't regret prioritizing this part of your life.

Chapter 11: What is Tantric Pleasure?

Pleasure is the most talked-about aspect regarding tantra. After all, what point would there be to tantra is there wasn't any pleasure involved?

The fact of the matter is pleasure is the core of the entire tantra practice. Pleasure is of the utmost importance. So, that's why we are going to have an in-depth discussion on pleasure and what it means to give it and receive it.

As we have stated numerous times in this book, tantra is a two-way street. As such, tantra is both about giving and receiving. Unlike other approaches in which students are taught to either give or receive pleasure, tantra is about reciprocity. This means that you should get as much as you give and vice-versa. If you feel that you are giving more than you get, then something is not entirely right. Good tantra practice means that you are able to feel as satisfied as your partner.

What is tantric pleasure?

Now, the question begs: what is pleasure?

Generally speaking, pleasure is a feeling of goodness in your physical body. This feeling is the result of engaging in a pleasurable sexual activity. The degree of pleasure that you are able to feel depends on your partner, the activities you do, and your ability to actually feel pleasure.

This is important as there are many folks out there who have trouble feeling pleasure. A common issue with feeling pleasure is generally associated with the feelings you might have about the activities in which you are engaging. For some, sex is synonymous with impure activities. For others, they may feel guilty about feeling pleasure.

While it is not our intention to explore the causes of being unable to feel pleasure, we are looking to establish that pleasure is about feeling good when engaging in sexual activity. Pleasure derived from traditional sex is limited to the physical body. This means that you are able to feel pleasure though it doesn't go beyond a temporary feeling of satisfaction.

For men, pleasure is generally derived from penetration or oral stimulation. For women, pleasure is also derived from penetration or oral stimulation though it should be noted that there is an emotional component that also provides pleasure.

In addition, sensory experience also produces pleasure. Visual stimulation is key while olfactory and auditory stimulation also plays a key role. On the whole, you should strive to combine as many senses as possible during sexual encounters. This will enhance the overall feeling of pleasure derived from the sexual act itself.

Yet, we haven't defined "tantric pleasure."

Tantric pleasure is the result of feeling pleasure at a physical, emotional, and even spiritual level. This type of pleasure is the result of your ability to connect on a deep level with your partner. As such, you are not merely finding physical gratification. You are entering a realm of profound connection that goes beyond the mere physical encounter.

When you hit this level, you are not only satisfying the physical, instinctive desire, but you are also nourishing your spiritual and emotional need for connection. When you really think about it, this is why many folks say they are left with an empty feeling after sex.

What's the reason?

The lack of emotional connection with their partner!

Now, you could develop a strong, emotional connection with someone you've just met. This can happen simply based on the fact that you have an open mind. In other words, you are open to communicating with someone on a deeper level. While this isn't something that happens with everyone you meet, it is something that can certainly happen when you know what you are looking for.

All about physical pleasure

The first step to tantric pleasure is physical. This is the starting point. As such, we can't ignore this point. In fact, if you try to skip physical pleasure and go straight to an emotional connection, you are missing a very important component.

Physical pleasure is vital as this is what fosters the overall enjoyment of the sexual encounter. Even though it's true that you can have a tantric experience without sexual intercourse, there is still a strong physical component. For example, when you have a tantric massage, there is a strong physical connection. Just the fact that you are doing the massage is enough to get you to really feel good at a physical level.

Also, physical pleasure is vital is generating the positive energies that course through your body. Without it, it would be very hard to achieve a sense of wellness. The key here is that there is a clear mind-body-spirit connection. So, you cannot ignore the physical. It is important and must be given its proper place.

Another important aspect of physical pleasure is the sensory experience that goes with a tantric session. You see, we perceive the world around us through our senses. As such, we can't expect to have a full tantric experience without being cognizant of the role our senses play. In this regard, setting the scene is pivotal in ensuring that you, and your partner, get the most out of your experience.

Establishing an emotional connection

As far as emotional connections go, it's not always easy to develop one. If you have ever been with a person in which your relationship did not involve any kind of feelings, then you can appreciate how empty this type of relationship can be. When you are devoid of emotional connections, you can't fully appreciate the level of passion between two people.

That is why tantra focuses heavily on developing intimacy. As we have stated on several occasions, tantra is not necessarily about sex. It's about creating an emotional connection through intimacy, which can bring you and your partner together. When you make a point of executing the exercises we have presented, you can build intimacy with your partner at a very deep level.

Please bear in mind that intimacy is built on trust. When you build trust, you can create a feeling in which you are certain that every encounter with your partner will be a memorable one. Even if there is no sex involved, you can be sure that it will make your life that much more enjoyable.

Emotional connections are also built outside of the bedroom. The overall tantric experience can carry over into your everyday life. If you are in a committed relationship, you can see how the small things truly add up. For instance, showing genuine concern for your partner breeds the type of trust that cannot be easily matched. In addition, your attention and devotion to your partner will signify how much they mean to you.

Does that mean you need to spend every waking moment with them?

Of course not.

But it does mean that the time you devote to them must count. There is no point in spending time with them for the sake of spending time, as this will not foster the type of relationship you are looking to build. That is why your dedication to building intimacy is crucial when it comes to tantra.

Here is an important reflection on intimacy: intimacy is a hard thing to build. It generally takes a long time to build, but it can be easily destroyed. Your actions can quickly undermine the intimacy you have worked hard to build. This is why it's always recommended that you, and your partner, take the time to work out any unresolved issues between you. Such issues create a wedge in between you. So, it's best to get them out of the way so that there is nothing lurking in the shadows.

Building a spiritual connection

Once you have built a strong physical connection and a deep emotional bond, you can then move on to building a spiritual connection. This connection is not easily attained. It is generally the result of trust and understanding. That is why you can't expect to skip a physical and emotional connection in order to get to a spiritual connection.

However, there is a "chicken or the egg" dilemma that arises when considering spiritual connections. Does the spiritual connection happen first, and that leads to a physical connection, or does the physical connection happen first, and that leads to the spiritual connection?

This dilemma can be answered in the following manner:

It depends on the circumstances.

There are times when two people have an instant physical attraction. This is commonly called "chemistry." So, when you see two people have chemistry, they quickly develop a strong physical bond. This bond may be expanded to include an emotional component. For instance, a purely physical relationship can develop into a romance. This romantic nature is when people "fall in love." Thus, it should be noted that falling in love is a question of a deep emotional bond that cannot be cast aside. Then, the relationship may evolve into a deeper spiritual connection. This is commonly seen in those couples who claim to know what their partner is thinking. Such relationships are rare but do provide an interesting point of view on going from a physical to a spiritual connection.

The flip side of this question is when two people are drawn to each other for some mysterious reason. This can be seen in the way "opposites attract," or someone has that "X factor." When you see these relationships, there is a deeper bond that cannot be easily ignored. The spiritual bond can then evolve into a deeper emotional and then physical connection. The end result is a platonic relationship that morphs into a physical one.

In either of these cases, there is a logical process in which the two parties move through a natural progression. It's not the type of thing in which you are hitting things off one day, and then deeply in love the next. Also, you can't expect to admire someone for immaterial reasons and then jump in the sack with them. There has to be a natural progression through the various stages of a deep and meaningful relationship. Granted, there are times when things happen very quickly. However, it's not the type of thing that can happen overnight.

Using tantra as a means of deepening connections

Can tantra be used to help a couple progress through the various stages of a relationship?

We thought you'd never ask!

Tantra is perfect for helping couples go from one stage of their relationship with another. In particular, tantra can help those couples that have been in a relationship for a while but seem to have lost that spark. As such, it's a great way or rekindling that passion that may have been lost over the years. As a matter of fact, tantra has been known to help couples rediscover each other in ways that they may have forgotten. If this sounds like you, then you must try tantra right away.

In the event that you are in a new relationship, tantra can help you settle into a dynamic in which you can go about discovering everything about one another. It can help you set the tone for your relationship moving forward. As a matter of fact, it's a great way of bonding especially if you've had negative experiences in the past. Tantra can deepen the bond between you while also helping you find a balance between the physical and the spiritual.

If you are single, then take this opportunity to wrap your mind around the tantra philosophy. You will find that being alone gives you a good opportunity to assess the situation you are in and make any changes you see fit moving forward. That will enable you to become the best version of yourself. That way, when you are ready to be in a relationship, you can make the most of your time with your new partner.

What could be better than that?

Chapter 12: The Male Orgasm

In a nutshell, the male orgasm is commonly associated with ejaculation. There would be no need to write any more about it if we kept this narrow perspective. However, when we take a broader perspective on this subject, we can see that orgasm and ejaculation are two completely different concepts. Yes, they are linked; however, they are not mutually bound to one another. This implies that men can have orgasms, multiple orgasms even, without the need to ejaculate.

If this is something that surprises you, then you might be surprised to find that an orgasm is not necessarily a physiological response to sexual arousal. Rather, it is an electrochemical reaction in the brain, which triggers the sensation of pleasure.

How does this work?

In order to fully understand how the male orgasm works, it's important to understand the entire dynamic that goes on within the male body and how this pertains to the ultimate climax of pleasure.

How arousal works

Men are predominantly visual creatures. This is the direct result of evolution. The male brain evolved in accordance with the needs and the environment in which early humans developed. Since the traditional male role was that of hunter-gatherer, the male brain developed a much broader set of skills related to vision. Consequently, males are much more inclined toward visuals rather than other senses, such as hearing.

Over the centuries, this visual nature has not diminished. Men are still predominantly visual. This is why many of the typically male professions deal with the measurement of distance and space in addition to calculations of speed, volume, mass, and so on. While this doesn't mean that women cannot do these professions, men are more biologically suited for them.

That being said, arousal in males is typically a visual event. Therefore, males are far more attracted to a visually esthetic female than females would be to a visually attractive male. As such, males tend to focus on a certain set of features that are considered to be attractive. For example, males find a youthful look much more appealing as it signals an instinctive reaction indicating that the female is apt for procreation.

When attraction, at a physical level, takes place, the brain signals the body to start moving blood flow to the genital area. To do this, the heart needs to work a little bit harder to ensure that blood flow is sufficient. In addition, the heart works harder, but blood vessels also need to widen in order to accommodate the increased blood flow. This is what eventually leads to an erection.

Now, let's assume that sex is about to take place. While arousal is happening, there is no sensation of pleasure yet. After all, if there is no "action," then there cannot be any presence of pleasure. This is where traditional sex gets it wrong.

In traditional sexual culture, men are taught to stimulate their genital area in such a way that pleasurable sensations are sent throughout the body; the brain decodes it and floods the body with feel-good chemicals such as endorphins. However, when the arousal stage moves into actual sex, if there is no control over the psychological aspects of the event, then what you end up having is the male ejaculating. This reaction is often confused with orgasm. Yet, it is a known fact that ejaculation and orgasm are two separate phenomena.

Why?

You see, ejaculation is a physiological response that is associated with procreation. Naturally, this function has to feel good. Otherwise, why would humans procreate if sex was unpleasant? Mother nature needed to make sure that it felt good so that the species could reproduce and thrive.

With that in mind, arousal leads to orgasm when a male is able to separate ejaculation from pleasure. When a male is engaged in tantric sex, his focus is moved away from the various aspects of sexual relations to the more emotional and even spiritual aspects of it. As such, his focus is moved away from feeling good physically, to enjoying the overall experience of it.

Many tantra practitioners say that they feel a greater sense of arousal and stimulation by letting go of their physiological sensations and focusing more on the sensory experience. This includes breathing and touching. Also, very powerful emotions are unleashed when males are able to focus on their partner's pleasure in addition to their own.

Getting to the big "O."

At this point, the big "O" becomes a question of the brain being able to process the sensory perception in such a way that it releases massive amounts of endorphins (among other substances) into the bloodstream. There is a cocktail of brain chemicals such as adrenaline and serotonin. The interaction of the chemicals in the brain leads to the overall feeling of pleasure. However, the interaction of these chemicals leads to overloading the nervous system to the point where an incredible sensation of pleasure takes over the entire nervous system in a wave-like manner.

This is an orgasm.

Guys who feel these orgasms during sex report they feel their erections getting stronger without the need to ejaculate. While the pleasure signals are there, they are not directly linked to the overall feeling of needing to ejaculate.

This is how you can separate one thing from the other.

In theory, this sounds all well and fine. But being able to achieve it is an entirely different ballgame. The challenge here is to overcome the conditioning instilled during adolescence. In many cases, adolescent boys learn that "faster is better." Sadly, this is a tremendous disservice that is done to mean as they grow up without being able to truly enjoy sex for what it's worth.

By fostering the erroneous perception that finishing fast is the best way, men are taught to deprive themselves of the magical experience that comes with truly enjoying sex with their chosen partner. When a man is able to achieve true orgasm, there is no comparison. This is why tantra is such a seemingly mysterious art form.

The good news here is that anyone can achieve true orgasms. Best of all, any man can achieve multiple orgasms while only needing to ejaculate once. If this sounds new to you, then do read on as we will describe the steps that you can take you to achieve this.

First, it's time to dissociate orgasm and ejaculation. They are two separate concepts. Orgasms are electrochemical reactions in the brain, while ejaculation is a physiological response to arousal and stimulation. The sooner you are able to separate these concepts from your mind, the sooner you'll be able to truly enjoy the time you spend with your partner.

Next, let go of the idea that the ultimate goal of sex is... sex. Of course, the main point of sex is to engage in intercourse with your partner. However, it is focusing solely on sex that makes it hard for a man to truly enjoy the situation. Generally, there is so much pressure to "perform." As such, this creates unneeded pressure. Why would you put so much pressure on yourself to do something pleasurable? Do you put so much pressure on yourself to eat properly? If you did, you wouldn't know a bit of anything you ate.

The same goes for sex. So, take the time to enjoy and savor all of the emotions, sights, and experiences that come with being someone you are attracted to, or even someone you love. This makes the entire experience much more rewarding.

Now, when you are in the midst of intercourse with your partner, try your best to remove your mind from what you are doing. This sounds paradoxical but the fact that is that if you concentrate on "doing it," then you end up getting caught up in not finishing too soon. Plus, your mind begins to play tricks on you. You start to wonder if your partner is enjoying it or if you are doing it right. These tricks are highly detrimental to your level of satisfaction while limiting the amount of enjoyment the both of you can derive from an encounter.

This is why tantra is about slowing the pace of the game. When you slow the pace of the game, you have the option to exert more control over the situation. If you feel that you are about to lose control, you can slow things down or even stop altogether. Some men find it useful to pull out and focus on touching, kissing, and caressing their partner while things settle down. Again, if your goal is to give your partner an orgasm, then you only see half of the picture. But if your goal is to give your partner the best possible experience, then you are on the right track.

Lastly, use your mind to focus your energy. This means that you ought to use your mind to move your energy throughout your body. Imagine your energy flowing throughout your body, nourishing everything in its path. This energy not only serves as a means of charging the body, but it also serves as a means of helping your body heal and repair itself. That might seem a bit strange. However, sex is known to promote healing energy within the body.

Additionally, you can recycle that energy between you and your partner. This is an energy that you are both sharing as a result of the mutual pleasure that you are sharing. When you both take the time to really savor your encounter, you will find that the "pressure" builds up. As this pressure builds up, the release of energy is an amazing feeling, unlike anything you've felt before. These are the mind-blowing orgasms that come with tantric sex.

Making sense of male pleasure

There is nothing wrong with feeling pleasure. It's a logical consequence of sex. If you believe that feeling pleasure is somehow wrong, you are only hurting yourself insofar as depriving yourself of wonderful experiences. In addition, you are also depriving your partner of having a wonderful experience alongside you.

So, finding true tantric pleasure is about framing your mind in such a way that you can enjoy the situation by taking in all the senses. Therefore, you can't rush this process. This isn't the type of process which you can complete with an egg timer. This is the type of process in which you need to be present at the moment things are happening. If your mind is wandering off, then you can't really make it work. By the same token, if your mind is focused on "performing," then the chances of you actually enjoying your encounter is far less.

Experienced tantra practitioners know that sex isn't about keeping score. There isn't some magic number that you need to hit in order to considered "good." What you will find is that there is a threshold in which you know you are moving in the right direction. This threshold is different for everyone. Nevertheless, your partner will be quite clear in showing you where they are going. If the experience is pleasurable for them, they will surely make it obvious.

So, if you are putting pressure on yourself to perform, it's time to drop those expectations and focus on sex for what

424

it is. Take the time to assess your expectations and bring them into perspective. Your job, if you will, is to create an experience that your partner will thoroughly enjoy. This includes everything around you, from the scene, the sights, smells, sounds, and of course, sex.

Beyond that, please keep in mind that sex is a work in progress. You can't expect to hit the heights of tantric sex right away. While the guidelines we have laid out will make an immediate impact, you can't expect to hit the heights immediately. It takes time to really click with your partner. Of course, it doesn't take years, but it does take a concerted effort to make sure that you and your partner get what you want about of your sex life.

Chapter 13: The Female Orgasm

In most literature, it seems that the female orgasm is shrouded in mystery. Some so-called experts claim that it's quite easy to find multiple orgasms. They make it seems as though there is some kind of switch you can simply flip and off you go.

Other gurus make it seem like it some kind of unattainable phenomenon that can only be uncovered by the proprietary method. As such, you stand no chance of achieving orgasm unless you follow their time-tested, patented moves.

The fact of the matter is that the female orgasm works in the same way that the male orgasm does. The female orgasm is an electrochemical reaction that releases all of the chemicals that produce the wonderful feelings that come with having a good time in bed.

However, it is also important to point out that the road to the female orgasm is different. Even if the overall reaction is the same for both men and women, getting there is a bit different. This means that you need to focus on the various components that lead up to the big "O."

In this chapter, we are going to be focusing on the elements which lead up to that big "O." In particular, we're going to be discussing the main reasons why reaching orgasm can be difficult. With the ideas that we will present, you'll be able to get a much broader perspective on the limitations that you may be encountering.

Arousal in women

Unlike men, women are not predominantly visual. Yes, women find visual stimulation highly enjoyable. Women value the visual esthetics of an attractive individual as much as men do. The difference is that women do not value visual attractiveness above everything else. In fact,

426

women tend to value visual symmetry a lot more than men do.

When talking about symmetry, it's important to keep in mind that women enjoy men who look proportionate. That is why most women don't find bodybuilders particularly attractive. The same goes for men who are too thin or those who are obese. The secret is maintaining a proportionate look in terms of height and weight. This means that while men don't need a chiseled body to be attractive, trying to maintain proper proportions makes a huge difference.

The way arousal works in women is that you have an overall sensory experience that leads to a set of emotions. It is this emotional connection between sex and emotions that leads to a pleasant sexual experience. In a manner of speaking, if your heart is not into it, then arousal can be hard to pursue.

Of course, there is instinctive arousal which is mainly driven by the need for physical intimacy. However, this need for physical intimacy is often confused with sex. Sadly, culture has reduced intimacy with sex. The reality is that sex is only one part of intimacy. This is why we have made a strong case for the need to incorporate intimacy in your life without making sex the main priority. When you take the need for sex out of the equation, you are left with the entire scene around you. When this scene isn't there, then you have no choice but to build it.

Fostering arousal should then become about creating a safe atmosphere in which you feel comfortable being yourself. Now, this is crucial as feeling uncomfortable, in any way, can be a huge detrimental factor in limiting your ability to truly enjoy sex. When you feel comfortable with yourself and everything you are doing, then you can certainly make things work as best as it can for you.

What's holding you back

Inexperienced individuals tend to relate the inability to orgasm to physiological factors. They believe that there is something physical that affects your ability to orgasm. The fact is that there are many more psychological and emotional factors that affect your ability to orgasm. That's why the exercises in this book have been presented so that you can put yourself in the proper frame of mind. When this occurs, you are able to truly make yourself feel open and liberated. When you find this sense of liberation, you can then go about enjoying yourself to the fullest.

So, what's holding you back?

The fact is that there is any number of issues which can wreak havoc on your mind at any given point. In particular, being uncomfortable with your body can play a largely detrimental role in helping you liberate yourself. You see, we tend to compare ourselves to certain standards all the time. We compared ourselves to "good" mothers, "successful" professionals, or "good-looking" people.

When it comes to you, and your physical appearance, there is no need to compare yourself to anyone else. Sure, you might be keen on improving your physical conditioning and fitness. But that doesn't mean you are not attractive. If your partner values you for who you are, then you already have the most important aspect of attractiveness. This is why it's important to let go of such hang-ups in the bedroom. Being too overly focused on this aspect will limit your ability to truly enjoy yourself.

Also, stress plays a huge factor in holding you back. When stress gets the best of you, it can be nearly impossible to shut your mind off. If anything, you'll be faced with nagging voices in your head that won't leave you alone. You might be really enjoying yourself when you are suddenly hit with a flood of thoughts regarding any number of things. These thoughts can totally undermine your ability to truly enjoy yourself.

To combat this, the breathing and relaxation techniques we have presented are highly effective. In addition, making time for yourself and your partner means that you have the freedom to enjoy yourselves without being concerned with other things. Just being able to forget about your phone for a while is enough to get you feeling completely liberated from the world around you.

Another crucial factor is to address any issues that may be driving a wedge between you and your partner. Unfortunately, all couples have issues, especially if they have been together for a while. Often, unresolved issues fester beneath the surface. So, you don't really see them superficially. But below the surface, they are clearly affecting the way you interact with your partner. As such, if there is anything that is affecting your relationship, it's important to deal with it, get it out of the way, and move on. If you let it sit there, it will gnaw at you. This will become evident as you engage in tantric practices. You might start okay, but if such thoughts should hit you, you won't be able to recover. You'll have no choice to get over it or struggle with them throughout your tantric sessions.

Getting to the big "O."

There is a general misconception that it is hard to get to the big "O." The fact is that it's neither easy nor hard. It's just a question of knowing how to go about it. This implies that when you are committed to the experience you are living, you can find the pleasure you seek. Many times, it's just a matter of getting lost in the moment. This is why we have mentioned the need to live "in the now." When you manage to get everything out of the way, you can find the path to true pleasure and ecstasy.

Unfortunately, the big "O" seems like an elusive target. This occurs when you are completely focused on getting there without really taking in the entire experience. This puts unnecessary pressure on you. After all, why make orgasms the main attraction to sex when there are so many other things happening?

This is an important consideration as sex is filled with various situations and occurrences. You have intimacy, touch, sights, scents, and also your role in giving your partner pleasure. With all of those things happening all at once, there is no reason why you should become fixated on just one.

When you let go of your pursuit of the big "O," you will find that everything becomes much more enjoyable. You won't find yourself completely focused on getting there. Rather, you will enjoy the journey, so to speak. It's a means of enjoying the read even if you don't reach the final destination. Sure, it would be great if you did, but if you don't, it wouldn't be the end of the world.

Something else to consider is that tantra allows you to build up enough experience so that you can learn exactly what buttons to push and when to push them. The various exercises that we have presented throughout this book will enable you to find the right spots for you. This means that you won't have to guess. You'll know exactly where the road will take you. Ultimately, this is a comforting situation as you won't have to doubt or second-guess yourself.

The path to the big "O."

Here is a very simple exercise which you can do to get you to the big "O" every time.

First, think about the road you will be traveling on. This could be a massage, a massage followed by sex, or perhaps just a moment of intimacy with your partner. When you visualize what you are about to do with your partner, it builds anticipation. This anticipation plays a nice erotic game with you as you become expectant of what can happen. When you build up with anticipation, you naturally become aroused. Unless you're not feeling up to it, just the sheer anticipation of a sexual encounter is enough to get your curiosity moving.

Next, see with your eyes what your partner is doing. Take in the sights, sounds, and scents of what's going. This could be a massage, cuddling, or intercourse. It really doesn't matter. The idea is to take in everything that's happening.

Then, close your eyes and try to "see" it in your mind's eye. Try to visualize everything movement, touch, or thrust. In a manner of speaking, you are translating what your body feels to what your mind can see. If you wish, you can limit your visual capabilities. For example, a blindfold or sleeping mask can work quite well.

Since your mind is occupied trying to recreate a visual from what you are feeling, you are more concentrated on taking in the sensory experience rather than actually seeing the events unfold. As you render these images in your mind, you will find that the sensory experience builds up.

After, try your best to anticipate the next move. If you are in control, say in a cowgirl position, try to anticipate your next move. In a manner of speaking, you are planning what to do next as you go. When you do this, you are building up even more anticipation. As such, you are avoiding a mechanical motion by transforming in order to into a fluid movement.

Lastly, as you feel the pressure building up, don't try to chase the big "O." Instead, picture that energy coursing through your body. Imagine how that energy can race through every fiber of your body. When you feel it rushing toward you, don't try to catch it. Just let it come to you. If you try to pursue it, you'll end up disappointing yourself as you may not end up catching up to it. In fact, orgasms can be quite elusive once you are really close. However, when you don't make a point of trying to catch it, then you'll find that it will simply come to you. And when it does, you'll know it's there. You'll be able to relish in the feeling that comes with experience full-on pleasure. In the end, you won't have anything to surpass the feeling that comes with finding yourself completely immersed in this kind of experience.

If that isn't enough for you, then don't worry. There is still more to come!

Chapter 14: Individual Ecstasy

Thus far, we have presented an extensive approach that can lead you, at your partner, to find pleasure and ecstasy. In a manner of speaking, this is about working in tandem to reach this goal. However, pleasure is an individual feeling that may, or may not, be easily achieved. It's important to take this into consideration as it's not always easy to find the bliss that you seek. If only it were as easy as turning on a faucet.

This is why experienced tantra practitioners are just as able to find pleasure themselves as they are able to help their partners find it. This becomes even more important when an experienced tantra practitioner finds a partner who is new to it. By virtue of their experience, they can help the newcomer find the heights of sexual pleasure.

In this chapter, we are going to take a look at how you can help your partner find pleasure and ecstasy, especially in those cases when it is hard for them to focus, enjoy themselves, and make the most of your experiences together.

Helping your partner find ecstasy

There are times when, for any number of reasons, your partner just isn't getting there. This could be due to something like being unable to forget about a stressful event, or perhaps having trouble reaching the big "O." This is where both of you need to keep in mind that the goal is not to find the biggest possible "O" or to last for four hours. The main idea here is to enjoy each other's company. This ought to be at the forefront of your mind all the time.

As such, you and your partner need to drop all of the expectations and focus on being together. That's all. All you need is to focus on the moment by savoring all of the emotions that come with enjoying the time you spend together. When you look at things from this perspective, you can't possibly go wrong.

Consider this situation:

Your partner's head is just not in it. They had a hard time at the office or perhaps some work-related problems. They are upset and can't seem to relax. Consequently, they just can't seem to enjoy themselves. Now, the worst thing you can do at this point is to assume that it's something related to you. In other words, take it personally.

Why would you?

Unless the issue is between the both of you, there is no reason why you should take it personally. Sadly, some folks think that they're partner isn't into it because they aren't attracted or don't like sex anymore.

This could not be further from the truth.

In this regard, it's important to take the pressure off as much as possible. In fact, there are times when you might have no choice but to just shut things down. You may end up simply cuddling. There may be times when all your partner needs is reassurance. Sure, this sounds easy, but it can be really tough when you have your motor firing on all cylinders. In that case, you can make a game of it. Perhaps your partner might find it relaxing to watch you taking care of business yourself.

The point here is to eliminate pressure. Tantric sex is not the type of practice you can master when on the clock. Relaxation and focus are essential to making it work. Otherwise, it would be nearly impossible for you to find the way to ultimate ecstasy.

Please try to make sure that you have zero expectations when going into the bedroom.

How so?

434

If you enter the bedroom thinking, "I am going to have five orgasms today," then anything short of that will be a disappointment. If you change that attitude to "I am going to enjoy my time with my partner," then you are setting a different kind of expectation. You are focusing your mind on what truly matters, which is, enjoying the moment with your partner.

Relaxation is the key

Stress and anxiety are mojo killers. You don't need to be stressed out about anything in particular to kill the mood. The regular stress of day-to-day life is enough to bury arousal and pleasure. This is why relaxation is a fundamental tenet of tantra. You cannot expect to have a full-blown tantric experience if you are not relaxed and fully prepared to enjoy this experience.

Nevertheless, finding the ultimate relaxation isn't easy. In fact, it can be nearly impossible to settle down and find the right path toward peace and calm. Here is where you can see that tantra is not about sex. If you reduce your encounters to merely sex, then you are missing the point. Sex is the ultimate byproduct of the intimacy you have built with your partner. If you can't enjoy that, then you ought to reassess your priorities.

What to do if your partner just isn't into it?

At first, it might be really disappointing, especially if you are all fired up and they are not. This can be especially frustrating if you don't have much time to spend together. Yet, getting upset is the last thing you want to do. Instead, trying to foster an atmosphere of relaxation is key.

When you set the stage for your tantric encounters, you have any number of tools at your disposal. You can rely on a quick massage to help your partner calm down. Or, you can practice breathing in tandem. And then there's meditation. Often, just lying down together and guiding them through a visualization exercise can help lighten the mood.

Here is a quick visualization exercise that you can do with your partner:

First, lie in bed together. It's best that you don't cuddle or hold each other as you want your partner to settle down. But, if you feel inclined to do, then that's fine, too.

Then, sync your breathing. You can count out loud using the 1,2,3,4 technique. Take three shallow breaths and then one deep breath. As you exhale, try to picture the air leaving your lungs and floating off into space.

After, take your partner through a visual journey. You can describe anything you feel your partner will enjoy. If you want to describe an erotic situation, that could work great, as well. The point here is to help your partner calm down by using any means at your disposal.

If you happen to fall asleep, that's great, too. Just the fact that you fell asleep is signal enough that the experience was relaxing.

Ultimately, being patient with your partner is paramount to achieving the level of intimacy and connection you seek. Plus, who knows when you might be the one who needs a helping hand. In that case, your partner's patience would certainly be most welcome.

Being supportive and understanding

Perhaps the most important thing you can do when things aren't going too well is to be supportive of your partner. After all, if you weren't feeling your best, you would expect your partner to be understanding and supportive, right?

This is the reason why you need to focus on helping your partner feel as comfortable as possible, especially when things aren't going smoothly. In fact, just being there can be enough to give your partner the reassurance they need to feel better.

In contrast, if you get upset and make a big deal out it, then you can be sure your tantric session will go down the drain.

Consider this situation:

The male partner is having trouble getting an erection. This situation can be a potential dealbreaker. That is true if your only purpose is to engage in penetrative intercourse.

But then again, what if you threw that out of the window?

What if you figure out other things to do?

This is where being supportive and understanding play a huge role. After all, the male partner is already under enough stress. So, removing the pressure and replacing it with understanding is the best way to make things work.

Now, let's consider a different scenario:

The female partner can't seem to focus. Things are going as planned, but she just can't seem to settle down enough to reach the big "O." It seems that no matter how much effort is put into, she just can't seem to get there. This can be common especially in situations of high emotional stress.

So, the male partner, rather than feeling disappointed that his partner wasn't able to get there, can turn things around and help her relax. For instance, slowing things down by cuddling, kissing, and touching can all help reduce stress. Of course, this isn't a full guarantee that everything will suddenly turn around. But just being supportive and understanding is enough to get the female partner in the best possible frame of mind.

Please keep in mind that one of the core tenets of tantra is to help your partner reach their pleasure. While it is true that you are not responsible for their feelings, it is important to consider the vital role you play. You can be the guide that leads them down the path they need to take. All you are doing is facilitating the way. You are, by no means, the one who is responsible for their pleasure. As we have stated numerous times, this is a journey in which we must all go through. But your support, understanding, and patience are all key to helping your partner get the emotional connection you both seek.

It's a two-way street

Indeed, tantric sex is a two-way street. It's important to bear this in mind as "traditional" sex isn't always a two-way street. In fact, traditional sex is generally about one of the partners enjoying themselves while the other may, or may not, get something out of it.

This is very common when male partners are inconsiderate of their female partner's pleasure. By the same token, this can occur when females put unnecessary pressure on their male partner. As such, the female gets the attention she seeks while the male is under stress to perform.

These situations all reflect cases in which mutual pleasure is not the main focus.

Think about that for a minute…

When you are convinced that the goal of sex is to simply enjoy yourselves, you'll find that getting to the big "O" is not nearly as hard as you might think. But then again, the big "O" isn't the only thing you can shoot for. Just being there for one another is the most important thing that you can do to foster the intimacy you seek.

Ultimately, it all boils down to knowing that tantric sex is about giving and receiving. You ought to be cognizant of how important it is to play on both sides of the ball. When you are perfectly aware that it is just as exciting and pleasure to give as it is to receive, then you will uncover the true nature of tantric sex.

As a matter of fact, experienced tantric sex practitioners will tell you that there is an incredible rush that comes from seeing your partner reaching the heights of ecstasy because you led them there. The same can be said about the type of ecstasy you can achieve as a result of being with your partner. This type of satisfaction is unmatched.

Lastly, helping your partner find their ecstasy is not your responsibility. In fact, none of what happens in the bedroom is anyone's responsibility. This is what makes tantra so great; you are doing things because you want to, not because you have to. There is nothing that says that you have to help your partner reach the heights of ecstasy. Your role is to be the guide for your partner, especially when they are going through a rough time.

When you are able to do that, the level of connection that is built cannot be questioned. This is the type of rock-solid intimacy that builds strong couples regardless of whether they are in a committed relationship or not.

Chapter 15: Couples Ecstasy

By now, you are fully prepared to take intimacy to the highest possible level. This means that you are now ready to make the best of your experiences by sharing in the sheer pleasure that comes with enjoying time with your partner. You now have the tools to make the most of your encounters. This means that all you need is to take the time to put the exercises into practice. That is why we have stated multiple times throughout this book that the most important thing is to focus on what you are experiencing at the moment, the "here" and the "now."

With that in mind, this chapter is about enjoying tantra as a couple. However, this chapter goes beyond what we have already discussed. We are going to see how you can enjoy ecstasy as a couple, particularly during sexual encounters. This means enjoying some "Os" while also enjoying the pleasure which you can derive from your partner's satisfaction.

Taking turns

A common misconception in the world of tantra is that true mastery of tantra implies that the couple orgasms at the same time. While this is certainly an amazing feeling, the fact is that it is quite difficult to accomplish as men and women have differing rhythms. Consequently, you might be building up unrealistic expectations when assuming that you must both orgasm at the same time.

When looking at tantric pleasure, there is nothing wrong with taking turns. In fact, taking turns can be a rather liberating experience.

How so?

By taking turns, you are essentially freeing yourself up to fully enjoy pleasure. This means that you don't necessarily have to focus on your partner. You can let yourself go freely. This will open up the road to mind-blowing orgasms.

Of course, there is no need to feel guilty. This is hardly selfish as you are not taking your partner for granted. All you are doing is going with it. Then, you can totally devote your focus on your partner. This will allow them to experience the same kind of pleasure you have.

The opposite also works very well.

Perhaps you are inclined to pleasuring your partner first so that you can free yourself up for the big one. Ultimately, it doesn't really matter who goes first. The only thing that matters is that you are both on the same page. It could be that on one occasion, you hit the big "O" before your partner does. On another occasion, it could be that your partner gets there ahead of you. As such, it doesn't matter. What does matter is that you both take the time to make your encounters as pleasure able as possible.

There is one caveat to taking turns:

Please don't feel that you are entitled to receive or obligated to give. In this regard, taking advantage of your partner can be dangerous insofar as creating feelings of neglect. Your partner may feel that you are only taking advantage of them while they don't get their fair share. By the same token, if you feel that you are only giving and not getting your fair share, then try to avoid feeling resentful or even cheated.

The key here is to foster communication at all times. When you foster proper communication, you are giving yourself the opportunity to be on the same page all the time. This is especially important when something doesn't go right. Rather than blaming each other, you can figure out what didn't work right and seek to rectify it. Over time, you will get into such a groove that you won't have to think things through. You will know exactly what to do and when to do it.

Reaching the big "O" together

One of the most challenging things about tantra is reaching that big "O" in unison. While difficult, it is not impossible. All it requires is careful pacing and synchronicity. Some couple strive to achieve this ability. They feel that being able to reach that big "O" together, even after multiple "Os" before that, can truly foster the intimate tantric experience.

Now, if you don't reach that big "O" together, it doesn't mean that you didn't shoot through the roof. But by reaching the big "O" together, you can make the most of a unique experience that is quite uncommon among average couples.

Here is an exercise which you can do to help you reach that big "O" together.

First, it's important to recognize each other's rhythms and patterns. Generally speaking, one partner tends to reach the big "O" sooner than the other. This is regardless of whether it's the male or female partner. Although males generally tend to climax sooner than females. As you become aware of these individual patterns, you'll be able to recognize the pace for each partner.

Next, sync your breathing as much as possible. When the action gets hot and heavy, it can be hard to keep the same tempo. The partner that is getting closer to the climax will generally breathe a lot faster than the other. As such, the partner who is breathing slower must help the other to match the slower pace. This is helpful in controlling orgasm, particularly in men.

Then, as your breathing syncs, you can then match your movements accordingly. In particular, if you feel that you are losing control, slowing the pace of the game down is essential. As you match your movements, you can regain that flow thereby matching each other's arousal. As you feel the tension build up inside one another, you can increase the tempo as desired.

After, talk to each other. You can develop a code word to signal your partner where you lie. A color code is usually the easiest. For instance, "green" means things are going well but not quite at the climax. "Yellow" can be used to indicate you are close while "red" means you are getting ready to blast off. The goal here is for both of you to stay on the same color. That way, you can increase or decrease tempo as the color code demands.

Lastly, don't try to time the big "O." Most of the time, one will get there slightly before the other. In fact, many couples indicate that one's big "O" is triggered by the other's orgasm. In a manner of speaking, one's pleasure gets the other over the edge.

What could be better than that?

After the grand finale

What do you do following the grand finale is just as important as everything else that happened prior to it. Lots of couples enjoy lying in place when engaging in intercourse. They purposely make a point of not pulling out as this helps foster that intimacy between them. This is a perfect time to continue breathing in sync while taking advantage of the opportunity for kissing and touching. Many times, the emotions are so intense that it takes a while to recover from it. As such, pulling out immediately after the big finale tends to be a mood killer.

Once you have decided to pull out, it's important to savor the moment. While you might hear a lot of experts say you need to cuddle, spoon, or remain physically close, the fact is that it's up to you. You can choose to cuddle or perhaps just lie together. Sometimes, emotions are so intense that you're practically speechless.

Some couples like to shower together afterward. This provides even more opportunity for intimacy. Others would rather just cuddle up and spend time together. Others still like to spend some time just talking. You might find that these are moments in which you have the most heartfelt talks with your partner. This is why "pillow talk" has become synonymous with pouring your heart out.

Ultimately, it doesn't really matter what you choose to do. The important thing is to savor the moment with your partner. The last thing that you want to do is get up, shower, and get dressed immediately following a powerful moment.

Sure, you might experience some unusual feelings. There are cases in which folks mention that emotions get all stirred up, especially if you are going through a tough time. This can happen. But that's when both partners need to be on the same page. Often, you don't have to say a word. Just taking a minute to live the moment is enough to truly nourish your soul.

One final consideration

For those who believe that tantra is a set of rules which you must follow to the letter, they could not be farther from the truth. The fact is that tantra is a discipline which has a set of guidelines that you are completely free to mold in your particular means and ways.

After all, humans are all different. There is no question about that. The core issue lies in the fact that you need to discover what works best for you. This is why tantra is best practiced with a partner whom you have a relationship with. And while it's true that we have stated the fact that you can have a tantric experience with someone you have recently met, the best results come from practicing tantra with a partner whom you have full confidence in.

When you have full confidence in your partner, you are psychologically free to explore everything there is to explore your sexuality. To sum things up, anything goes! Yes, really, anything goes. This is why you need to go about finding what really makes you and your partner tick.

If you are into BDSM, that's fine. You can have a full tantric experience within the domain of BDSM. There is nothing in the tantra philosophy that says you can't engage in BDSM and have the full tantric treatment.

If your idea of having a tantric experience is to go out to a club and then hit the sack, that's perfectly fine, too. The point here is to find that balance that will help you reach the mind-blowing heights that you wish to reach.

For couples with kids and an overall busy lifestyle, reconnecting through tantra is a must. Try your best to clear your schedule, make time for each other, and just forget about the world. You don't need to run off on vacation for two months. Even a single afternoon can do wonder for your relationship. By being able to let go of everything around you, you can find the peace you need to really get in touch with your sexuality. Best of all, this isn't the type of practice you need to spend money on. You can set the stage in a very simple manner, have the house to yourselves, and have at it.

Tantra is about finding the zone that will eventually lead you to that impressive feeling of lust, connection, intimacy, and pleasure. In the end, you don't need to have a complicated set of positions and rituals. With tantra, what works for you is what works best. Please resist the temptation to compare yourself to others. They do what works for them. You do what works for you. Ultimately, this is the goal of tantra. In the event that you have multiple partners, then you will realize that different approaches work for different couples. As a result, becoming familiar with the person you are with is the fundamental axiom of tantra.

Conclusion

Thank you very much for taking the time to read this book. We hope that you have found everything you wanted to know about tantra and how you can make it work for you and your partner.

Now, you might be asking yourself, "what's next?"

If you haven't already started trying out the exercises we have laid out in this volume, then the time has come to do so. If you feel your partner is on the fence, talk to them! Ask them to read this book, too. It could be that they just need a little more information about the topic.

Once you are ready to try things out, the most important thing to keep in mind is to go slow. Don't rush things. The biggest mistake that couples make when starting out it to rush things. Allow things to flow naturally. Eventually, you will find your own rhythm. By then, you will have the experience you seek to find.

Please keep in mind that anything goes with tantra. As long as you follow the main guidelines we have set forth in this book, you will find the overall tantric experience to be the most rewarding of your life.

So, what are you waiting for?

The time has come for you to savor the most amazing sexual experience of your life. You will find that once you go tantra, you won't go back.

Thank you once again for taking the time to read this book. If you have found it to be useful and informative, please tell others about it. We are sure they too, will find it useful.

See you next time!

FEMDOM

Dominant Sex With a Dom Female. How to Make Him Your Sex Slave. Turn Your Man Into a Quivering Sub.
BDSM, Spanking Tactics...

contained within this document, including, but not limited to, — errors, omissions, or inaccuracies.

Table of Contents

Introduction

Welcome to the FEMDOM world! If this is your first time experiencing this type of relationship, then you are in for a treat. You will find that embracing your dominant nature is one of the most liberating experiences you can have in life. It's a means of acknowledging who you are, and most importantly, giving yourself the chance to express who you really want to be.

In this book, we are going to explore the FEMDOM dynamic, what this type of relationship is like, and how you can take your male partner from where they currently stand and turn them into your personal plaything. If that sounds too good to be true, then rest assured that it is far more common than you think.

If you have experienced the FEMDOM dynamic but want to explore it further, you will find a trove of information in this book that you won't easily find anywhere else. This book is meant to help you put the pieces together of a FEMDOM puzzle that will lead you to your ultimate desires.

We are going to explore what FEMDOM is, what it is all about, and how you can transform your man into an obedient sub. The fact of the matter is that there are no limits here. We will be testing your limits and those of your sub.

This volume is intended for women who are looking to embrace their dominant side. The techniques outlined in this book are meant to take your dominant self and put it to the test. While we won't be talking about purposely hurting your partner, we will be talking about inflicting as much pain as they can tolerate.

Don't worry; we won't be dealing with brutal, medieval torture. But we will be talking about the ways in which your man will gladly take pain and humiliation all because they enjoy it. If anything, they enjoy making you happy, and whatever makes you happy makes them happy.

This is quite a power rush.

So, if you're ready to explore your dominant side, then keep on reading. This book contains a progressive list of techniques that are meant to test your male submissive's limits. With each technique, you will grind their willpower into dust. Eventually, you will have a fully compliant submissive that will stop at nothing to please you.

If you believe that's too good to be true, you'd be surprised to find that it's actually quite common. There are plenty of men out there who wish for nothing more than to have a truly dominant woman do with them as she pleases. But in order to deliver on your expectations, you need to understand the ways of the FEMDOM dynamic. That's why this book is your ultimate guide to FEMDOM.

Please bear in mind that anything goes in the FEMDOM world so long as both partners mutually consent. This isn't about forcing your partner to do something they don't want to do. This is about getting them to willingly accept your dominance over them... and love it!

Part I: Getting Started With FEMDOM

Chapter 1: What Is FEMDOM and What it Is Not

There is a great deal of ideas surrounding FEMDOM in popular culture. In film, you generally see a leather-clad female pummeling a puny and insignificant male. In pornographic films, there is a varying degree of violence inflicted upon male submissives. Moreover, you find that these "subs" actually enjoy the pain they are receiving. In fact, it seems as though male subs seem to welcome the pain they feel.

The fact is that FEMDOM is a type of power dynamic that isn't necessarily like the depictions you see in film and pornography. FEMDOM is based on a power dynamic that is typical of all human relations. When you think about it, human society is based on hundreds of these power dynamics. These dynamics receive the name of "dominance hierarchies."

A dominance hierarchy implies that there is someone who controls others. Traditional hierarchies, particularly those seen in male-dominated societies, put women in a position of inferiority. This leads to women being subjugated to the will and desire of the males who control society. While discussing the abuse that women are subjected to in male-dominated societies is beyond the scope of this book, it's worth pointing out that modern society is geared toward giving women their rightful power back.

As such, FEMDOM is a dominance hierarchy in which a dominant woman exerts her influence over a submissive man. It is also important to point out that in this book, we are going to focus on a dominant female controlling a submissive male. This is an important distinction as there are FEMDOM relationships in which it is a dominant female and a submissive female. However, we won't be doing down that path in this volume.

Dominant-Submissive Relationships

Generally speaking, all male-female relationships have some kind of power dynamic. As such, one of the partners is naturally more dominant than the other. When a dominant person enters a relationship with a naturally submissive person, the power dynamic tends to balance out. So, the naturally dominant individual has no trouble getting along with the submissive partner. In fact, the submissive partner welcomes the control that the dominant individual holds.

Regardless of whether the dominant individual is male or female, a relationship among a natural dominant and natural submissive makes things work out well enough. Things get complicated when two dominant individuals enter a relationship. This dynamic creates a power struggle in which both individuals want to subdue the other. This is quite common with a dominant female and a "regular" male. Even if a regular male isn't a naturally dominant, there is always a degree of resistance on their part to the dominance exerted by the female. This is both instinctive and culture. After all, it's not "cool" to accept, as a man, that they are dominated by a female.

This power struggle generally leads to the deterioration of the relationship unless the female gives up trying to be dominant, or the male accepts that they are not naturally dominant and should assume a more submissive role. Such outcomes are hard to come by, particularly as a dominant female should not have to compromise for the sake of making an insecure male "happy."

What Is a FEMDOM Relationship?

So, defining FEMDOM takes us down a path of the sexual dynamic that occurs between males and females. Typically, males are expected to be dominant in the bedroom. Now, this by no means implies that violence by a male on a female is justified. What this does imply is that the male is expected to lead the interaction among the couple during sexual intercourse. When the male is unable to lead, then the female is left with the task of leading the way. If the female is not naturally dominant, then this might create serious issues for the couple in question.

Generally speaking, the power dynamic from the relationship itself tends to carry over into the bedroom. This means that if the male is naturally dominant and the female is naturally submissive, then this dynamic will carry over into the bedroom. On the contrary, if the female is naturally dominant and the male is naturally submissive, then this dynamic should also carry over into the bedroom.

The challenge then becomes to get the submissive male to embrace the fact that they should follow the lead of a female in all matters sexual. This female dominance can be reflected in something as simple as having the female initiate intercourse. Furthermore, it can be expanded into something as broad as female dominants exerting violence and pain into their submissive male.

The FEMDOM relationship is born when the man accepts that they are submissive and that their female dominant (also referred to as a "dom" or "dominatrix") is the one in charge of the entire sexual dynamic. This dynamic can then extend to whatever levels the couple feels comfortable with. In some cases, submissive males simply seek a female dom as a "power figure." Other male submissives (henceforth referred to as "subs") seek a maternal figure. In other words, they want to be "babied" by their dom. This is seen in some films in which the male dresses up as a baby and crawls around on the floor.

Also, FEMDOM relationships can extend into the world of BDSM. This is a domain which we will explore in this book with great detail. It should be noted that the typical definition of a dominatrix is a female who literally reduces a man into dust. This is where BDSM can be used to practically humiliate a man into the lowest common denominator. Of course, we're not espousing violence or belittling anyone. Yet, the power dynamic that emerges between a dominatrix and her subs takes on some very wild overtones. And yes, professional dominatrices tend to have multiple subs.

The psychology of FEMDOM Relationships

A FEMDOM relationship is predicated on the psychological factors that lead a male sub to accept their submissiveness. By the same token, a female dom must embrace her dominance. This implies breaking the traditional societal role that places women as the "weak" sex. Women can be just as dominant or even more so than men. As such, female doms must embrace their dominance so that they can fully derive the pleasure that comes with exerting their dominance over males.

As for males, the first step is to acknowledge their submissiveness. This step is by far the most significant step that a man can take in their journey toward becoming the sub that they truly are. Then, a female dom can go about teaching a male sub in the ways of becoming a true sub.

At this point, we will look at two different perspectives.

First, let's consider a committed relationship (boyfriend-girlfriend or husband-wife). In this type of relationship, the male accepts that their female partner is the dom. As such, the male then relinquishes their control over to the female with the understanding that she has his best interest in mind and that everything that happens between them is of mutual consent. This is very important as the intention here is to break down the male's resistance. If the male is not completely on board, then the chances of the relationship working out are slim. Of course, there is always some kind of resistance at the beginning, but then again, that's what the exercises in this book are all about.

458

Second, let's consider a non-committed relationship. Under this concept, we can take those relationships in which the interaction is solely based on sex or those relationships which are casual, a type of "friends with benefits" arrangement, so to speak. In this type of relationship, the interaction is based solely on sex, and thus the female dom must be ready to exert all of her influence on the male sub. In these types of relationships, males tend to purposely seek out female doms so that they can directly engage in this type of relationship. In some cases, inexperienced male subs may seek out an experienced female dom to "teach" them the ways of being a sub. Under these circumstances, the male sub will be far more willing to accept being submissive.

Whether you are in a committed or non-committed relationship, it's best to lay down the ground rules first. There needs to be a clear consensus about what the relationship entails, and most importantly, how far the male is willing to go. Limits and boundaries are important. However, it is just as important for males to accept that they must be willing to push their own boundaries.

A good way of looking at boundaries in a FEMDOM relationship is by comparing them to a regular BDSM relationship. Both the dom and the sub have their boundaries. These boundaries must be respected at all times. Anything beyond that can be agreed to mutually. This is important to ensure both safety and pleasure.

What a FEMDOM Is Not

A dom-sub relationship is not synonymous with an abusive relationship. A first glance, the boundaries between a dom-sub relationship and an abusive one tends to be quite blurry. But when you drill down, you will find that there is a clear distinction.

An abusive relationship is generally defined as one partner, causing harm to the other. This means that the abuser says and does things to the victim, which causes them physical and psychological harm. This includes assault, sexual abuse, and psychological distress. Such relationships are unacceptable and should be ended immediately. Sadly, traditional cultural perception places a sub-dom relationship, such as BDSM, as "mutually-agreed violence."

Consequently, FEMDOM is not some type of weak justification for a female to purposely harm males. Yes, there is a high degree of aggression involved, particularly in torture techniques. And yes, there is a high degree of masochism on the part of the sub, but at the end of the day, both parties are perfectly aware of the events taking place and are in perfect agreement. This is why consent is fundamental. In some cases, paperwork is signed in order to ensure mutual consent.

FEMDOM relationships are also a means of allowing both males and females to explore this sexuality. As such, a FEMDOM relationship is not a female using "mind control" over a male. This may be hard for casual observers to understand. Deep down, subs want to be dominated. They want to be humiliated. They want to be tortured. In a manner of speaking, it's like deriving pleasure from pain. By the same token, the dom has a sadistic side to them as they derive pleasure from inflicting pain on their sub.

Sure, we could go into the psychological and emotional causes of this behavior. But the fact of the matter is we are simply acknowledging reality. A female dom derives pleasure from exerting their influence over a male, while a male sub derives pleasure from being subjugated to the will and desire of a female.

One rather interesting explanation for this behavior lies in the fact that people who are in positions of power tend to become overwhelmed with responsibility. As such, having intimate encounters in which they are free to surrender power over to someone else can prove to be liberating.

However, there is a caveat here: anyone who is truly dominant will do anything in their power to avoid relinquishing power. As such, they will try their hardest to keep control. Often, this implies going to great lengths in order to remain in control of the situation, and the people, around them.

Ultimately, a FEMDOM relationship is about what both partners want to get out of it. For one, it's the rush of power, while for the other, it's the pleasure of being dominated. And while this is clearly a balance of power dynamic, at the end of the day, if it makes all participants happy, then so be it. Who are we to judge what makes others feel good about themselves? The goal here is to provide useful information that can lead to a happier and more enjoyable sex life.

Chapter 2: Why Turn Your Man Into Your Plaything?

As a woman, exploring your dominant side may not be the easiest thing to do. After all, social conditioning has forced women into the submissive and agreeable role even when they are not naturally inclined to be that way.

As a matter of fact, being a dominant woman can be hard, especially when considering how insecure men turn out to be. This makes it tough for men to accept their submissive nature (unless they are naturally dominant). Now, it should be noted that by "dominant," we mean that a man is not only comfortable in their own skin, but they are also naturally inclined to lead. This has nothing to do with being the loudest guy in the gym or the meanest dude on the block.

That being said, your desire to embrace your dominant nature means that submissive men will naturally gravitate toward you. Even "dominant" guys will gravitate toward you when they see that you are naturally dominant. But what should you do with a guy like this?

It really depends on what you want to get out of a relationship. For some ladies, being in charge is enough of a power rush. They feel satisfied in knowing that they are in control of their partner. For others, they feel satisfied bossing their man around. This feeling is especially heightened when they are able to get him to do what she wants when she wants it.

But then, there are women who want more. They may be in full control of their relationship, but there is always something more that they would like to get out of it. That's why we are going to discuss five reasons why you should go all the way into turning your man into your personal plaything. After all, if you are both down with the dom-sub power dynamic, then why not go all the way?

Reason #1: You Both Enjoy It

As with any type of sexual relationship, there needs to be consent from both parties. If this is the case, then there should be no reason for either of you to hold back. If anything, you both ought to embrace a FEMDOM dynamic.
Why not?

If he is at least willing to give it a try, then there is no reason why you shouldn't pursue it further. The fact is that a man who acknowledges that the woman in his life is the "boss" isn't far away from being a good sub. Given the fact that a FEMDOM relationship is essentially an emotional and psychological bond, you both have everything to gain from this type of relationship.

In addition, dom-sub relationships generally involved a sadistic/masochistic component. As such, both partners get intense pleasure from the relationship itself. The difference lies in the perspective of the relationship. As a result, the sub derives their pleasure from seeing their sub go through any number of situations while the sub feels pleasure from being subjected to the treatment their dom inflicts upon them.

Now, there is an important element here: the sub is not attracted to the treatment per se; they are attracted to being treated in this manner by the dom. It's kind of like enjoying a cheeseburger, but it isn't just any cheeseburger; it's the cheeseburger from a specific restaurant.

This is exactly what happens in a FEMDOM relationship. You man isn't attracted to pain, humiliation, and torture itself. He is attracted to YOU, inflicting this type of treatment on him. This is what makes it so pleasurable. While he might be willing to engage in this type of relationship with someone else, to him, it's doing it with you that unleashes the full submissive experience.

So, as long as you are both enjoying the dynamic, then have at it! There is no reason for you to hold back. If anything, resolve to try new things. Make a concerted effort to push your boundaries as much as possible. You never know what heights of pleasure you can hit.

Reason #2: He Asked for It

Every time a man enters a FEMDOM relationship, it's because he asked for it. A man is never forced into a FEMDOM relationship. Even if he is a victim of sexual assault of some nature (which usually happens at the hand of another man), he will seek to be in a FEMDOM relationship. This is something that he wants, even if he can't consciously articulate.

This implies that your man, while perfectly willing to be in a FEMDOM relationship with you, won't come out directly and say, "Hey babe, I think it's time we had a FEMDOM thing around here." So, he may not necessarily say it with words, but he will totally say it with his attitude and his behavior.

How can you spot this disposition?

There are a number of subtle and not so subtle clues that will tell you what's going on in his mind.

First, you can easily tell a man is submissive by the way he lets you lead things in the bedroom. Often, submissive men allow women to dictate what happens during intercourse. This can be something as simple as letting her decide when penetration occurs when oral play happens, or even when he orgasms. In other cases, submissive men are perfectly comfortable with letting the woman make demands from him no matter how outrageous they may seem. These are the guys that are willing to dress up a clown if that turns his partner on.

464

Next, submissive men show some kind of fear toward women. Now, this isn't the type of fear in which they hide under the bed (at least not early on...), but it does become manifest when things get hot and heavy. For instance, these types of men are unable to react appropriately when a woman shows signs of arousal. They are simply unable to take charge and lead the way. In fact, they may sit there waiting for orders.

Lastly, dominant women are a turn on for these kinds of men. The turn-on occurs when the woman exerts her influence on the man through any number of ways. For example, these men are happy to be penetrated by their female partner. These men find pleasure and satisfaction in being penetrated by their female partner through the use of a strap-on or dildo. You might think that these men are really homosexual. However, we're talking about perfectly heterosexual men who enjoy the submission that occurs when they are penetrated by a woman.

So, don't be surprised to find your man asking to be dominated. The signs are there. All you have to do is be on the lookout for them.

Reason #3: Power Is Addictive

There is a reason why dictators go to great lengths to hold onto power. It's because they become addicted to it. Simply put, power is intoxicating. It produces an overwhelming feeling of superiority over someone or something. This feeling might be a bit too much at first, but over time, the rush that comes with having control makes it impossible to let go.
The same goes for the FEMDOM world. When you experience the rush that comes from completely and utterly dominating someone, you become addicted to it. While it's not like getting high on drugs, it certainly produces a need for more and more of it. This is where doms are tempted to push their subs farther and farther. In general, subs go along with it because they won't really

question what their doms want, that is, unless they feel threatened.

Also, FEMDOM relationships offer something that "traditional" relationships don't offer: a balance of power. There are women who are constantly competing in a "man's world." Often, this constant competition leads to a feeling of exhaustion. After all, it's not easy having to justify being in a position of power in the business world all the time. So, the FEMDOM dynamic affords you the opportunity to be in charge without being questioned by others. There is no second-guessing in FEMDOM. Your sub is perfectly willing to go along because they trust you and follow you. As such, you can really be yourself without the need to justify it all the time.

Reason #4: You Are Comfortable With Running the Show All the Time

Being a dom means you have to be in charge all the time. That's just the nature of the game. If you have a sub at your feet, your sub won't move a finger unless you tell them to. This can be tiresome, especially if you are meticulous and want to plan everything down to the slightest details.

There are some women who are just like that. They need to have everything planned out to the slightest detail. They cannot afford to let anything escape their attention. As a result, being in charge of everything, all the time, can be draining.

You see, there is no such thing as delegating responsibility in the FEMDOM world. You are in charge of everything, and your man has no choice but to go along for the ride. Otherwise, they can hit the road. It's as simple as that. So, you must be comfortable with the idea of being in charge of everything, even if it means be overburdened at times by it.

Consider this situation:

Your partner is fully committed to letting you run everything the way you see fit. As such, you need to tell your partner what they are going to wear, how they are going to please you, and what they need to do in order to be pleased. For example, you must tell your partner when to perform oral sex on you and when they can penetrate you. While this may sound scripted (to a certain degree it is), the truth is that you can't really improvise. Otherwise, you run the risk of missing out on a truly pleasurable experience.

In addition, holding power also means protecting your partner as well. Since they are in a vulnerable position all the time, you need to make sure that whatever happens needs to as safe as possible. For instance, if your partner likes choking, then you better be sure you don't take it too far.

Reason #5: It's just fun

Then, there is the simplest reason of them all: it's just fun being in charge. After all, who doesn't like being the boss?

It's fun to be the one who dictates what is to be done and when it should be done. If you can't find pleasure in holding someone's entire life in your hands, then FEMDOM might not be the best for you. In fact, you have so much power over your sub that you could basically kill them without any resistance.

This is where the essence of the power rush comes from.

Yet, it's so much fun to know that during that encounter, you are the master of your corner of the universe. The best part of all is that your partner is perfectly willing to remain powerless. They are perfectly comfortable with the idea of relinquishing any kind of resistance. They know that by submitting to you, they will obtain the ultimate pleasure they seek.

Now that is powerful stuff.

At the end of the day, the FEMDOM dynamic is fun for both the dom and the sub. As long as both parties are perfectly clear on the nature of the dynamic, there should be no reason why the both of you can't have the time of your lives. Each encounter is meant to give you the opportunity to explore your innermost nature. It is during these encounters that you have a safe space in which you can be yourselves. There is no one judging what you are doing. This is incredibly liberating.

So, if you are truly into FEMDOM, then go for it! The last thing you want to do is to spend your life trying to play a role you weren't to play.

Chapter 3: Are You Ready for FEMDOM?

Being the dom in a FEMDOM relationship sounds pretty simple. If anything, it sounds exciting to be the one in control all the time. At this point, it might sound exciting to have a puny little man groveling at your feet while they are compelled to cater to your whims.

However, that's only a part of the game. Being a dom is so much more than that. It's not merely a question of having sex slaves doing your bidding. It's about using your dominance in such a way that the relationship is self-sustaining and provides both of you with the pleasure you seek. That's why being a dom is much more than just wearing leather and walking around with a flogger.

By definition, a dom is someone who is powerful, imposing, and relishes in taking control of a situation. A true dom doesn't need to be led by anyone. A dom instinctively takes charge of a situation even if they don't know what to do. You see this type of behavior all the time in all facets of life. In business, doms let their character shine as they naturally draw others around them. These are true leaders who others tend to look to.

This type of personality easily translates into the bedroom. In the bedroom, true doms are able to take their partner on a journey of pleasure. Regardless of the nature of the relationship, the sub is perfectly willing to be led as they trust their dom's judgment.

However, doms tend to be confused with bullies. Often, you see films in which there are "doms" beating up defenseless subs such as in BDSM. This gets worse when the sub is forced into doing things they are not comfortable with. This is abuse and must not be tolerated. You can't expect to be a dom by forcing someone to do something they don't want to do. You can't be considered a dom simply because you are in a position of power.

A true dom is always concerned about their sub's wellbeing. In some BDSM relationships, the dom is in charge of every aspect of the sub's life. This includes making sure they eat properly, get enough rest, and exercise regularly. It may sound like a parent running a child's life, but the fact of the matter is that a true dom is committed to making sure that their sub is safe and feels secure.

We won't be going that far in this book. The scope of this book is not focused on the dom-sub relationship outside of the bedroom. But we do want to emphasize that being a true dom means that you are willing to act in a way that will always ensure your sub's wellbeing while respecting whatever boundaries you have set.

With that in mind, here are five ways to recognize if you are a true dom.

Sign #1: Most People Let You Take Control of Things

A true dom is a leader in all aspects of life. The true dom is perfectly comfortable with taking responsibility. So, people recognize this and automatically let the dom take over. You see, being dominant is about taking responsibility for the circumstances surrounding a situation. In the workplace, true doms take on the responsibility of getting a job done on time, even when they are not the supervisor. If anything, the supervisor might be a "fake dom," that is, they hide behind their job title to boss people around. But they are not a true dom as they would rather delegate responsibility on others.

In the bedroom, a true dom takes responsibility for their pleasure and that of their partners. This is important to bear in mind as a common misconception of a dom is that they seek selfish pleasure.

That could not be farther from the truth.

Another common misconception is that the sub is actually suffering while in the submissive role. Observers believe that a sub who is being humiliated is being forced into something they don't like.

That's completely false!

A true sub enjoys being subjected to a lower rank. They derive pleasure from being put into a position of inferiority. Otherwise, they wouldn't willingly accept this kind of relationship. Moreover, they would run away as fast as they can the first chance they got.

So, embracing your true dominant personality means that you are perfectly willing to lead your partner(s) to their own pleasure while you help them pleasure you. It's a win-win as everyone derives the pleasure they seek from the FEMDOM dynamic.

Sign #2: You Have Power Even When You Are Not in a Position of Authority

Contrary to what most people think, power isn't something that you can just grab. You might be able to take on a position of authority by force, but people will never recognize your power. Power is something that people willingly relinquish to someone else. This is why charismatic leaders have a huge following. It seems as though people gladly acknowledge they hold the power.

In a FEMDOM relationship, you don't need to beat your partner senseless in order to get them to acknowledge your dominance. Male subs automatically acknowledge their FEMDOM's power over them. It's a natural occurrence. You don't need to threaten male subs. They will willingly go along with you. There is no need for any external coercion. It may seem paradoxical, but it's just a natural process.

Now, you might encounter men who are attracted to the idea of being a sub. But, they are either wrestling with internal issues with regard to this, or they are simply not ready to let go. This is where the training process you can provide for them is intended to progressively let them get over their hang-ups in such a way that they can progressively embrace their submissive nature, until one day, they are nothing more than your personal slaves.

However, this is a personal process. You can't really force anyone to be a sub. Yes, you can force them into a submissive role, but they won't enjoy it. If anything, you'll probably kill them first before they are truly able to respond to your dominance. Sure, there are folks (male and female) who get a twisted pleasure from harming others. However, the truth FEMDOM gets her pleasure as a result of the pleasure subs get from feeling pain, humiliation, torture, and so on. If you are familiar with BDSM relationships, then you can totally appreciate this dynamic.

Sign #3: People Look to You When There Is Trouble

This sign isn't directly related to the bedroom, but it's a great way of telling just how dominant you really are. When people automatically look to you when something is wrong, it means that people recognize the fact that you have power. These folks understand that they can count on you as you are not afraid to take the lead. Also, it is because you have demonstrated that you have taken on responsibility at various points in your life.

When you meet new potential sexual partners, they will automatically sniff out your dominant nature. As such, the "dominant" males (not the true dominant males) will try to avoid you. Fake doms are generally insecure males. As such, they will try to avoid you as much as they can.

However, those males who are already cognizant of their submissive nature will gravitate toward you automatically. But this doesn't mean that they are weak.

In fact, they could be highly competent men. What it means is that they simply seek a female dom who can provide them with the female force they seek.

Plain and simple.

If you are in a relationship at the moment, don't be surprised if you are the one who makes all the decisions. If you find that your partner is perfectly willing to follow your lead, then don't be surprised to find that they will not object to an increasing level of submission. That's where this guide can help you take your man further and further down the road to full submission.

Sign #4: Your Sexual Partners Don't Resist Your Lead

When you find yourself having intercourse with a male partner, you might be surprised to find that they offer very little resistance to your lead. For instance, when you ask them to perform oral on you, they willingly oblige. Then, when you ask them to penetrate you, they gladly do it. After, you ask them to pull out and touch you, and they quickly follow suit. This type of attitude is a clear indication that you are dealing with a submissive man. The situation is heightened when the man simply stands by until you command them. In fact, some men will even go as far as resist orgasm until the woman tells them it's okay to do so.

If that seems strange to you, perhaps you haven't really taken the lead in your relationships.

When you consciously take the lead, the man in your relationship will either try to fight back or give in. Now, if you are dealing with a naturally dominant male, he will not give you much of a chance to lead. He will automatically take charge, and that's that. At that point, it's up to you to follow his lead or offer resistance of your own.

Naturally, dominant males like to lead all the time. They have no trouble in taking a woman by the hand and leading them on the journey to mutual pleasure. A naturally dominant male will do everything he can to give his partner the best experience possible.

This doesn't happen with "fake doms." Fake doms like to boss girls around in pursuit of their selfish pleasure.

The dame dynamic applies to true FEMDOMS. The true FEMDOM simply takes charge and doesn't ask questions. The male can then follow suit or find someone else. When you really think about it, it's really that cut and dry.

Sign #5: You Don't Have a Big Ego

One of the key characteristics of a fake dom is that they talk a big game. These are the types (both male and female) who like to brag about their experience. They like to boast about how they don't put up with crap from anyone, blah, blah, blah.

A true dom doesn't have to say much to make their presence felt. They also don't have a big ego.

Think about that for a minute.

If you don't have a big ego, you don't have the need to talk a big game. You know who you are, what you are capable of, and you are confident you can deliver all the time. Your partner(s), in turn, will quickly acknowledge this. They will seek you out because they know that they are guaranteed to have a great time every time they are with you.

This isn't even about looks. Sure, it helps to be attractive, but then again, what good is a pretty face if they are shallow and selfish?

This is why the true dom makes their presence felt just by being who they are. There is no need for any fluff. It's all substance. This is why there is no need for a big ego. If anything. A big ego is just a means of overcompensating for shortfalls. While this is rather common among men, women are also guilty of this from time to time.

So, it's always a good idea to keep your ego in check. You don't need to pretend to be humble or even submissive. All you need to do is let your actions speak for themselves. The rest will fall into place. At the end of the day, you know who you are and what you are capable of. You are interested in attracting men who want the same things as you. So, don't waste your time with people who are pretending to be something they are not.

Chapter 4: Is Your Man Ready for FEMDOM?

Is your man, or any man in your life, for that matter, ready for FEMDOM?

That is a very interesting question...

It might be hard to tell. In fact, you may never really know until you actually go down that road. You see, most men, while willing to go along with a FEMDOM relationship, may have never actually experienced one. So, they won't really know what to look for.

In some cases, you might find a man who already has experience in this type of relationship. In that case, it's easier to deal with them. It could be that they've tried it, but never really had someone to lead them and teach them the ways of FEMDOM.

You can't expect a man to know what to do unless someone teaches. FEMDOM is not the kind of thing that you can learn on your own, at least from the sub's point of view. This is the type of thing you need to learn on your own. As a matter of fact, even if a man is an experienced sub, doms have different attitudes and personalities. As such, this means that you need to mold your man, or men, into the way you want them to be. This is why there can never be two identical FEMDOM experiences for a male sub.

This means that it's your job to take your man and turn him into the male sub you want him to be. However, you need to keep in mind that he needs to be ready to give in and embrace his role as a sub. You can't force him to accept this role. Otherwise, you would be breaking his will. This would lead to disastrous consequences as he wouldn't relish the role that you would put him in. The whole idea is to turn him into a willing sub. Thus, he needs to see how much pleasure he can derive from pleasing you in every possible manner.

So, in this chapter, we are going to take a look at five signs that will tell you if your man is really ready to become your sub.

Sign #1: He Doesn't Question Anything You Say or Do

This sign applies to every aspect of your life. While it doesn't mean that your man has blind faith in you, it just means that he's willing to accept anything you say and do without putting up much of a fight.

With this sign, there is one important element.

When you are a highly competent woman, you're much more likely to make smart decisions and avoid making major mistakes. While nothing is perfect, you get it right most of the time. This builds credibility and reliability on your end. So, your man won't have much to complain about the way you go about life.

A great example of this is money management. If you find that you are much more efficient at managing money than your partner, and he does not question any of your decisions, especially because you have shown to be competent, then you can be sure that he will go along with your decisions in the bedroom.

While money is just one of the many examples in which you can see just how much influence you have over your partner, it goes to show that he is ready to be led... by you. It's important to note that he may never be able to have a FEMDOM relationship with anyone else by you. You see, he trusts you. He follows you. So, he may never have the same type of feelings toward anyone else. He'll be willing to open up to you. But you must show him the way. His naturally submissive nature will not allow him to discover

FEMDOM on his own. If anything, he'll be afraid to go outside of your relationship out of fear of upsetting you.

In the event you meet someone new, you can easily tell if they are submissive. All you have to do is boss them around. It could be that they will go along with everything you say out of desperation. But then again, if you find that he is unable to look at you straight in the eye, he can't interject during a conversation, and can't seem to work up the nerve to ask you about anything, then it could be that you have a natural sub on your hands.

It would then be up to you to pursue a dom-sub relationship further.

Sign #2: He Accepts Orders

This sign is pretty straightforward. You are the boss, and he obeys orders. Now, we're not talking about bossing your man around. We're talking about commanding him as if you were in the army. It's one thing to tell your man to do something he's been putting of for a while. And, it's another entirely different thing to command your desires.

For instance, during sex, you tell him exactly what you want him to do. You tell him where to touch you, how to touch, and when to touch you. And he is perfectly fine with this! You don't see him trying to go for his pleasure ahead of yours. If you ask him to sit by the bedside and wait until you are ready for him, he will gladly do it.

Some folks confuse this attitude with a lack of character. They make it out to be that he is "not a real man" or that he is "pussy whipped." Unfortunately for most men, the typical male stereotype of the "macho alpha" isn't really applicable. The vast majority of men will never truly exhibit the traits of the so-called "alpha male." In fact, the alpha male is a superior kind of male that isn't easily bred. This type of male is not the biggest, loudest, and strongest (at least not physically). This is the kind of man that isn't afraid to be vulnerable, yet strong enough to deal with life's adversities head on.

Do you see where we are going with this?

So, if your man isn't exactly alpha male material, it does mean he isn't a "real man." It's just that his personality is not suited to be the one leading the charge.

This is where you come in. You have total control over the dynamic in your relationship, and if he is perfectly fine with accepting a submissive role, then so be it. Take full advantage of your dominant nature and his submissive demeanor to build a dynamic in which he doesn't have to pretend to be strong, and you don't have to pretend to be weak.

Sign #3: He Always Puts Your Needs Ahead of His

While it is true that dominant men are perfectly capable of putting others' needs ahead of their own, a submissive man will never go out of his way to satisfy himself without your approval.

Consider this situation:

A submissive man will not dare go out to boys' night because he is afraid that you won't approve of his friends. Now, the difference here is that a weak man is just afraid of standing up for himself. A sub will think about pleasing you first, and then if you approve, he will go out with his friends.

Do you see the difference?

When you translate this attitude into the bedroom, your sub will always be at your beck and call. If you ask him to give you oral first until the cows come home, he will gladly do it. Then, you can "reward" him by doing what you know he likes. In this case, you are not doing what he wants; you are being generous enough to grant him what he likes. He'll be perfectly happy to work hard for his reward because, in his mind, your happiness and satisfaction are first.

Perhaps the biggest difference between a dominant and submissive male is that a truly dominant male will put the wellbeing of others before his. However, the dominant male understands that it is important for him to take care of himself for the sake of those he protects. As such, a dominant male is protective. The submissive male seeks protection. It may not be physical, but certainly emotional. This is where the emotional connection of a FEMDOM relationship is so strong.

That is why you should not frown upon your male sub's need for protection. If anything, you lose nothing by giving it to him. All he wants is to know that you have everything under control in such a way that he can let go of himself and be free to enjoy his sexuality.

Sign #4: He Seeks Your Approval During Sex

This sign ties perfectly well into the previous one. A naturally submissive male will always ask for your approval during sex. Whenever he does anything, he wants to know if this is something you like, something that you enjoy. So, he will constantly seek validation during intercourse.

In this case, you often get questions like, "am I going too fast?" or "do you like what I'm doing?"

Now, you might be thinking, "just shut up and do it!"

But don't get upset. In fact, cut the poor guy a break. He just wants to do things right by you. He wants to make sure that you are enjoying things as much as he is. The difference lies in the fact that he either doesn't know how to go about things or would much rather have you tell him what you want, when you want it and where you want it.

If you are comfortable with giving him a blueprint to your body, then the good news is that you will be guaranteed a good time, every time. Even when he can't "rise to the occasion," you can always find something for him to do. Oddly enough, that is liberating for men.

Think about that for a moment.

In those times in which a man cannot have an erection, it can be liberating to know that the female will not chastise him for his lack of virility. In fact, she will find alternatives for him to get the job done. In these cases, "punishment" is used. One such example could be a humiliating activity like licking the soles of your shoes.

So, cut your subs a break. They just want to please you.

Sign #5: He Is Willing to Accept an Open Relationship

This has got to be the biggest sign of them all.

Why?

Well, because he is willing to go along with an open relationship on your end, but not his. He is not allowed to see anyone else unless you approve of it. However, you do not need to seek his approval to see someone else.

This is where dominatrices end up having relationships with multiple men. All men know that the dominatrix has other men (perhaps they just don't know who they are), and they are perfectly fine with it.

A great example of this is cuckoldry. In this technique, the female dom has sex in front of her sub. This technique is used as a means of humiliation. The male sub has no choice but to sit by and watch. Depending on how far the female dom wants to take it, the male sub might be required to perform sexual acts on the other male. This is particularly humiliating if the sub is not homosexual or does not enjoy sexual activity with other males.

Ultimately, if your sub will not question you for having an open relationship on your end, then you know you have a truly submissive male on your hands. So, do take the time to pose this situation on the table. If you find that he will not put up resistance, then just make sure that you acknowledge his feelings by giving him the reassurance that he needs. Mainly, if you are in a committed relationship, make him feel safe in that you won't leave him for someone else. All you are doing is just having some fun in your free time.

Part II: Easing Into FEMDOM

Chapter 5: Basic FEMDOM Tactics

One of the most important roles of any FEMDOM is to groom her male subs the way she wants them to be. Since male subs aren't born knowing how to be the right sub, they need to learn how to become one. And even if you found an experienced sub, he'll be molded to his previous dom's ways. Needless to say, your ways are naturally going to be different.

Also, if you happen to have a newbie on your hands, then it's up to you to train him in the way you expect him to act. You can't just expect him to figure out what to do. As such, it's part of your role to set the rules, establish guidelines, and enforce them.

At this point, it's important to note that there needs to be consequences every time your sub transgresses your wishes. To provide "punishment," you can implement any of the tactics we are going to describe in the remaining parts of this book.

However, one very powerful tactic is to withhold what gives him the most pleasure. For instance, if your sub enjoys penetrating you, then you can choose to withhold this from him until he is fully compliant. In a manner of speaking, it can serve as a treat for a job well done.

In that regard, you too, will learn to recognize your sub's demeanor. As you see what really gets his motor running, you will be able to use it as both an advantage and as a means of controlling him. Please remember that the name of the game is control. If you do not assert your dominance from the get-go, you will never be able to fully master your sub.

In this chapter, we are going to start things off slowly. We are going to describe tactics that are more psychological than sexual. These tactics are meant to assert your position and teach him the rules of the game. You can then choose if this will lead to sex, or just remain as part of the training. If anything, you could ask him to please you while he has to wait his turn.

Teaching Your Sub Some Manners

What is a FEMDOM relationship without proper manners?

Your sub needs to understand that you are the master and should address you accordingly. The use of proper manners is a powerful psychological technique that is intended to instill in him the respect that he must observe for you. You cannot expect him to automatically address you and treat you the way you desire. This is something that he must learn. So, you are there to gladly teach him. In addition, never forget that he's there to please you at all times...

A good way to get things started is to let him know he must use "please" and "thank you" at all times. He will not be allowed to do anything unless he politely requests permission. **This is very important**. He cannot be allowed to do anything unless he requests and is granted permission.

For example, if he wishes to touch himself, or you, for that matter, he must ask for permission. If he touches himself in an attempt to pleasure himself, that would be considered a transgression, and a penalty would ensure.

If he is granted permission to touch himself, say to masturbate, he must thank you properly for allowing him to do so. Otherwise, he would be nothing more than an ungrateful worm of a man.

Additionally, make sure he addresses you the way you wish him to do so. Some common ways are "mistress," "ma'am," or "madam." If you choose to take up a dom name, say "Madam Pain," then make sure he addresses you properly. Otherwise, it's going to be time-out for him!

Serving You

Another important part of being an obedient sub is to serve you just the way you like it. A good way to kick things off is to have him serve you food and drink. He can play the role of the slave serving their mistress.

Now, you can take this as far as you would like. You can give him explicit orders about what you want him to do for you. You can ask him to paint your nails or shave your body. You can even take it further and add humiliating requests such as cleaning up a bathroom mess. Remember that he must obey your orders to the letter. In exchange, he might get a small treat, say masturbation, or perhaps pleasuring you.

However, don't allow him to enjoy himself at first. As such, try to avoid intercourse during this time. Otherwise, it will build an expectation that he will get sex every time. That is clearly not the case; you will not allow him to do what he likes just because he did what you said.

That is expected of him. After all, it's the least he could do.

Sissy Play

This is the first time we are going to explore sissy play. In essence, this technique involves getting him to do "girly" things. One easy yet effective way of getting a sub to learn his place is to have him wear make-up. Of course, you won't be doing any of it. He'll be doing it himself. So, he had better learn how to do his make-up properly.

Once he has done his make-up, you can be the judge. If he has done things to your satisfaction, you might consider giving him a treat. It's entirely up to you. Another interesting tactic is to have him watch a guy on guy porn with you. This is especially useful if he has not shown any interest in men. This will allow you to create an interesting visual for yourself while he gets to take a walk down his sissy side.

Please keep in mind that male subs fantasize about their feminine side. Some might act upon it, while others may not feel entirely comfortable. So, if you give him the chance to explore his girly side, it could end up being a huge turn-on for him. As such, don't be afraid to encourage his girly side. The likelihood that is a closet homosexual isn't very high. Otherwise, he would have sought a male dom and not a FEMDOM.

Later on, we're going to be revisiting sissy play at a more advanced level. For now, keep things relatively simple by letting him explore his feminine side.

Pet Play

Role plays are quite common in dom-sub relationships. Some are rather "traditional," such as patient and doctor. However, FEMDOM is all about taking things a step further. One such role play that takes things to another level is pet play.

In this tactic, your sub is your pet. You can choose to make him an animal pet, or just a "human pet." Now, keep in mind that you are essentially reducing him to an animal. So, he can't think for himself. He needs to be given commands just like you would a dog, for instance. As such, he cannot do anything at all. He must be obedient to your every command.

This tactic is essentially meant to be a training tool. However, you can use it as part of foreplay if you wish. You can have him run around like your pet, perhaps with a leash around his neck, which can then lead to some type of sexual activity, such as performing oral on you. If he is a good boy, he might be able to get a treat, such as watching you masturbate or touch himself.

Other variations of pet play include riding him like a pony. While the point is not to actually ride him like a pony, what you achieve with this is to assert a dominant position over him. Consequently, he will get the idea that you are "on top"; hence you are the mistress.

Another great idea is to give him a pet name. Now, we don't mean things like "sugar" or "honey baby." We mean real pet names like "marbles" or "fuzzy." Using pet names can be a fun part of humiliation tactics. In such cases, the names you call him are meant to humiliate him without actually demeaning him.

Treating Him Like a Child

There are some men who have severe mommy issues. As such, they like to be treated like children, or even babies for that matter. One interesting fetish that some guys have is being breastfed. Others like to dress up in diapers and prance around like babies. Some will even go as far as ask to have their diapers changed and get their bottle.

This particular tactic really depends on you. If you like, you can use it in combination with other tactics. For instance, if he is a good boy and serves you properly, you can breastfeed him is that is what he likes. Another interesting variation is a mother-son role play. For some guys, getting it on with mommy is the ultimate fantasy. But since they are subs, they need to do everything mommy says. Otherwise, they can't get what they want.

Not all FEMDOMS are into this kind of role play, but if you are up for it, it's definitely worth giving it a chance. Not all FEMDOMS like the idea of mothering their subs, but it might end up creating an interesting dynamic for both of you.

Making Basic Tactics Work Effectively

The tactics which we have discussed in this chapter as pretty beginner-friendly. They don't require a great deal of sacrifice and are suited just fine for the novice sub. If you are not very experienced as a FEMDOM, it's also a good way for you to gauge what you want out of a relationship. Please keep in mind that subs don't need to know how experienced you are. But it certainly helps too if you know what you're doing.

In the event that you are in a committed relationship with your man and you are both exploring this kind of relationship, then you can both explore these tactics together. This will enable you to develop your own dynamic, as a couple, without having to consider any possible third parties. This type of journey can really bring you together as a couple and solidify your relationship. In addition, quite a few male subs have a hard time asking for it. They may hint at it through their actions and attitude but may never actually come out and say it.

Also, if you are contemplating having multiple subs, then these tactics will be essential in building the type of relationship you want with each of your subs. You can tweak them to suit your individual needs and the various personalities of your subs. Ultimately, you need to figure out what works best for you. That way, you can provide your subs with the guidance they need in order to fulfill your wishes.

Lastly, please keep in mind that this is a learning process. As you embrace your inner FEMDOM, you too, will begin to discover what turns you on the most. It could be something as simple as being served, or it could expand into something much larger such as BDSM.

In reality, it's all up to you!

In this world of FEMDOM, no one is here to tell you what to do. You are the mistress of your domain. And even if you decided to team up with other FEMDOMS to make a large event, there is no one who can tell you what to do. Your sub is your sub, and that's the end of it. You have the right to do whatever you want. After all, your sub is with you because they want to. You are not forcing them to be with you through brainwashing or anything like that. As such, you have every right to be who you want to be. It's your domain.

Chapter 6: The Use of Physical Aggression in FEMDOM

Some form of violence is generally involved in dom-sub relationships. The level of violence depends on what both parties agree to. If violence, such as physical aggression, is utilized without the full consent of both parties, then essentially what you have is assault. In such cases, the victim needs to leave the relationship at once. If there is serious harm committed, then charges may have to be pressed.

That being said, the use of physical aggression can be a wonderful tool to assert your dominance over your mal sub. In fact, it is especially powerful as men are considered to be physically superior to women. As such, the act of having a woman physically hit a man is more powerful psychologically than it is physically. You don't need to beat your man to a bloody pulp in order for him to get the point. If anything, the threat of aggression is enough to render him helpless.

If that seems unbelievable, then you have seen nothing yet.

In this chapter, we are going to explore how the use of physical aggression can help you assert your position as a FEMDOM. Since we are still in a "training phase" so to speak, we are not going to look at physical aggression in bondage. This is something that we will be exploring later on. For now, we are going to focus on how you can use this tactic as a means of laying down the ground rules for your FEMDOM relationship.

Using Your Hands to Assert Your Dominance

The level of force used in FEMDOM relationships largely depends on how much your sub is willing to tolerate without it becoming physical assault. Generally speaking, most male subs tolerate spanking, slaps in the face, or squeezing of the genitals (this is a torture technique we will look at later on). We don't advise you to kick your sub, especially when they are on the ground, as this could be potentially dangerous. Now, it's a completely different story if you place the soles of your feet on their back. This is more of a dominant gesture than aggression as such. Also, please refrain from punching as that may also cause serious harm, especially during the heat of the moment.

Now, it should be said that some men actually enjoy being beaten. This appeals to the masochistic side of a sub. In fact, plenty of men find it exciting to be beaten and then engage in sexual activity. However, please bear in mind that you are the dom, and as such, need to ensure your sub's wellbeing.

Additionally, please bear in mind that your sub will generally be in a vulnerable position. They may be on the floor, bound, or blindfolded. So, you want to make sure that they feel safe. Otherwise, the fear of actual bodily harm may end up spoiling the moment and turn you into a big bully.

So, don't be afraid to slap your man around. In doing so, he will learn his place, especially when he transgresses any of your rules. You man needs to know who's in charge, and you need to let him know that you run a tight ship. If he can't deal with it, then it's too bad for him. You're the boss, and you are going to make your presence felt.

Using Artifacts to Assert Your Dominance

This is where it starts to get kinky. Devices such as floggers, whips, ropes, chains, and sticks are all used to hit subs. Many times, carrying a device around, such as a flogger, is mainly intended to be a display of power. The fact that you carry it around with you during sex play means that you are in charge. Furthermore, it is a great disciplining tool, especially when you are training a novice sub.

To use a flogger as a training aid, all you need to do is strike your sub every time they do something you don't like or if they do something wrong. For instance, if your sub does not address you properly, this would earn him a flogging in the back or butt (avoid flogging to the face as it could be quite dangerous). However, if the sub has done something right, it could earn him a tickling with the flogger as a reward.

Other devices, such as whips, are generally used as part of torture tactics. Yet, they could be used as a training aid, as well. Sticks come in various forms, sizes, and shapes. They can be used to both strike as well as poke your sub. Make sure you don't use sharp sticks to poke. However, poking can provide you a gentle nudge to your sub that they must do what they are expected.

As for ropes and chains, these are mainly used to restrain subs. Nevertheless, they could also be used to strike your sub. More than the actual pain ropes and chains can cause, it's the psychological impact that these devices have. After all, what good can come from being struck by a chain? Plus, chains are useful devices during pet play. You can walk your sub around like a dog, and if he misbehaves, a playful whack will serve as a kind reminder of what is expected of him.

Kicking, Pushing, Wrestling and Other Kinds of Physical Aggression

For some guys, there is a rush in being dominated by a woman. This is quite common among larger women and smaller men. This type of situation creates arousal. There is something about being unable, or at least unwilling, to physically dominate a woman. Now, the average man has a greater brute physical force than the average woman. Yet, there are women who are substantially stronger than some men. It is this difference that makes men seek physically strong women.

As a matter of fact, it's quite tempting for female bodybuilders and exceptionally tall women to become dominatrices. Under such circumstances, it would be quite hard for a weaker man to put up any kind of resistance. This would constitute the ultimate turn on for a lot of guys.

However, you don't need to be physically superior to subject men through physical force. In fact, it's normal to see rather petite women engaging in the role of dominatrix without having to be physically superior. All they need to do is push the right buttons. For instance, having a good understanding of martial arts or self-defense can be enough to deter a man from trying to physically attack you. If they can see that you mean business, they won't try to put up a fight. They know that you can handle yourself.

Of course, not all FEMDOM relationships reach this point. However, it can be an interesting angle to pursue should it come to that point. Hey, if you're a bigger gal, you might even be able to manhandle a puny guy. He would love that, and you certainly would get a kick out it!

Spanking and Genitals

Let's take things up a notch here. For some guys, getting hit in the genitals can be a turn on. In a manner of speaking, it's pleasure through pain. While getting nailed in the nutsack can be painful, when it's part of a FEMDOM dynamic, it can produce a feeling of pleasure and release. Often, you will find that most guys don't have an erection while getting hit in the genital area, but there is a good deal of logic to it, causing arousal.

You see, any type of hitting, spanking, or slapping in the genital region causes increased blood flow to this area. As a result, it is a good way of stimulating the blood that feeds the penis. This, in turn, promotes a strong erection.

This is a good technique to use, especially if you want your sub to penetrate you, but he might be having a bit of trouble getting things along. But keep in mind that we're not talking about some gentle tapping, here. We're talking about doing it hard enough to where he can wince in pain.

Additionally, genital spanking can be used as a punishment. To do this, a flogger, or perhaps a paddle, can be used. If your sub doesn't do as he is ordered, a nice tap in the genital area can be used to remind him of his duties.

However, there is one word of caution, though: the genital area can be quite sensitive. So, make sure that you don't go overboard and injure your sub. While you would have to strike him pretty hard, things can get out of hand in the heat of the moment. So, it's best to make sure that you don't overdo it. Otherwise, you may leave your man incapacitated (at least in that region) for a while. Plus, blunt force trauma in the genital region could lead to health issues. That's why it's best to take it easy.

Beyond that, your man should know that you are not afraid to resort to physical punishment if he is unable to live up to expectations. He needs to understand what your expectations are, and if he can't perform up to your standards, then there will be consequences.

Physical Punishment

Okay, so now we're getting serious about punishing your man. While you may use psychological means of punishing your man, such as withholding gratification, insulting, name-calling, and perhaps sissy play, there needs to be some sort of physical punishment that you can use to assert your dominance.

In this regard, spanking is not the only thing you can do. While spanking (or any other type of physical aggression can be used), the truth is that there are other creative, less violent ways to make your man get the message. These tactics can be humiliating, or just play physically exhausting.

So, here are a couple of ideas.

First, make your man carry something heavy. A good trick is a bag full of pennies. Pennies, or any coins of that matter, can be quite heavy. Now, while the average guy would be able to pick them up easily, it's no so easy to hold a bag of pennies for a long time. This tactic works by having your sub extend his arms while holding a bag on pennies in each hand. After a few minutes, his arms will begin to tire. At this time, he cannot let go of the bag until you authorize him to do so. If he drops the bag, then he must not only pick it up but may be subject to additional punishment. You could spank him, or even humiliate him. After all, shouldn't a man be strong enough to hold a bag full of pennies? Additional ideas are a stack of books, dumbbells, or any other heavy object which he can hold in one hand.

Next, a great idea is to have your sub kneel on a pencil. That might not sound like such a bad thing. But after a few minutes of kneeling on a pencil, the pain can be nothing short of agony. To make things fun, he could kneel on a pencil while giving you oral pleasure. The punishment can end when you orgasm. If that takes a while... then too bad for him!

Lastly, why not make your man drop and give you 20? If he isn't very physically fit, it'll be tough for him to do 20 pushups in one go. If he can't do it, then further punishment may ensue. If you have a military streak about you, pushups, jumping jacks, or any other kind of physical exercise can be used as a punishment. This tactic is actually more of a reward as he would actually get in shape!

496

As you can see, physical aggression is more about causing a psychological impact on your sub rather than actually physically harming him. So, don't hold back and be creative. Just make sure not to go too far... at least for now!

Chapter 7: Dressing Up for FEMDOM

Clothing is just as important as any other part of the FEMDOM dynamic. Typically, images of leather-clad women with whips come to mind. On the flip side, you see mean dressed in ass-less chaps while wearing a leather mask.

However, the truth is that dressing up for FEMDOM is about whatever you want it to be. You don't have to dress in a latex dominatrix suit to be a badass dom. After all, this may not be your style. The best way to go about clothing is to choose whatever makes you feel comfortable. This is about what makes you happy. Along the way, you might get some requests from your subs. This is important as FEMDOMS, who have multiple subs, may either choose to have on style across the board or perhaps dress in different styles to suit the fantasy the sub wants to be a part of.

This opens up two possibilities.

First of all, you are a FEMDOM, you have a style, and anyone that wants to be with you has to get with the program.

Fair enough.

Please keep in mind that you are a dom. You don't have to justify your style to anyone. If anything, subs need to explain themselves to you. They need to convince you to accept them in your life. Otherwise, you can kindly reject being with a sub simply because he doesn't suit your style.

For example, you could be the leather-clad type that has whips, floggers, and chains. While this is a more stereotypical BDSM set up, it's what a lot of guys want to experience. So, you can deliver that experience to them while satisfying your own power streak.

Also, you could be more into the mothering role. So, you would present yourself as a mother. This might imply babying your subs so that they are completely dependent on you. This may include activities such as diaper changing, breastfeeding, and treating your sub like an infant.

Another interesting twist is going goth. The whole dungeon set up can be quite exhilarating for some guys. They would rather get it on with a goth dungeon mistress than with a latex-clad dominatrix. While the dynamic might essentially be the same, the visuals and the can vary.

The second possibility can be found in a committed relationship. Let's assume that you and your partner are looking to explore the FEMDOM dynamic. So, you might end up having multiple roles that you can play. Perhaps your man wants to experience a doctor-patient environment. Or, he wants to be babied. In addition, he might be into the whole dungeon setup.

Now, it should be noted that you are not pleasing him. If he wants to be babied, then he has to earn that privilege. He needs to pay his dues before you can satisfy his mommy fantasies. If he wants to go into the dungeon, then he needs to pay his mistress respect before he can have the privilege of being accepted into the dungeon.

In this arrangement, the FEMDOM dynamic is fully under your control. The only thing different is that you are giving you male sub an incentive, something to look forward to, in a manner of speaking. He knows that if he is perfectly compliant, he will get to experience the situation that he longs for. Simply because he gets the chance to be who he wants to be, he will go along with whatever games you want to play with him.

It should also be said that mixing things up a bit is always fun. Perhaps you're not always in the mood for the dungeon. Perhaps you are in the mood to be the boss who takes advantage of her employees. Maybe you want to become a police officer that humiliates a criminal. Or you might be in the mood to be a military drill instructor who puts her new recruits through the wringer.

All of these scenarios are mere examples of the plethora of possibilities you can explore. However, whatever scenario you explore, they need to be set up in such a way that you retain control while making your sub earn his right to be a part of it. If you allow him to feel like you are giving him what he wants, then you are giving away your power. If he has willingly accepted to give his power away to you, then there is no reason why you should do anything to surrender an iota of it.

Choosing the Right Dress for Your Sub

Choosing the proper outfit for your sub largely depends on your style. Generally speaking, most FEMDOMS have a number of different outfits their subs are expected to wear throughout their time under her command. This also depends on the type of game you want to play.

Let's consider this situation.

You have a new sub in your life. As such, he is automatically assigned to the lowest possible rank. This implies that he can expect nothing more than to be treated as the lowest piece of dirt (well, that's just us getting carried away a bit). So, he also needs to dress the part.

Now, you could just have him running around naked. That's pretty harsh on a new sub. It makes them feel vulnerable and weak. Psychologically, being naked exposes you so much that you don't really have a sense of power. In a way, you are already breaking his will.

Let's assume now that while you are "breaking in" your new sub, you want to have some pet play. Well, why not have "fluffy" or "fifi" wear a dog collar? Alternatively, he could wear a saddle so you can ride him. If you really wanted to ramp it up, there are butt plugs that have a tail on the end. Using this type of device serves both a practical purpose (anal play) and a psychological purpose (the animal tail). Plus, if it's a cute foxtail or something, it adds a sissy component to it.

As you can see, it's really a question of being creative!

Perhaps the only restriction to keep in mind is anything that would be degrading on the basis of cultural or religious reasons. Beyond that, there really shouldn't be any kind of restriction in your dress ideas. After all, he's your sub and has to get with the program.

Costumes and Role Plays

This is a very common situation that arises in the FEMDOM world. When you get into role plays, you would naturally think about using costumes as a part of the scene. This is perfectly natural. After all, what would a good role play be without the use of costumes?

However, if you are so inclined to use costumes, there are a couple of things to keep in mind.

Firstly, what do you want to achieve? That is, your role is to dominate him. Therefore, costumes and role plays are not about what he wants. It's about what you want. So, it doesn't matter if he likes seeing you in any given outfit. If you don't want to wear it, there is no reason why you should.

Secondly, it's all about domination, right? So, wearing outfits that don't assert your dominance is not necessarily the best way to go.

Think about this situation.

Your sub may think you are looking absolutely smoking in a schoolgirl outfit, but how does that assert your dominance over him? That's the type of question you need to be asking yourself. Moreover, how does the costume fit into the overall powerplay you are seeking to make? If the costume does not contribute to asserting your position of power, then there is no reason for you to wear it

Lastly, any costumes your sub wears should not give him any power whatsoever. If anything, his costumes should reaffirm his submissive nature. So, if you are going to be a police officer, a prisoner outfit might be the best way to go. But if you are going to pretend to be a sexy cop and he's the big bad thief, then that is not really going to work out in your favor.

Costumes can also be used to humiliate your subs. If your sub likes dressing up in women's clothing, perhaps giving him a total girly outfit would provide him with the ultimate experience. Combine that with humiliating treatment, and you might have yourself one heck of a session. The main point here is to do anything, and everything you can, to show that you're the boss.

No questions asked.

Common FEMDOM Dress Up Ideas

What you choose to wear should make you feel as comfortable as possible. It should be about you feeling good about yourself while also making you feel sexy. There's nothing worse than wearing something that doesn't necessarily flatter you. Nevertheless, there are some universal looks that will never go wrong in the world of FEMDOM.

So, let's take a look at some of the classic items you can wear during your FEMDOM sessions.

- Knee-high or thigh-high boots. These are classics. They look great and assert a position of power. The high-heel boots really make a statement, especially if you want to degrade your man by stepping on him. They come in different colors, so these can be used in a variety of situations.

- Latex suits. Latex suits are practically a cliché in the FEMDOM and BDSM world. Still, they are timeless and serve to really drive your point home. Plus, most men fantasize about this type of outfit. So, it would certainly be worth giving it a go. Just make sure you are not allergic to latex.

- Anything that's leather. This is another classic style. Black leather is the industry standard though varying colors can also create an interesting combination of visuals. Red and white are very common colors and stand out very well in a dark setting.

- Lingerie. This is a bit tricky. If you wear lingerie, such as bodysuits or thongs, it is because you want to. This isn't meant to be a treat for him. Of course, he will be turned on by the fact that you look good, but that's just an added bonus for him. As far as you're concerned, you're not catering to what he likes. This is about what you like, and that's that.

- Corsets. Corsets are a staple of FEMDOM. They look good, and they are practical to wear. They allow you a free range of motion. This is important, especially if you are going to be engaging in bondage or any other type of physical activity. If you would rather have something looser on your body, a bustier might be a good option. Again, it looks good and provides you with the range of motion you would be looking for.

- Bodycon dress. These dresses have become very popular in recent years. They not only flatter your figure, but they also create the visual effect you want. Combining a bodycon with boots or stiletto heels creates the ultimate male fantasy.

- High heels. On the subject of heels, stilettos are another staple of FEMDOM. They create a wonderful image and go well with virtually any type of outfit. Stilettos work really well with skirts and dresses. However, if you choose to wear leather or latex pants, they can also complement your outfit very well.

- Stockings. These are a great complement to any outfit. Stockings are definitely sexy and are always in style. You will never go wrong with stockings. Fishnets work really well too. Plus, if you choose to undress, wearing stockings creates an interesting visual.

At the end of the day, whatever you choose to wear ought to make you feel comfortable and secure about yourself. The last thing you want is to go for a look that isn't you. Please remember that you don't have to look a certain way to be a knock-out FEMDOM. Your sub will go wild in anything you wear. So, don't hold back. This is your time to feel empowered.

Chapter 8: Setting the Stage

FEMDOM is all about the ambiance that surrounds the practices you want to engage in. So, setting the scene is an important aspect as creating an environment that can assert your dominance is key. What that scene looks like is entirely up to you.

When going about setting the scene for your FEMDOM encounters, you must consider what you want to get out of it. This means that you must consider the way in which you wish to assert your dominance. One classic example is the dungeon motif. This scenario is conducive to pulverizing your subs if they choose to enter.

However, it's not always entirely possible to have your own dungeon. This is especially true if you don't have a place devoted exclusively to your encounters, and you have a house full of kids. Still, that doesn't mean you can't set things up just the way you like them.

That's why this chapter is focused on setting the stage for your encounters in such a way that you won't have any trouble making a considerable impression on your subs. Most importantly, it can become the type of scenario you enjoy most. This is the kind of situation in which you can feel comfortable, thereby giving you the greatest amount of pleasure.

Privacy Is Key

Perhaps the biggest concern for FEMDOMS (and their subs, especially) is privacy. When you think about this aspect, it's important that you consider the need for a space that is away from prying eyes. This opens up a number of possibilities which you ought to consider.

First of all, does your current place of residence offer the option of setting up a room devoted exclusively to your escapes? Perhaps a basement or an extra bedroom could do the trick. This is particularly important if you're into the whole BDSM or dungeon setup. Thus, privacy becomes an important consideration.

There are other alternatives if you can't devote a specific place to your FEMDOM tactics. Lots of couples rent out hotel rooms. And while hotel rooms can't be easily converted into a dungeon, at least it provides a reasonable amount of privacy. Please keep in mind that just about every male sub is not keen on being publicly recognized as a sub. They may have no issue with being your sub, but they may have issues with everyone at the office knowing about it.

Also, renting out an apartment solely for the purpose of your encounters is also an option. However, this could be an expensive arrangement, although there is one alternative here. There are men who are willing to pay for the experience of being dominated. Now, this doesn't mean paying for sex by any means. There are guys who are perfectly willing to pay for a dominatrix to pound them. As strange as that may sound, there are plenty of guys who just want the experience of being manhandled by a woman. It may sound paradoxical, but they are not necessarily interested in the sexual experience. After all, you can decide to let them engage in sexual activity or not. In the end, it's your decision to pursue this avenue.

Creating the Fight Environment

The whole dungeon motif is practically cliché in the world of FEMDOM. In addition, it should be noted that not all guys who seek the FEMDOM experience have the dungeon in mind. What they really want is the domination that comes from being reduced to dust by a dom.

So, this implies that your environment doesn't have to be converted into a torture chamber. You can outfit them with the toys and devices that you plan to use. In fact, there are many couples who carry out their FEMDOM dynamic is a regular apartment. There are instances where you find a leather-clad FEMDOM sitting in an armchair getting a pedicure from her pet sub.

What this means is that you don't need to have your house renovated to suit your FEMDOM preferences. Other couples who are in committed relationships make tweaks to their bedroom to suit their activities. For instance, they install heavy curtains to ensure privacy while arranging furniture to suit the types of activities they engage in. This may include keeping a closet, or chest, readily available (this is where the goodies can be hidden).

Another important consideration is sound. Lots of couples make sure that they are at liberty to make as much noise as they please. This not only applies to other household members, but also to the neighbors. After all, you don't want the neighbors to overhear what's going on...

As for lighting, this is also an important part of setting the stage. Plenty of couples prefer a darker environment. So, they might go ahead and install dimmers or even colored lightbulbs. Again, these types of tweaks enable you to set the mood just the way you like it.

With regard to scents, this aspect should ideally reflect what you like. Perhaps there are certain scents that please you. Or, you might be inclined to use foul smells, especially as part of humiliation tactics. Ultimately, it really depends on what you want to achieve with your experience.

Lastly, it's important to consider other people who may participate in your escapes. For instance, if you plan to engage in cuckoldry, you might want to make allowances for an additional person in your space. If you also plan to have multiple subs at the same time, then you should also keep those spatial considerations in mind.

At the end of the day, setting the scene largely depends on each person's circumstances. If you have the money and room to create your own dungeon, then by all means. But if all you want is a private area in which you can let your imagination fly, then there are plenty of minor tweaks you can make to suit your personal needs and style.

What About Props?

This is a common concern when it comes to setting up your personal space. Many FEMDOMS use props in their encounters. This includes whips, chains, handcuffs, and so on. So, if you happen to use a good number of props, what do you do with them?

Now, if you have a dedicated space for them, then there's really no issue. You can just keep them in the same spot. That way, you won't have to search for them when you actually need them. Things get a bit trickier when you don't have a dedicated space.

Earlier, we mentioned keeping them in a closet or a chest. However, you may not be keen on spending time on setting things up before and organizing after every session. But don't worry, there are alternatives.

The most common storage solution is a "toy box." These boxes are disguised to look like a closet or a footlocker. They come in various sizes and can hold the toys and props you wish to use in your encounters. Plus, they are an inexpensive solution as they can be accommodated inside a closet or kept under the bed. The best thing about these boxes is that they don't take up a lot of space.

Another interesting storage alternative is a suitcase. These come in all sizes. They are great because you can travel with them as well. They can fit the number of toys and props you need while keeping them handy. This is important as you may not always have time to set up every prop you plan to use. In addition, if you get creative, your toys will always be on hand. That's what makes these types of suitcases so convenient.

Also, there are cloth rolls which you can use to store essential toys. These rolls look like the ones used by old-school doctors. When you unroll them, all of your toys or torture devices are revealed. They are great if you are not packing a lot, or just want the essentials on hand. Additionally, they are great if you are just starting out and don't have a lot of props, yet. They are easy to store and give you the option of carrying stuff around with you should scenes be carried out in various locations.

All About Furniture

This is where things get really interesting.

If you the option of setting up a dedicated space for your FEMDOM scenes, then there are a number of options from which you can choose your furniture. The most common is just a plain table with stirrups or straps. These tables are plain wood though we would recommend going with stainless steel, kind of like surgical tables, just in case there are bodily fluids expelled at any point in time.

Having a dedicated table can help you with torture tactics. As a matter of fact, some gals like to set up their place to look like a workshop. So, the place a table in the middle with shelves and hooks holding up all the goodies. This type of setup doesn't exactly look like a dungeon. If anything, it looks like something taken out of a horror movie. But, if you're into it, then it certainly works for a terrifying experience.

Another very interesting piece of furniture you can use looks like a dentist's chair. You'll find them under the name of "facesit" chair. They are designed so that you can sit on your sub's face while they lie down. While the chair isn't exactly designed with your sub's comfort in mind, it's intended to avoid suffocation. It can also be used as means of torture as it gives you access to your sub's lower body without them being able to see what you are doing.

You will also find a chair that resembles a regular chair, like the kind you would have in your dining room, but without the bottom. This chair is generally used for torture tactics. The sub sits in this chair, usually bound or restrained so that the genital area is exposed. This type of chair is used in cock and ball torture, or just for the purpose of giving a couple of friendly whips.

Lastly, you will find an assortment of couches and sofas, which can also be used as part of your FEMDOM tactics. Of course, you can use a regular couch, in particular, the armrests, to bend over your sub. However, one popular type of sofa-like piece of furniture looks like an "m." This is used to bend the sub over. It's great for penetration, such as with a dildo or strap-on, and also allows for restraint. It is also a fun place to sit and relax if you should so choose.

A Word of Caution

Perhaps the biggest mistake when starting out with FEMDOM is rushing out to get a bunch of things. The fact is that it's always best to refrain from making significant purchases at first. The reason for this is that you might get stuff that doesn't really go with your persona. This is why it's always recommended to purchase your gear as you find your identity in the FEMDOM world.

For example, you might be gung-ho about the whole dungeon setup but then realize it's not really you. So, you end up spending a bunch of money on a number of things which don't really suit your style. On the contrary, you can experiment with various things and move on from there.

One simple idea is to get an old chair from a garage sale or thrift store, cut out the bottom and use that as a facesit chair. You don't spend a great deal of money, and you are able to experiment with something specific. In anything, it's probably best to get old furniture as your subs may end up having bathroom accidents while on the chair. So, you don't want a nice piece of new furniture being spoiled.

On the whole, you can turn any space into your personal lair. All you need is to find your identity and take it from there!

Chapter 9: Accessories...
Accessories... Accessories...

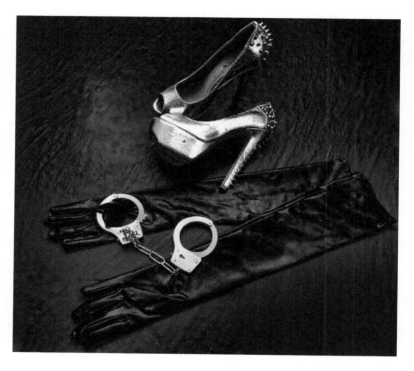

Throughout this book, we have mentioned toys, accessories, and other goodies. So, the time has come to drill down and focus on what these toys are and how you can use them in your FEMDOM scenes. The main thing here is to look at the array of options and then choose the ones that suit your preferences best.

Now, it should be noted that there are all kinds of kinky toys out there. Some of them look like they were pulled out of a medieval torture chamber. Others are just plain and straightforward stuff you see in movies. Ultimately, it depends on how far you want to take things and how much you want to push your subs.

It should also be said that you don't really need toys to make your presence as a FEMDOM felt. In fact, there are FEMDOMS out there who make a name for themselves by using household stuff. That can add a really mind-bending dimension to your games.

In this chapter, we are going to focus on the main types of toys that you can use and how they can be implemented to really get the most out of your FEMDOM role plays.

Whips, Ropes, and Chains

These artifacts are typical of BDSM. They are used to restrain subs while also inflict pain upon them. Of course, we're not talking about torturing people to death. We are making a point though of how you can use these artifacts to give your subs the experience they have been looking for.

First off, whips are quite common. They are used in a plethora of situations. Most commonly, they are used to discipline subs. When a sub gets out of line, cracking the whip becomes a must. Whips are also one of the staples in the dungeon or goth setup. They are cool and can really create the effect you are looking for.

Also, the use of floggers is common. For most FEMDOMS, some kind of combination of whips or floggers gives them control over their subs. This is especially important when you think about how much subs relish in their pain. Plus, it's a relatively harmless way of giving subs what they deserve.

Now, here's a good way in which you can subject your subs to some kinky pain. Sit your sub on the bottomless chair. You can use a rope to restrain them, or perhaps a chain for greater effect. Now, take the whip or flogger, and hit them under the chair. This will land the blow right on the testicles. The pain that this tactic causes can be quite considerable. The only thing to be careful with here is to avoid hitting them too hard. A good rule of thumb is to start off easy and ramp it up as much as the sub can take it. The use of a safe word would come in handy here if you should so choose.

In addition, using handcuffs is useful when looking to keep your sub from moving about. Police handcuffs work well though you need to be careful you don't lose the key. Alternatively, shackles can create a seriously mind-bending experience. The leather shackles seem to work best as they won't purposely damage your sub's wrists. However, you might have subs who are into the full-blown experience. If that's the case, then why not indulge your sub?

All About Masks

We could write an entire book about masks!

Seriously, masks play such a prominent role in BDSM, FEMDOM, and dungeon scenes. The main attractiveness to them is that masks offer a degree of anonymity to both sub and mistress. Mainly, it allows subs to feel even more submissive as they are reduced to a faceless element.

As for the mistress (or master in any event), it allows for a psychological effect based on the power dynamic that you have chosen. Some FEMDOMS would rather not wear a mask and simply go for gothic makeup. Some FEMDOMS won't wear anything at all. As always, it's a question of what you prefer.

First off, there are masks that are intended to block the sub's visuals. These masks may resemble blindfolds or sleeping masks. They don't do much in the way of fomenting submission but can be a good means of getting newbies to settle in.

Then, there are full-face coverings. The classic mask is the one with the zipper for a mouth. If you search for a "gimp" mask, you will find an array of full-face coverings that resemble medical face masks, military gas masks, or the kind that have the zipper for a mouth.

These masks are used to indicate silence. As such, the sub has no means of uttering a sound. In the event that subs cry out in pain, these masks muffle sounds. So, they also serve this purpose. However, care needs to be taken that the sub does not suffocate. This can become an issue, especially if they are restrained. That's why it's best to check to make sure your sub can breathe alright.

There are other types of masks that are basically animal faces. These are used in humiliation tactics. For instance, you are treating your sub like the animal that they are. So, it is only fitting that they actually look the part.

As for military gas masks, some FEMDOMS and BDSM practitioners are into the whole Nazi setup. So, the old-style WWI gas masks add a touch of horror to the entire situation. For example, the FEMDOM can wear one to create a scene of panic while the sub may wear a plain full-face covering. Another twist is a surgical face mask that makes it seem like the FEMDOM is a demented doctor. The sub has no choice but to swallow their fear.

Please note that there is a myriad of masks to choose from. So, it really depends on what you like and what you feel is fitting for your sub(s).

Dildos and Strap-ons

Now we're talking about anal play. This is big-league stuff for most guys. While new subs may not be into this much, at least not right away, you will find that most subs are actually yearning for some kind of anal play. As such, you can use these artifacts to your advantage.

Let's start with dildos. There are many kinds of dildos out there. You can find some really creative ones while others that are out of a horror film. However, when it comes to male subs, dildos don't really need to be creative. They just need to get the job done.

For most subs, though, they may have very little anal play experience. So, you might want to ease them a little bit. To this end, butt plugs may serve best. Butt plugs are shorter and are built to facilitate penetration. They are made out of glass or rubber. If your sub is completely new to anal play, a rubber butt plug might be your best choice.

Butt plugs are very useful when training your sub as you can require them to have one inserted throughout your time. Stricter mistresses require subs to wear them throughout their regular day. If your sub is compliant with this, then you may have yourself a fully trained butt slave in short order.

As for dildos, glass dildos may not be your best choice with inexperienced subs. You might want to try rubber ones as they provide the easiest experience. They come in all shapes and sizes. So, having a couple in different lengths and circumferences can help create an interesting experience for your sub.

Also, vibrators can work well, too. While they don't create the same effect as they do in women, vibrators can offer a different kind of sensation for your sub. You will find that your subs will gladly accept dildos as part of their training at one point or another.

When it comes to strap-ons, you will find these to be the ultimate power rush. When you have a sub, who is bent over and practically helpless, penetrating them can provide you with a rush of adrenaline while the sub learns his place. Like dildos, strap-ons come in all shapes and sizes. So, you can choose the one that best suits your preferences.

Additionally, anal beads are quite popular when training subs. These are a bit uncomfortable at first but can provide you with the training your subs need if you are planning to go deep with them. They come in various sizes. So, you can start off with a smaller size and work your way up.

Trying Out All Kinds of Goodies

In the world of FEMDOM, there are all kinds of goodies you can try out. These all depend on how far you plan to take things and what your subs can tolerate. There are cases in which your subs can only take so much. So, it's a good idea to go easy on them. In other cases, your subs might be able to handle a lot more. That can be your cue to really turn up the heat.

One goodie you might want to try is the cock ring. These rings are placed around the penis when it is flaccid. Then, as the penis grows in size, the ring constricts around the penis. This makes it painful to get an erection. This forces the sub to cool it. Similarly, ball rings constrict the testicles. This creates an overall sensation of pain while cutting off circulation. These are used as a common torture tactic.

Ball gags are also used during kinky play. They can be an interesting alternative to masks. There are ball gags that give the sub something to bite down on or just a regular gag, which is meant to both muffle sound and restrict breathing. Care needs to be taken with these so that the sub doesn't suffocate during an encounter. It's always important to be sure your subs are safe as they fully trust you.

Clamps are also commonly used in BDSM and FEMDOM play. Clamps are usually placed in very sensitive areas such as the nipples, penis, or tongue. They are meant to cause pain while providing your sub with stimulation in certain areas. Placing clamps on testicles can be used as a torture tactic.

You will also find some extreme toys such as needles. Using sharp objects are truly extreme. We don't recommend the use of these types of torture tactics as they can put your sub's wellbeing in danger. The same goes for full-body latex suits. They can cause your sub to suffocate. As such, it's best to avoid using these types of devices until you are fully aware of what you are doing.

Choosing the Right Toys for You

At the end of the day, choosing the right toys should be about finding the best ones to suit your individual tastes. If your sub is yearning for anal play, then, by all means, oblige him. This is why we have repeatedly stated that this is your domain. Any sub that chooses to enter must know what they are up against. Consequently, they must deal with whatever you throw their way. This will not only help you assert your dominance but also give you the pleasure that comes with inflicting pain and torture on your subs.

So, do take the time to go over what's available on the market. Since it may be hard to choose, you might want to start out with the essentials and take it from there. Also, don't be shy about trying household items out. For instance, using an old electrical cord as a restraint is a weird but effective idea. Old paintbrushes are great for teasing while clothespins make fabulous clamps. As such, you don't need to spend a great deal of money to really spice things up. A little creativity can go a long way, especially when your subs are begging for more!

Part III: Basic FEMDOM Tactics

Chapter 10: Humiliation Tactics

Humiliation is a common tactic used in FEMDOM. Just about every kind of blog, book, or program you see about FEMDOM includes humiliation as its main focus. However, we are not going to focus this book solely on humiliation. In fact, it's just one of the tactics you can use to dominate your male subs.

Does that sound interesting?

Indeed, you can use humiliation as just one means of exerting your dominance. Most importantly, there are a number of various tactics that you can put into practice. So, it's not that there is just "humiliation." There is a number of ways in which you can put humiliation into practice. By following these tactics, you will surely drive your main point home.

The Main Purpose of Humiliation

The main purpose behind humiliation is not to debase de human condition of your subs. This is something that perhaps gets lost with a lot of the websites and videos you find nowadays. The point of humiliation is to subjugate your subs to your command. As such, they need to understand who is in charge and what this represents to them, and to you. So, the use of humiliation tactics is intended to further break the sub into a submissive role.

Moreover, you can easily see how subs settle into a subservient role by the way the faithfully execute your orders and commands. Consequently, you don't need to denigrate your subs in order to get them fully immersed in a submissive role.

Additionally, humiliation tactics are quite broad. They can go from rather basic elements such as sissy play to more graphic situations like bathroom play. Ultimately, it's a question of seeing how much your sub can tolerate. If you find that they can handle their fair share of humiliation, then you can be certain that you will find a good balance between dominance and submission.

Sissy Play

The first tactic we are going to look at is sissy play. Earlier, we talked about how sissy play is one of the first things that most subs experience. When you are looking to use it as part of humiliation, sissy play can be seen as a means of putting your sub into a deeply submissive role.

The first step to sissy play is cross-dressing. Some guys love to dress up in girls' clothes, or perhaps have a fetish about it. So, you are only too happy to oblige. With sissy play, you can use your imagination. For example, your subs can wear female panties while they prance around for your amusement. In other cases, they can wear makeup and dresses. Some cross-dressing play includes dressing up like a doll.

If you feel inclined, a gimp mask can add an interesting touch to your sub. If you wish to take photos to use as humiliation material later on, just make sure you don't capture your sub's face. The last thing you want is to have intimate photos leaking out. Nevertheless, using photos as humiliation material, later on, is quite useful. You can have your subs go through this humiliation and then use the photos as a means of blackmail if they should ever get out of line.

Another component of sissy play is anal play. With anal play, your sub is placed in the role of receiver. As such, you are treating them like a sissy because they secretly enjoy being penetrated. You can use dildos or strap-ons for this purpose. However, more extreme domination games include another male penetrating the sub. While this may be taking things a bit too far, you may be surprised to find your subs agreeing to this.

Lastly, sissy play is a psychological tactic in which roles are reversed. So, the FEMDOM takes on the traditional male role while the male sub takes on a traditional female role. Thus, your sub is well aware that they don't have much power while in your presence. This means they can either deal with it or get out.

Shaming and Name-Calling

FEMDOMS love to assign pet names to their subs. Now, by "pet names," we don't mean "boo" and "honey." We mean things like naming your sub as you would a pet. This is important for two reasons. First, you avoid using your sub's real name, thereby ensuring discretion. Second, you are creating an alternate person for your sub. As such, they might be Mr. Smith, sales manager, out there in the real world, but inside your domain, they are "Fifi" or "meatball." This type of tactic ensures that subs are certain to remember who they are in your presence.

Also, name-calling extends to making specific references to their physical appearance. A chubby sub may be referred to as "fatso." Perhaps your thin sub might become "skinny" when being referred to. Again, the idea here is to force your sub to remember who they are at all times. Perhaps the only limit here would be to refrain from mocking a physical disability. Doing so would be downright mean. Although it really depends on the dynamic that you have. Still, it's best to avoid shaming a sub if they clearly have a disability.

That being said, shaming also extends to open chastising your subs for their behavior. For instance, you allow your sub to touch themselves while you torture them in some manner. As the play proceeds, the sub ejaculates. Consequently, you proceed to shame your sub for doing so. Some mistresses can be quite strict and shame their subs for even getting an erection without being told to do so.

Additionally, shaming can be used constantly as a means of reminding subs of their place. For example, if they are big and tall, you might use shaming like, "you're a big tall guy out there but nothing more than a sissy in here." This type of shaming has a practical, psychological effect on the sub. Therefore, the sub is reduced to a clearly submissive role.

Shaming is also commonly used when subs don't follow orders or don't meet expectations. Let's assume you command your sub to shave you. But they hurt you in some manner. Depending on your style, you can verbally lash out at your sub for nicking your skin. You can use all kinds of verbal jabs like "you're so useless" or "your absolutely worthless." While such statements would be completely cruel in the real world, bear in mind that this isn't the real world!

Humiliation As Punishment

Another interesting angle is to use all of the tactics that we have mentioned earlier as a means of punishment. So, any of the tactics we have mentioned in this chapter can be used as a manner of disciplining your sub. Let's say that your sub doesn't particularly enjoy sissy play. Well, that's what they get if they don't live up to your expectations. Perhaps you can put a leash on them and take them around for a walk if they don't follow your orders to the letter.

Another punishment tactic is to use specific name-calling to remind the sub of their transgressions. When the sub messes up, a particular name is used. For example, you may not use an animal name during regular interaction. But as soon as your sub makes a mistake, then this name is used. A name such as "bobo" (you can come up with your own, for sure) would be used to remind the sub that they messed up, "you're useless bobo, aren't you?) this is a powerful humiliation tactic that can really drive a point home, especially when subs don't really seem to follow your orders.

Also, this is where you can bring out humiliating videos or photos. If your sub doesn't seem to get it, they can be reminded of the consequences unless they shape up. A powerful tactic is to take pictures or videos of them being penetrated. It can really drive the point home should they not follow your orders to your liking. Again, just make sure your sub's faces aren't visible. Trust us; it's best to play it safe with this kind of material.

Cuckoldry

We saved the best for last.

Cuckoldry is derived from a medieval word that was used to denote men whose wives cheated on them with another man. The key here is that the man had some kind of knowledge about it but didn't do anything. This term was coined from birds who would raise another bird's eggs in their own nest. It was kind of like raising children that were not yours biologically. While being a stepparent is nothing to be ashamed of in human society, it is in the animal kingdom. Consequently, the term was used to denote men who were cheated on by their wives. During medieval times, a cuckold was generally the last guy to find out about it. The entire town knew who the cuckold was except the cuckold himself.

Translate that concept to our day and age, and you get a man whose wife (or committed partner) openly cheats on him with another man. Now, there is a difference between cuckoldry and swinging. Swinging implies consent among both parties. Also, swingers open exchange partners. This is the main difference with your average cuckold. The cuckold cannot have any other partners. They are forbidden to have another partner lest they incur the wrath of their mistress.

Now, let's take a look at the various dimensions of cuckoldry.

There is cuckoldry within a committed relationship, such as marriage or a long-term stable relationship. In this scenario, the mistress openly brings in other men with whom she engages in sexual intercourse. This is important as the humiliation increases in proportion as the mistress has sexual intercourse with the third party. It should be noted that the third party is not necessarily a sub. Otherwise, the cuckoldry scenario doesn't play out well. In fact, the mistress may have open displays of affection to the third man. Moreover, the mistress may even pleasure the man in order to increase the level of humiliation of the cuckold.

The most common level of cuckoldry is forcing the sub to watch. This is humiliation enough. However, humiliation can increase considerably. In order to further humiliate your sub, you can ask him to participate in the sexual act. For instance, the sub may be forced to masturbate the third man. This is particularly humiliating if the sub doesn't have any attraction toward other men.

Additionally, the sub can be humiliated by being the recipient of the third man's ejaculation. For instance, the third man may engage in sexual intercourse with the mistress and then ejaculate on the sub. Generally, the ejaculation is shot off on the sub's face. The sub may even be asked to swallow the semen.

Perhaps the ultimate level of cuckoldry is having the third man penetrate the sub. This can be done after being forced to watch the mistress engage in sexual activity with the third man. Naturally, this is especially humiliating for the sub, particularly if they are not attracted to men.

As you can see, cuckoldry is, in many ways, the ultimate form of humiliation. However, if you are not in a committed relationship with your subs, then you might find that the more extreme forms of cuckoldry are suitable. The use of masks might be your best option in order to ensure the privacy of all parts, especially if there is a video taken of the events. Nevertheless, cuckoldry can turn out to be the biggest power rush you can get in the FEMDOM world. Oh, and don't forget that cuckoldry is an effective means of punishment, especially if your sub decides to engage in sexual activity with someone other than you. So, if you are able to find willing participants, why not give it a chance? Subs who are not your committed partners will find it humiliating to be manhandled by another male while you are running the entire show!

Chapter 11: Oral Play

What would FEMDOM be without some good oral play?

Now, please note that we are not talking about you, the FEMDOM, engaging in oral with your sub. That's the last thing your sub deserves. This is about your sub taking the time to please you orally. Therefore, you must make sure that your sub knows the rules of the game. Otherwise, there will be consequences to face.

Oral play is an essential part of the whole FEMDOM dynamic. It can be used as a part of your regular scenes while it can also be used as a form of humiliation. As such, it is quite versatile and provides FEMDOMS with any number of options to make their sub's life quite interesting.

In this chapter, we are going to explore the role of oral play in the FEMDOM world and how you can make the most of this fun experience for both you and your sub(s).

Oral Play Fun

Oral play is commonly used to have the sub pleasure of the FEMDOM. This is really the only way you can really consider oral play to make sense within the FEMDOM domain. Now, you might perform oral on your sub, but as part of teasing torture (more on that in a bit).

So, things can get pretty wild from here.

Let's start with the basics. Firstly, you can have your sub perform oral on you by simply pleasuring you with their mouth. It's up to you if you would like to have your sub perform oral on you until you orgasm. Regardless, the sub is there to please you no matter what the circumstances.

When performing oral on you, you must command the sub so that he can perform it in the manner you prefer most. This could be through the use of the mouth, lips, and tongue. If you would like the sub to use their fingers, that could work, too.

One of the fun twists of this tactic is to have a whip or flogger. That way, you can direct your sub to do things as you like. This means that if the sub isn't meeting your expectations, you can give him a gentle nudge to remind him of the way you enjoy doing things.

Now, oral play is part of the FEMDOM power dynamic. Therefore, your sub must be in a position of inferiority. So, this generally positions the FEMDOM sitting on a bed, couch, or chair while the sub is generally kneeling. Earlier, we mentioned how kneeling on a pencil as a torture tactic. Well, this is a great moment to put that tactic into practice. If you take your sweet time enjoying the oral play, then the discomfort would be prolonged for the sub.

Also, you can break out your facesit chair. This is the perfect time to use it. You can comfortably sit in the chair while your sub takes care of business. As you can see, this is why facesit chairs are so popular. Alternatively, a bottomless chair can work just fine. The only issue here would be to make sure it's the right height. That way, your sub can do the business without making too much of a fuss.

You may choose to require your sub to use toys are part of oral play. If you are inclined to do so, then you must give your sub explicit instructions on how you wish them to use the toys you provide. Most commonly, subs are required to use vibrators in addition to performing oral play. In doing so, you must rid your sub of any restraints. At the very least, they would need to be able to use their hands. Please keep in mind that any use of toys is done with the sole purpose of pleasuring you. Don't think for a moment that your sub has the free rein to cause any kind of discomfort to you. This would be grounds for punishment. So, it's important that your sub is reminded of that.

Oral Play Teasing Torture

You may want to use teasing as a means of torturing your sub. To achieve this, you can resort to oral play. Now, the last thing your sub can expect from you is for you to go out of your way to please him. That is why this teasing torture is all that more powerful. You are essentially giving your sub a glimmer of hope, yet you yank it away just as easily.

Oral teasing torture is generally used when the sub is bound. You can tie up your sub to a table or a chair. Then, you can really turn up the heat. For this torture, a feather duster works really well. It is especially cruel if your sub has an erection. You can use the duster to tickle sensitive areas while giving him some dirty talk. You can make your sub beg you to touch them. Then, as you make it seem like you will be giving him oral pleasure, you can move away. Doing this multiple times can really drive your sub nuts. Some even ejaculate from the excitement. If that is the care, the shaming, name-calling, or some other type of punishment may ensure.

Some FEMDOMS may actually perform some kind of oral on their subs but generally when they are in a committed relationship. You can do this as a means of showing some kind of appreciation for your sub, who is also a life partner. In such cases, you might be inclined to give your sub a thrill or two.

Oral Play Humiliation

This part is quite interesting and entertaining. Oral play can be used as a means of humiliating your sub, especially if you want to punish them. It's quite interesting to see how they react, particularly when asked to do something they are uncomfortable with.

One of the most common oral play humiliation tactics is to do oral on a dildo or strap-on. At first, it might seem a bit strange to your sub. After all, it's not that common to fool around like that with a dildo. However, the fact that it's shaped like a penis makes it psychologically intense. To take this exercise further, you can make your sub suck on the dildo or strap-on in order to lube it up prior to anal play. Then, the sub must suck on it to keep it lubed up so the anal play can continue.

This tactic can be taken further if you have multiple subs. One sub can suck on the dildo or strap-on, which is then inserted into another sub. It can make for a very intense experience, especially if you have brand-new subs.

Another interesting part of oral play humiliation is to have your subs lick your shoes and boots. Specifically, you can have your subs lick the soles of your footwear. This may not have any practical purpose as far as sex goes, but it serves quite well to create a strong effect of submission. This is quite commonly done when training new subs. So, do make sure to incorporate it as part of your new sub training regimen.

Also, for the foot fetish fans, subs can be required to kiss your feet, lick your soles or suck on your toes. Now, you might also ask them to paint your toenails, but that would be a fun little reward for them. So, if you, or your sub, happen to have a foot fetish, this is the way to go. You will find that many FEMDOMS make a point of having their subs perform oral play on their feet. While it's not quite humiliation (especially if they like it), it can be pretty rough if your sub isn't into feet. Additionally, you may require your subs to wash your feet, give you a pedicure, or just massage your feet after a long session of dominating subs.

If you are looking to take it up a notch, performing oral on another male is essentially the limit for a lot of subs. This exercise can be a part of cuckoldry or just plain humiliation.

In cuckoldry, the cuckold will most likely be required to perform oral play on the third male. While this is not always the case, it's generally part of the ultimate experience the cuckold is asked to go through. Should the cuckold refuse, then there may be physical punishment to be had. If the sub definitely refuses to go any further, then you may have to reconsider their commitment to being a sub.

When cuckolds perform oral on a third male, the cuckold may be required to receive the ejaculation from the third male or simply perform oral prior to, or after, the third man has penetrated you. Also, the cuckold can be required to perform oral play multiple times throughout penetration. One other angle is to have the cuckold lick the third male's testicles while he is penetrating you.

In the event that you have multiple subs on board, they may be required to perform oral play on each other. However, you can limit just how much fun they have with each other. For instance, you may keep them from ejaculating, or you may require them to finish off the other sub. Some FEMDOMS use this tactic as a means of providing their subs release, especially if they have been subjected to teasing torture.

This tactic can be further enhanced by the use of masks. So, if a sub is unable to see the other sub on whom they are performing oral play, they may be less inclined to feel weird about it. At the same time, the lack of visuals can create a very eerie scenario for your subs.

And then, there is rimming. Rimming consists of performing oral play on the anal region of another person. As such, rimming offers a number of interesting alternatives. For starters, your sub may be asked to perform rimming on you. This can be done while you squat on his face or while sitting in a facesit chair. The sub can use the mouth or tongue to perform the rimming action.

Also, you can have subs rim one another, especially if you are prepping them for anal play. For instance, one sub may be asked to rim the other prior to your penetration of them with a dildo or strap-on. This works quite well in a group setting, especially when you are running a dungeon with multiple subs.

If you are engaging in cuckoldry, you can have the sub rim the third male either as part of the humiliation exercise or perhaps while he is penetrating you. In this case, the sub may be lying on his back while you squat over him in a reverse cowgirl position. This would leave the sub's face exposed to the third male's testicles and anus. You can even throw in some teasing torture just for good measure.

Lastly, oral play can lead to humiliation when you have your subs lick the floor or any other surface. While this may seem unclean, well, your sub really has no choice. Of course, you are not going to ask him to lick the garage floor, but just having them lick the floor as part of their training is enough to set the tone for their experience. Some FEMDOMS like having their subs kiss the ground they walk on. It's a metaphorical way of forcing your subs to worship you as their mistress.

As you can see, oral play has many different facets to it. You can be as creative or as extreme as you like. We have explored many different ways in which oral play can become a part of your domination tactics. So, it's always good to start off easy and then ramp things up to the point where your subs can handle things. You'll be surprised to find your subs handling a lot more than you think!

Chapter 12: Getting Messy

In FEMDOM and BDSM, "getting messy" can get, well, messy. By "messy," we're referring to bathroom play. Now, bathroom play can cover a lot of different areas. Generally speaking, bathroom play involves humiliating your sub(s). As such, you can take this as far as you want. This means that your subs may be in for quite a messy time.

It should be noted that bathroom play isn't for everyone. It's a very specific fetish that some people really enjoy while others would rather avoid it. Depending on your personal tastes, you may want to engage in it or not.

In this chapter, we are going to take a look at bathroom play, the various types of tactics you can employ within the realm of bathroom play.

Bathroom Play 101

In essence, bathroom play can involve anything related to the bathroom and activities conducted in the bathroom. One of the simplest activities in engaging in sexual intercourse in the bathroom. But that would be something that regular couples would do. As such, FEMDOM takes things to a whole new level.

When looking at bathroom play, you are really going to test your tolerance levels. If you are squeamish, this may not be the best type of tactic for you. Yet, if you are not afraid of pushing the envelope, then by all means.

If you are really into pushing things to the extreme, you will find that "toilet slavery" is one of the most extreme activities you can enjoy. The main reason behind this is that it pushes the limits of your tolerance. Since we associate the bathroom with dirtiness, it can be quite hard to get over the psychological barrier pertaining to this. Consequently, you may find it hard to engage in bathroom play. Yet, as we have mentioned, this is a bit of a niche fetish. There are some subs who are perfectly willing to go along with it.

Now, one word of caution. Make sure you have the means to keep everything tidy when engaging in this type of play. The issue here is that if things get really messy, then cleaning up may get pretty rough afterward. Sure, your sub is there to do the dirty work, but you may end up with a bigger mess than you had bargained for.

Golden Showers

One common bathroom fetish is known as "golden showers." In essence, "golden showers" refers to the FEMDOM urinating on her sub. This is primarily done as a humiliation tactic, though it can be used as a means of satisfying a fetish.

It should also be noted that golden showers differ from a squirting orgasm, that is when females urinate following an orgasm. These types of orgasms are common in porn films and are generally seen when the female is in a submissive role. In this case, golden showers are a means of showing dominance over a sub.

The most common practice is to have the FEMDOM simply urinate over the sub. This can be done by simply squatting over the sub, or by way of sitting in a bottomless chair. At this point, things can get really kinky.

Firstly, you can simply urinate over your sub's body. Really, anywhere on his body will do, although you may find that the chest area is the most common. The sub may be restrained in some form or simply lying down. In most cases, the sub is restrained in one manner or another.

Secondly, an even kinkier twist may include the FEMDOM urinating on the sub's face. The sub may be required to swallow or simply take the blast. Masks may or may not be used though they generally are. The sub is not usually allowed to wipe anything off. As such, they may be required to lie there in a pool of urine. This is why we recommend that you make sure cleaning up afterward doesn't pose a bigger problem.

Some fetishes involve drinking urine. For instance, the sub may be required to collect the urine in a container and then drink it. Also, the sub can be required to lick or perform oral play on the FEMDOM after urination, thereby licking off the excess urine.

As you can see, golden showers are part of a fetish, which may or may not be used as a humiliation tactic. Golden showers among subs are not commonly used, and it is not generally seen as a part of cuckoldry. Although, anything goes as long as all parties are involved.

Scat/Toilet Play

Things get really messy here. Scat or toilet play (also know was "toilet slavery") involves feces. Like golden showers, subs are required to receive feces from their FEMDOM. When you think about this type of play, you really have to be open to anything. After all, you may not be entirely comfortable with defecating on your subs. Nevertheless, some subs relish in this type of play as it is one of the most extreme fetishes.

Basic scat play generally involves the FEMDOM defecating on the sub on any part of his body. The sub may be restrained in some manner, as is usually the case, though he may simply lie on the floor. The FEMDOM may defecate by squatting over the sub or use a bottomless chair. In some play, the sub may then be required to rub the feces all over his body. Pictures and videos of this can subsequently be used as a humiliation tactic, although it should be noted that most bathroom play involves the use of masks as a means of privacy.

To make things more extreme, the FEMDOM may defecate on the sub's face and mouth. This is really

535

extreme as the feces may then be smeared over the sub's face. In a very kinky, and perhaps nasty twist, the sub may be asked to eat the feces. As such, the sub is "eating out" of his FEMDOM's ass.

Another twist to this fetish includes rimming the FEMDOM after defecation. Needless to say, the sub licks the feces from the FEMDOM's ass. This is certainly extreme and even repulsive to some. Again, it's a question of seeing how far your subs are willing to go.

This is why scat is a very specialized fetish. Not all FEMDOMS do it, but those who do may find some very loyal subs. Subs who have this particular fetish relish in having their FEMDOMS dominate them in this manner. So, it's worth considering if you are inclined to such messy tactics.

Tips for Bathroom Play

As you can see, bathroom play can get pretty messy. After all, urinating and defecating on the floor can be quite tough to clean up. So, let's take a look at some helpful tips if you choose to engage in this type of play.

If you have a dedicated space, or room, such as a dungeon, you may be able to install a drain. This can really facilitate things as you can simply hose down the area afterward. This will avoid having to clean up and mop the floor. In particular, if you engage in scat, having feces on the floor is not a fun thing to clean up. Even if you get your sub to clean up after himself, it can still be a problem leaving the area neat and tidy.

Also, having a dedicated area can enable you to set up the gear you need, such as a facesit chair. This makes it easy to clean up should things get really messy. Otherwise, you may consider laying down a tarp beneath the chair to ensure that you have an easier time cleaning up afterward.

536

In cases where you don't have a dedicated space, some FEMDOMS prefer to use the bathroom itself. This can make sense as, well, that's what a bathroom is for. Some like to use a bathtub as it is quite easy to clean up after. Also, the bathroom floor is also equipped to handle such messes. So, you might find t easier to just go ahead and carry out your play right on the bathroom floor.

If you plan to do bathroom play in a hotel, stick to the bathroom. The last thing you want to do is make a huge mess in a hotel room. If you do, you might get nailed with extra charges for cleanup. Needless to say, that's not the best way to go about it. So, sticking to the bathroom is usually a good choice.

It's also important to have a shower available. Smells can get on pretty strong. So, it would be nice if all those involved had a chance to shower. You can make a game of it. If your sub wants to shower afterward, he will have to earn it. For instance, you could have him shave you while in the shower. Also, you could have him give you a bubble bath. You can always use your imagination.

Lastly, it's best to clean up any chairs you may use. Again, your sub will be only too happy to oblige. So, it's always a good idea to make sure that you keep any furniture you use nice and clean. That way, you won't have to regret any nasty smells later on.

What to Expect With Bathroom Play

Bathroom play is one of those extreme fetishes. Not all folks are inclined to it though most FEMDOMS experiment with it at some point. So, if you are grossed out by it, it's probably best not to engage in it. Also, you might want to refrain from getting too messy if you are sick to your stomach. After all, that could create a very nasty mess that might send everyone over the edge.

On the whole, bathroom play is the kind of kink you can use to humiliate your subs. Some FEMDOMS like to use it as an alternative to cuckoldry. Others like to include it as a part of cuckoldry. As you can see, the theme here is to use the tactics we have been presenting as you see fit. There is nothing wrong with using your imagination. Of course, if you have a sub that's begging for it, then why not give it a try? Some guys love this type of fetish. So, it only makes sense to try it out. Who knows, you might find something truly interesting!

Part IV: Advanced FEMDOM Tactics

Chapter 13: Torture Tactics

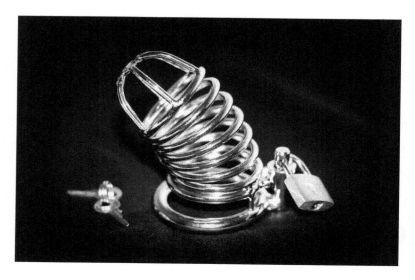

After mastering the basics, it's time to move on to some really heavy-duty stuff. In the world of FEMDOM, it's quite common to use torture tactics as a means of keeping subs happy. Many of the tactics used in FEMDOM are essentially the same as those used in BDSM. So, if you are familiar with BDSM, then you can appreciate the way FEMDOM uses them. The main difference is that you have a dedicated male sub on the receiving end of torture.

Torture tactics are used mainly as a means of arousal more than humiliation. Also, torture tactics are used as a means of punishing subs. When used as punishment, they need to be harsh enough to create a psychological impact on the sub so that they understand what the consequences of their misbehavior are.

That is why this chapter is focused on looking into the main torture tactics used in FEMDOM and how you can play around with them so that you can suit them to your individual style of play. Please keep in mind that these tactics can be customized to suit your particular preferences. As a result, there is no right or wrong way of going about it. They are just there for you to make them your own.

Bondage

We had to start here, right?

For newbies, bondage provides an enormous rush. This implies being tied up, literally, handcuffed and shackled. In some cases, mistresses simply tie up their subs and leave them there to contemplate life. Some mistresses slap a mask on their bound sub and let him sit there for a while.

Now, bondage can get as creative as you like it to. There are tables that resemble hospital beds. So, the rails on the sides can be outfitted with handcuffs or shackles. Leather shackles are far more comfortable than metal ones. In fact, metal shackles provide a more realistic experience if you will. Some more creative FEMDOMS like to get antique shackles. When it comes to antique shackles, the rustier, the better.

Then there are boards that can be used to tie up your sub. These boards can be upright so that your sub is standing, while others resemble a wheel. There are some which actually spin. These are pretty entertaining as you can place your sub upside down. They can be part of pretty gruesome torture as hanging upside down for a while can get pretty painful.

Also, subs can be tied to chairs. Earlier, we described the use of the bottomless chair. There are some chairs which are already outfitted for this purpose. However, you can just get an old chair and use ropes. If you prefer chains, then these will do perfectly fine. Some FEMDOMS like to leave their subs tied up in a chair as part of their initial training. It can be fun to leave a tied-up sub to figure out what to do.

If you have a dungeon area, then you can really get creative. For instance, old brick houses have pretty nasty basements. So, shackles can be outfitted to the wall. That will really give the impression that the sub is in a real dungeon. Alternatively, chains that are bolted into the wall can give the sub some room to move though they wouldn't be able to get very far. Additionally, you can shackle both arms and legs. Thus, you can fully restrain your sub.

Some FEMDOMS like to hogtie their subs. To do this, you can use a regular rope to tie your sub's hands behind their back and then tie up their legs with the same rope. This allows the sub to have both hands and feet bound behind their back. They can then be placed on their belly or on their side. If you add a mask and/or ball gag, you have a perfectly helpless sub. There are leather restraints that are already outfitted for this purpose. So, you can simply latch on the cuffs to hands and feet, and your sub is all tied up in a jiffy.

Cock and Ball Bondage

This is a very specific torture tactic. In this tactic, you are placing restraints on the penis and testicle area. Naturally, this sounds pretty painful. The sub finds himself literally bound by the balls. Depending on the type of device you use, this can get pretty painful.

For example, the use of a cock ring can cause quite a bit of pain. There are various sizes which you can use. So, the smaller kinds don't give the sub much room to maneuver. The larger rings are good for controlling erections. These rings can be quite painful if the sub gets hard because it constricts the penis. As a result, an erection can be quite painful.

One particular type of cock ring is called the "gates of hell." This is a device that has multiple rings that slide onto the length of the penis. These can be quite painful or pleasurable (depending on how you look at it) when the penis is fully erect. It is mainly used as a chastity device though it can be pretty painful if the rings are too small.

Cock rings slide on to the testicles. They create a great deal of pressure in this area. There are various sizes that can constrict the testicles to a greater extent. Thus, the pain can be quite unbearable. The most painful kind are the ones that separate the testicles down the middle. The pressure it creates by separating the balls can be rather uncomfortable after a while. As such, subs can learn valuable lessons through these devices.

Also, there are cages that you can use to fully restrict movement of the penis and create pressure on the testicles. These cages resemble various rings placed together in a triangular shape. This device is designed to constrict both the penis and the testicles. Needless to say, the use of a cage can make it quite uncomfortable for your sub.

Cock and Ball Torture

Alright, with this type of torture, you are actually getting pretty physical. Here, you are literally poking, pinching, stretching, piercing, and even stepping on the testicles and penis. If you combine this with cock and ball rings, you can practically demolish your sub's genitalia.

For starters, pinching your sub's balls can be a great place to start. This may include using your fingernails (especially if they are long) to pinch the scrotum, or devices such as clamps to actually squash your sub's balls. The use of clothespins can create a similar feeling. Additionally, you can use tweezers to pinch your sub's balls. One creative use of tweezers is to pull hairs out. This can be quite painful after a while.

Other forms of cock and ball torture include stretching. Stretching generally refers to stretching the penis though it can also be done to the testicles. This type of torture can get pretty creative as you can do something simple like using your hands, or a stretching device. Some of these devices resemble a vice. With such a device, you turn a knob or handle, and the device automatically stretches the penis and/or testicles. Another particularly brutal type of torture is to attach a weight to the genitalia. The naturally hangs down, thereby stretching out the testicles or pulling the penis out as far as it will go. Some of the more creative devices use a rope and pulley system. These are common in dungeons and create an interesting visual effect, especially for films.

Then, there is piercing.

Piercing generally refers to the foreskin and scrotum. It is not common to actually pierce the penis and testicles as this could cause severe injury. To do this, any number of devices can be used. The main point is to cause sharp pain in the area that is being pierced. Needles are a popular device used in this type of torture. For instance, regular sewing needles (not surgical) can be used to pierce through the foreskin (not the actual penis) or poke at the scrotum. Needless to say, this can be quite painful. Most mistresses like to put a mask on their subs during this type of torture in order to muffle sounds.

Also, other less conventional devices such as a staple remover can be used to both pinch and pierce through the skin. Some of the most creative torture tactics involve the use of nails (the kind that are used in construction) and staples. Imagine stapling your sub's foreskin to their scrotum!

Of course, it's important that you be careful as piercing may cause bleeding. So, if there is a lot of bleeding, then you may have to deal with the blood loss before proceeding. Also, it's a good practice to disinfect tools before piercing. The last thing you want to cause is an infection. Although, make sure that your sub doesn't know about it. After all, they are there to be tortured.

Anal Torture

Anal torture differs from anal play. Anal play is a fun activity in which subs get penetrated like little sissies, and that's it. They may be penetrated by a dildo, a strap-on, or even another mal. In this case, we are going to be looking at anal torture. So, we are going to take things to the extreme in this case. Please note that this type of torture can be really painful. That's why the use of masks is quite common. That way, your subs can scream out if they wish. Otherwise, the use of a gag may also work well.

Anal torture is generally caused by inserting some kind of device into the anus of a sub. Needless to say, this can be quite painful in subs who don't have much experience with anal play. Plus, anal play is rather humiliating to most subs. So, everyone wins.

The most common type of anal torture is penetration. However, this type of penetration can be done without lubrication. Needless to say, that is not fun. Without lubrication, the insertion of any object can be quite rough. If you are using a rubber dildo or strap-on, it can be quite tough to gain insertion. In the case of a glass or metal dildo, it might slide it a bit easier.

Also, the use of large devices is a good torture. For instance, large-size butt plugs can be quite painful. The sub must open up pretty wide to take the bulk of the butt plug and then hold it. A butt plug can be used in combination with cock and ball torture. Thus, this creates an excruciating experience.

Additionally, rough and/or violent penetration is a good way of showing dominance. You can ride your sub while wearing a strap-on or perhaps have another male penetrate them, such as in the case of cuckoldry. Rough anal play might not be as bad, but it does create a powerful psychological impact.

Subs may be placed on their hands and knees, that is on all fours, they may be restrained in some manner, or they may be placed lying face on a bed, table or couch. Generally speaking, there is some kind of restraint involved, though if your sub can handle it, they may be allowed to have use of their hands.

One interesting device which could be used is a fuck machine. This is a mechanical device that mimics the thrusting motion of a person during intercourse. When used for anal torture, a fuck machine can unleash a relentless assault on your sub. Naturally, this can get pretty painful after a while. You can combine this device with other types of torture or just use it for your own amusement.

Getting Creative

Ultimately, torture tactics are about being as creative as you can. Many FEMDOMS evolve their torture tactics to suit their personal tastes. Some like to claw their subs while others may use biting. Some like to pummel their subs by slapping or spanking them. There really is no limit to what you can do so long as your subs don't get injured. This is the main thing to keep in mind here. As long as you don't cause any serious harm or injury to your subs, they'll get over a few bruises.

The only practice we do not recommend is cutting. While some FEMDOMS may engage in this, we don't recommend it. Cutting can be dangerous, as you may cause severe bleeding, although it is quite common in some vampiric practices as it is a form of bloodletting. However, this can be dangerous for both the health of the sub and may cause infection. So, proceed at your own peril.

Beyond that, torture is the most exciting part of the FEMDOM experience for both subs and doms. Don't hold back as subs enjoy pain. They have a masochistic streak that enables them to get aroused from the whole ordeal.

And after some good old torture fun, you might be inclined to cap things off with a good round of sexual intercourse. Why not? You've earned it.

Chapter 14: Anal Play

Up to this point, we have discussed anal play quite extensively. We have discussed it as a means of humiliating your subs, punishing them, and even torturing them. As such, we will now focus on more specific types of anal play which you can use for your own amusement, or perhaps to further inflict torture on your subs. The best part of all is that you can use your creativity to suit your particular tastes.

With that in mind, let's get on with some interesting games you can play with your subs.

Anal Play Can Be Very Pleasurable

On the surface, anal play seems like it's all about domination and humiliation. And while that is true, it can also be quite pleasurable for a sub.

Allow us to elaborate on this point.

So, being penetrated anally can be quite humiliating and downright emasculating for a male. It makes them feel powerless while apparently stripping them of their masculinity. This is why you hear a lot about prison rape. When inmates are raped by other males, most people associate this with some kind of deviant sexual perversion. The fact is that there really isn't anything sexual about prison rape. It's mainly a question of asserting power among the prison hierarchy.

This is an important point to keep in mind. While engaging in anal play is about having fun and enjoying yourself, the main purpose of doing this is to assert your dominance as the FEMDOM. If we take it even further, it can be about completely stripping your sub of his masculinity. This is especially important when you have powerful men who like to be helpless sissies when in your clutches.

Surprisingly, anal play can be quite pleasurable for a sub. You see, the prostate gland can be stimulated from behind, that is, through the rectum. When this occurs, the stimulation to the prostate can lead to uncontrollable orgasm and ejaculation. In some sexual practices, females are taught to insert their fingers into the male's anus and stimulate the prostate. This is done as an alternative means of sexual pleasure.

In this case, you are actually giving your sub a welcome treat, and you can stimulate their prostate gland as part of the entire anal play dynamic. So yes, they do have to put up with the pain of the insertion. But ultimately, they derive a benefit from it. Because of this, you can use anal play as a risk-reward type deal. They must go through the pain of being penetrated, but the end result will be quite pleasurable.

To ensure that you hit the prostate, a longer dildo or strap-on would be needed. Short and stubby dildos or butt plugs won't do the job. You would need something longer, regardless of its thickness, to ensure that you hit the mark. You can tell if you're in the right spot as your sub will come to enjoy the effect.

Anal Training

When you're dealing with a new sub, they will most likely be unfamiliar or unaccustomed to anal play. There is nothing wrong with that. If anything, it just means that they don't have much experience with this type of play. In fact, you'll find that some guys ask their wives and girlfriends to engage in anal play with them. Most women are freaked out by a request of this nature. In fact, they may even suspect their man to be gay when, in reality, they are only seeking a different type of rush. This is why a great deal of subs seek out mistresses who can oblige them.

With that in mind, anal play can be quite fun for your sub(s), but you can't really expect them to handle everything you throw at them, at least not right away. So, here's are some helpful tips for anal training your new subs.

First, make regular use of butt plugs. At first, the shorter, thinner kind can work well. You can require your sub to wear a butt plug through their regular day. In doing so, you may even lead to bathroom control. For instance, the sub cannot go to the bathroom for a certain amount of time. This is meant to ensure that they keep the butt plug in place as part of their training.

Then, you may also require your subs to wear anal beads. These are inserted all the way up the rectum. At the tail end of the beads, there is a string that is pulled on to remove them. This helps to stretch out the anal cavity, thereby facilitating penetration. Plus, they can be rather uncomfortable, especially if you are sitting at your desk all day.

Anal beads and butt plugs come in all sizes. So, you can gradually move up from the smaller sizes up to the bigger ones. This type of practice can make it seems like your sub is "graduating" from one size to another. The great thing about this type of exercise is that you don't need to be there with them to ensure that they are training their butt hole.

While your sub is in your presence, you can devote specific time to training his butt. If the sub is clearly not ready for full penetration, you can progressively stretch out their butt hole by using a combination of dildos. Some mistresses like to start out their new subs with thinner dildos and progressively use thicker ones. As your sub's butthole gets stretched out, you can certainly make good use of bigger and bigger dildos. In fact, you may even use a larger dildo to pleasure yourself as a means of visual teasing, and then use that dildo on your sub. In a manner of speaking, it's like, "do you like what you see? Okay, now it's your turn!"

Lastly, be careful if you use other types of objects in your sub's butt. For instance, vegetables are commonly used though they may break during intense play. Also, avoid wooden objects as they may splinter, thereby causing injury. Anything that's sharp or pointed may cause internal bleeding. Also, anything that has a rough texture to it might also cause considerable injury. So, it's best to stay on the safe side.

Being Penetrated By Another Male

This practice can really drive your subs over the edge. Throughout this book, we have discussed this possibility as a means of extreme humiliation, such as in the case of cuckoldry. On the whole, having your subs penetrated by another male can be a pretty extreme form of punishment.

So, let's take a look at two scenarios here.

The first is to have another male (hetero, bi, or homosexual) join the fun. This male would be in charge of penetrating the sub(s). Now, it is important to note the presence of multiple subs as having the others watch what happens to one can create a pretty tough mental picture.

In this situation, you can even play games. For instance, you can draw straws or turn a roulette wheel. The sub whose number comes up would get the business. This can be quite exciting for spectators and pretty gruesome for the subs taking part. If you only have one sub present, you can spin the wheel to see if they get a dildo, strap-on, or the other male. This type of humiliation game can get even more extreme when engaging in cuckoldry. If anything, having a game such as a spinning a wheel can produce a humorous tone to what would otherwise be a pretty intense moment.

The second scenario would be to have the third male pick his sub. This works very well when the third mal doesn't know who the subs are, and while the subs are wearing masks. As such, the third male can take his pick of whoever he wants.

This particular scenario can be amplified to have a number of subs with multiple FEMDOMS and males present. In a manner of speaking, it's like having a FEMDOM party. There are some parties in which masters and mistresses come together to have their pick of subs. In fact, you might even enjoy swapping out subs for an evening. These types of parties are rather common and generally happen on an invitation basis only. So, if you get on well with other FEMDOMS or take party in a FEMDOM community, you may very well get an invite to one of these parties. However, if you are in a committed relationship with your sub, you might want to think twice about taking part in such a party.

At these parties, you'll find that masters enjoy penetrating multiple subs. This tactic is quite useful as part of a humiliation game, or just as a means for the master to please himself. Mistresses may also take the time to penetrate multiple subs. This could be part of a party game, or simply as part of a sub initiation. In such cases, some FEMDOMS require their subs to go through some sort of initiation ritual. In some circumstances, this may include taking part in a party and being "served" to others doms in their community.

What If Your Sub Is Not Into Anal Play?

By definition, being a sub means you are willing to oblige to anything your mistress wants. As such, subs can't really say no to much. This implies that they must be compliant, or else they would lose their sub status.

This opens up an interesting path.

There are some guys who only dabble superficially in the world of FEMDOM. So, they only seek a dominatrix to walk them around like a puppy and whip them up a couple of times a month. This means that they are not fully committed to being subs. In such cases, you may find that these are men who are only looking to experiment with the FEMDOM world.

When a man is only looking to experiment, they are most likely looking to see if it's right for them. If that's the case, then you can't really blame them for not wanting to engage in certain practices. This is what differentiates the true subs from the guys who are only experimenting.

So, if you have a sub who is willing to go along, but reluctant to actually open up, you may want to go easy on him. So, the use of butt plugs and anal beads can be a good introduction to the world of anal play. You might want to lay off the heavier stuff until they are truly ready to go that route. Please bear in mind that one of the roles a dom plays in any power relationship is to guide their sub down the path of both pleasure and pain. Consequently, you can instruct your sub on how they can learn to love the pain they feel.

In the event that you are in a committed relationship, then you can determine whether certain anal play tactics are off-limits. For instance, you may be perfectly comfortable with penetrating your sub yourself, but completely against having someone else do it. In that case, then you can set the boundaries as the FEMDOM.

Ultimately, your decision to engage in anal play largely depends on your personality and how far you want to take things. Some FEMDOMS are perfectly happy with having a slave who just wants to serve his mistress and take a dildo up the butt every so often. Then, there are situations in which you can really turn the heat up.

It's up to you!

There is no one here to tell you what you should do. It's all a question of doing what is most comfortable and natural to you.

Chapter 15: BDSM Play

Throughout this book, we have mentioned BDSM as part of the FEMDOM dynamic. While it is generally incorporated into FEMDOM, it's not a requirement to engage in BDSM as a part of FEMDOM. In fact, you can have a rather "light" version of FEMDOM in which you don't engage in any type of BDSM play. These types of "light" FEMDOM relationships may include humiliation tactics like cuckoldry and anal play but without the dungeon or bondage setup.

In general terms, BDSM stands for "bondage, discipline, submission, masochism." As you can see, it's a pretty large term that encompasses a number of practices. So, associating BDSM to just bondage is only a part of the story. When you "discipline" a sub, you are engaging in BDSM play. If your sub enjoys pain, then that's BDSM play as well.

On the whole, BDSM is characterized by bondage and torture. But then again, that's only one approach to the traditional way of approaching the FEMDOM dynamic. As such, the classic depiction of the latex-covered dominatrix is only one way of making BDSM work in practice.

In this chapter, we are going to look at the four components of BDSM and the various ways in which you can incorporate them into your usual FEMDOM practices.

Bondage and Restraint

Typically, bondage is seen as tying up subs in a dungeon while menacing doms torture them senseless. While that is only one way of going about it, there are many different ways of approaching bondage. So, let's take a look at them going from relatively mild bondage scenarios to rather extreme ones.

To get started, simple restraint tactics like handcuffing a sub to a bed rail can provide enough excitement. You may choose to restrain the sub's hands only or restrain both hands and legs. There are kits that can be retrofitted to any type of bed. Otherwise, you may purchase a bed frame that would specifically lend itself to this type of setup. Alternatively, a hospital bed with the rails on both sides serves this purpose very well. Some rather simple bondage scenes depict a sub handcuffed, or shackled, to the bed, wearing a mask, while the mistress has her way with the sub. This may seem rather mild compared to some of the stuff we have talked about throughout this book, but it's a fun scenario that regular couples love to explore.

Earlier, we mentioned the use of surgical tables. These tables can be used very well in a space where you can leave it there. For example, if you have a workshop in your garage, you can set up a table like this for the purpose of BDSM. Folks who outfit their basement for BDSM play like to leave a table in a corner where they can have their fun.

When using a table, it's important to make sure that it's pretty sturdy as it would have to support quite a bit of weight in addition to any struggling or squirming. So, using your kitchen table may not be the best option in this case.

Some bondage practitioners like to use old doctor's examination tables, especially the ones with stirrups. That way, you can have clear access to your sub's nether regions. They make for some very interesting bondage scenes, especially if you want to explore a doctor-patient bondage scene.

Then, there are chairs.

The basic, bottomless chair we have discussed earlier can serve quite well for bondage play. Older metal chairs, the heavier ones, work really well for this type of play.

Generally speaking, they serve very well when it comes to keeping your sub from moving around more than they should.

It's when you look at specially designed chairs that things get really crazy.

For starters, there are chairs that look like a demented dentist's chair. Some have stirrups while others have armrest with cuffs on them and chains for leg shackles. These chairs are reclinable and allow the FEMDOM access to all parts of the sub.

There are other chairs which have a "T" shape. The chair itself is a normal chair with leg restraints. However, the "T" shape is used to restrain the arm. So, you have the sub in a sitting position with arms stretched out. This allows for an excruciating position. Also, you have access to your sub's entire body.

In addition, you'll find a chair that resembles a throne. However, it's essentially a medieval torture device as it has armrests with restraints (some have restraints in the back so that the sub's arms are tied behind the backrest) and leg shackles. But here is where they get really insane. Some have the option of adding a dildo or other type of device on which the sub must sit on. Others have an open hole that gives access to the sub's genital area. These chairs provide very little comfort and are intended to increase pain after prolonged sitting.

Lastly, there are some chairs that are built so that the sub's front is tied to the backrest of the chair. Essentially, it appears as though the sub is sitting with the chair turned around backward. This position exposes the sub's backside, thus giving the FEMDOM free access. This position is very good for anal play. You could also engage in cock and ball torture if you fancy.

When using chairs, make sure that the chair won't slip or tip over. If it does, it could cause a great deal of damage to your sub. Needless to say, this is something that is best avoided. So, do keep this in mind when setting up your chair. In some cases, they are bolted to the floor, while in others, they are pegged up against a wall. That way, no amount of struggling would tip the chair over.

Discipline, Submission, and Masochism

By now, you are well-versed in the ways of discipline and submission. You know exactly how to treat your sub(s), and most importantly, how to discipline them should the need arise. It's important to note that when you threaten a sub, it's important to follow through. For instance, if you say to a sub, "don't do that or else," then you had better mean it.

Often, discipline is just a question of being firm in your decisions. When you threaten a sub and follow through, the sub will have no choice but to take your word for it every time. This can be a bit tough with new subs, as they may not be entirely clear on your expectations. This is why you must be tough on them at all times. Otherwise, your subs won't learn to respect your rules.

Additionally, subs are masochists. Otherwise, they wouldn't be willing to engage in the practice they are involved in. They enjoy the pain they feel. They derive pleasure from being pounded by a dominant figure. While it's true that some male subs seek a male dom, they also seek out female doms as this helps to fill a void they are missing. In fact, don't be surprised to find high-ranking folks, businesspeople, and rich individuals seeking out this kind of thrill. In many ways, it makes them feel alive. Also, it may just be that they are bored with their usual sex life and are seeking something new.

For what it's worth, you have something that these individuals seek. You can provide them with the ultimate experience. As such, don't go easy on them. Take your subs as far as they will go. You will find that subs can generally tolerate a great deal of pain and punishment.

Once they recover, they'll keep coming back for more. It might sound counterintuitive, but the average individual seeks the rush that comes with being manhandled by a dominant female.

As we have mentioned throughout this book, use your imagination. There is no shortage of ideas that you can come up with. If anything, subs will remain faithful to you, the more creative you get. So, go off the deep end if you wish!

Conclusion

Thank you very much for making all the way to the end of this book. We hope that you have been inspired by the ideas we have presented herein. The world of FEMDOM is an exciting domain which is so vast. There is no shortage of wonderful ideas which you can put into practice. In fact, don't be surprised if your sub(s) come up with some kinky ideas of their own.

At this point, you are ready to run your own show. If you are new or relatively inexperienced in this type of play, don't worry. The most important thing at this point is to develop your own personality. As you do this, you will find what tactics turn you on, and also, what tactics turn your subs on.

In the event that you are exploring FEMDOM as part of a committed relationship, it's always good to talk things over before truly committing to it. Often, being on the same page makes this experience the best that it can be. However, if you neglect to agree on the fundamentals, you might not get the results you seek.

On the whole, the FEMDOM dynamic is empowering and can help you truly explore your dominant side. As a female dom, you are the one in charge of running the show. As such, you have the power to turn any man into a quivering coward. Don't feel sorry for them. Many guys crave that experience. After all, they are truly subs. The thing is that they have been unable to let themselves express their weaker side. So, in the privacy of a FEMDOM dungeon, they can show just how weak they truly are.

We hope you have enjoyed this book. If you felt it was useful and informative, do tell others who may be interested in it. We want nothing more than the FEMDOM community to grow. There are plenty of powerful females out there and countless weak men who seek the control of a powerful female. If that sounds like you, then go for it! You have everything to gain from exploring your dominant side.

Kama Sutra for Beginners

The Sex Positions Bible to Drastically and Rousingly Increase Libido with Your Partner. Discover Secret Tips and Tricks from Ancient Times...

Table of Contents

Introduction

Congratulations on choosing this book and thank you for doing so! There are plenty of books on this subject on the market, thanks again for choosing this one! Every effort was made to ensure it is full of as much useful information as possible; please enjoy it! If you find this book useful in any way, a review on Amazon is always appreciated!

Disclaimer

Before we begin, there is one thing that I would like to mention. This book is not intended to replace medical advice. It is not responsible for the actions or the results of the reader. Please seek out the advice of a doctor before starting any health program. The author is not a medical doctor, and the information in this book is meant only to supplement your health decisions and actions, not dictate them. The wonders of autophagy are still being discovered as this book is being written. Please enjoy the information provided but also be wise in consuming it.

Introduction to the Book

The main focus of this book is to share strategies for maintaining a deep emotional connection with your long-term partner and how to accomplish this through the teachings of the Kama Sutra. Contained here are tips and suggestions on exactly how to continue to have an intimate and loving marriage for years and years from the perspective of the Kama Sutra.

What You Will Learn

In this book, we are going to delve into The Kama Sutra. This includes specific sex positions and techniques that you will learn about and can try with your partner in order to make your sex life more advanced than ever before.

I will begin by explaining what the Kama Sutra is, and I will share with you some ways that it can be incorporated into your own personal sex life. I will also share with you the other benefits of the Kama Sutra, such as how to increase intimacy, how to kiss and caress your partner, how to engage in rough sex and how a man can please a woman. After reading through this book, you will have a much deeper understanding of what the Kama Sutra can teach you about sex and love, and you will better understand the history of this guide.

Why This Information Cannot Be Found on Google

While there are many articles and blogs on Google that discuss the Kama Sutra, none of them are as accurate and as comprehensive as this book. Many online resources that focus on the Kama Sutra are only concerned with the sex positions, but there is so much more to learn and benefit from when studying this ancient text. In this book, you will find much more information than you would anywhere else. The Kama Sutra itself was not originally written in English, so this book is the best way to understand exactly what the teachings of the Kama Sutra entail.

As you will find out over the course of this book, the Kama Sutra is full of invaluable lessons that will change your sex life forever. Further, this book will not only improve your sex life but your relationship or marriage as a whole. The Kama Sutra is a book that contains deep and meaningful lessons about love, being in a relationship, sharing yourself with another person, different ways of demonstrating your love using physical touch, and much more. Through reading this book, you will find much more information than you would on the internet, as it breaks down the different sections of the Kama Sutra and presents them to you in a manner that is easy to digest, understand and implement in your own life. There is very little information on the internet regarding the Kama Sutra that goes as in-depth as this book does, and you will thank yourself for picking it up.

Chapter 1: What Is Kama Sutra?

We are going to begin this book by first learning a little bit about what exactly the Kama Sutra is. Then, we are going to learn a brief history of the Kama Sutra before we begin looking at how it can benefit you in the next chapter.

Firstly, what is Kama Sutra? When we say the term *Kama Sutra*, it is actually in reference to an ancient book. You may not have been aware of this fact, as most of the time we talk about Kama Sutra as a type of sex. While this book does guide you through sex by teaching you sex positions, it is actually a guide rather than a style of sex. Often, people will say "Kama Sutra Sex." As if it is a type of sex, when they are instead referring to a text. Throughout this book, you will see the term "The Kama Sutra," as I will be mentioning the book and its teachings.

You could say that the Kama Sutra is a guide to love and a guide to enjoying a pleasant life with your partner. This book can be seen as a guide to a long-lasting marriage that will help you to keep sex interesting. It will do this by showing you how to benefit from new forms of intimacy.

Common Misconceptions

Most often, the Kama Sutra is discussed in terms of wild and crazy experimental sex positions. There are numerous articles, blogs, and magazines that talk about the Kama Sutra in this way. The truth is, however, the Kama Sutra is a book that contains much more than just this.

You may have heard of Kama Sutra in conversations about sex or in articles that you read online. The truth is, however, this is a sacred book that was written long, long ago, which contains a guide for anyone who is looking to get more out of their relationship and their sex life.

A History of Kama Sutra

The book *The Kama Sutra* was written in Northern India. It was originally written in the language of *Sanskrit*. Sanskrit is an ancient Indian language. The original texts that gave rise to Buddhism were written in this language, which shows you just how much history is involved in the Kama Sutra. This book was written sometime around the second century AD, though nobody can be exactly certain of when.

The Kama Sutra is said to have been written by a man named *Vatsyayana*- who was an ancient Indian philosopher. It cannot be confirmed for sure if he wrote the entire book singlehandedly, but according to researchers, he made a significant contribution to the text.

The word *Kama* loosely translates to mean *affection, love, and desires*. This is quite telling, as the book is aimed at teaching the reader about all three of these factors. Affection, love, and desire are all very important when it comes to a long-term relationship or a marriage.

The Kama Sutra includes seven different sections or chapters. Each of these sections is focused on a different aspect of pleasure. These aspects of pleasure include both physical pleasure and emotional pleasure. Vatsyayana recognized that in a marriage, both forms of pleasure are equally important.

Only one of those seven sections contain sex positions, and the other six sections talk about a variety of other topics. These six sections each touch on a different category of sexual act or situation in which a couple can achieve a deeper level of intimacy. For example, kissing, touching, massaging, and so on.

Since the book was written in a time and place where it was surrounded by Hindu culture, it is considered disrespectful to the culture if the Kama Sutra is taken out of context. What this means is that it should not be read one single section at a time, rather it should be seen and consumed as a whole. This is because it was meant to be this way when it was written. The book is meant to be read all at once, from beginning to end. This allows a person to examine it in its entirety so that they can receive and benefit from the full scope of teachings that it contains.

What the Kama Sutra Contains

The Kama Sutra is a guidebook for love. Within the pages of this book are contained tips and tricks for everything involved in loving and caring for another person.

While the majority of times, the Kama Sutra is discussed in reference to the adventurousness of the sex positions it contains, this is only one small section of the book. The rest of the book contains a guide to many other forms of showing affection that does not include penetration. The Kama Sutra is said to be a guide to love, as it teaches its readers how to love and please their partner in a variety of ways.

The Kama Sutra was written with the intention that it would be read by men. This is likely because it was written so many years ago. The information that it contains pertains mostly to men who wish to attract and court a female partner. The book teaches men how to treat this woman whom he will eventually call his wife.

The Kama Sutra includes a guide to kissing, foreplay, loving touches, and other ways to achieve intimacy with your partner. These methods include bathing together and giving each other sensual massages- not necessarily the erotic kind.

The Kama Sutra also mentions same-sex relations in terms of one man having multiple women. It also touches on sexual encounters involving multiple men and one woman.

This book is full of information and tips for achieving a close emotional bond with your partner, which can be beneficial for any couple. As you can see, this book is much more than a book of wild sex positions.

When it comes to the section on sex positions, The Kama Sutra includes a variety of positions that range in difficulty level. It contains 64 sex positions in total. Later in this book, we will look at several of these sex positions in detail, including how to perform them and what benefits come of them. After reading about these sex positions and how to perform them, you can try to liven up your sex life by trying some of them out for yourself.

The Benefits

This book is full of information that can be useful in learning more about how to treat your partner lovingly in ways other than during sex. It can be useful whether or not you wish to learn more about sex positions in particular, as it can also help you to connect with your partner on a deeper level emotionally.

As your relationship progresses, it is important to keep sex and lust alive. When you become more and more comfortable with someone, the mystery and desire can begin to fade. This is completely normal. This happens because of the excitement of getting to know a person is no longer there. At the beginning of your relationship, everything you did together was brand new. At the beginning of a relationship, you are so eager to have sex with each other because the other person is new and hot and sort of like a novelty.

As you get used to being with your partner, it can be easy to lose those feelings of excitement and settle into the comfortability of your life together. This is by no means a bad thing. Getting to this point in your relationship is fun and comforting in its own way. This stage of a relationship is different from and in some ways, better than the early stages.

From a sexual perspective though, we don't want this stage of your relationship to bring with it the end of an exciting sex life. Introducing the concepts and lessons from the Kama Sutra can help you to maintain the lust and intimacy in your relationship. It can also provide you with new sexual adventures to take on together as an established couple.

The Kama Sutra contains a wealth of information about sex and different sex positions as well as including information about different positions from which to give massages, tips on kissing, and tips for men on courting women. There are a wide variety of sex positions included in this book, so there is no shortage of new positions to inspire you if you are feeling that your sex life is becoming stale. Information from this book can still be found to this day, even though it was written so long ago, not even in English!

The Criticisms

Though the Kama Sutra remains quite relevant to this day, several criticisms have been voiced regarding this ancient text and its contents, especially in recent years. In this section, we will examine three of the most popular criticisms that the Kama Sutra has received.

1. The Male Gaze

The Kama Sutra has received criticism for the way that it was written since it comes from the perspective of a man and discusses how to please a woman. Though this book mentions same-sex relations between two men, this is only in the context of men sharing one single woman. This can be seen as sexist to some.

2. Male Pleasure

Another criticism that has been voiced is concerning the way that this book discusses a man's ability to benefit from having many female sexual partners, and even mentions how he can have them all at one time. The Kama Sutra mentions that a man can have one wife and several mistresses, which is not a popular opinion in the year 2020.

3. Controversy

There has been debate about whether the Kama Sutra is a book that should be praised for the way that it teaches men how to prioritize intimacy and female pleasure, or whether it should be criticized for how it puts men in control in terms of sex. Even when it talks about relationships and love, it is written for a man who wishes to court his woman. Whichever way you view this book, it contains many valuable lessons. After reading this book, you are free to make your judgment about whether or not you think this book is still relevant.

4. Inclusion

Many people also think that the Kama Sutra should not be relevant anymore as it is not inclusive of different levels of ability and strength, as well as not including the potential for people with physical disabilities to try these positions.

5. Too Adventurous

For some, they may find that the Kama Sutra may seem like it is just a little too adventurous. Some people may think that this book full of positions that takes away from the deeper purposes of sex and simply wants to try to challenge the bodies of the couple during sex.

6. Realistic?

The Kama Sutra has been criticized for being a book that contains sex positions that are not realistic for the average human to try to recreate.

7. Sexism

This book has also been criticized for being sexist, as it is written for a man who wants to know how to please a woman physically and emotionally.

Chapter 2: Kama Sutra Tips and Tricks

Now that you have a solid understanding of what the Kama Sutra is and what it contains, we are going to go over some tips and tricks on how to get the most out of this book. After you read through this chapter, chapter three will focus on some of the specific techniques that the Kama Sutra contains and how you can begin to benefit from them.

What the Kama Sutra Can Do for Your Relationship and Sex Life

As I mentioned in the previous chapter, the Kama Sutra is not limited to the sex positions it contains. As you know by now, the Kama Sutra contains much more than this chapter alone. This is not to say that the chapter on sex positions is not of importance, as it can still provide you with a wealth of information about how to improve your sex life with your partner. For this reason, not only does the Kama Sutra give you tips and tricks for your relationship, but also some practical advice for trying new things in the bedroom.

How to Begin Talking About the Kama Sutra With Your Partner

It can be quite a difficult task, opening up to your partner about something that you wish to change about your sex life. This may be the first time you plan to have a serious conversation with them about sex. You may fear judgment or hurting their feelings, and you may fear that your partner will not be interested in what you are suggesting.

As we discussed in the previous chapter, your lust and desire for your partner may fade as time goes on. Using the information contained in the Kama Sutra can help you to keep your passion alive in the bedroom by providing you with new and exciting sexual adventures to embark on together.

You may feel unsure of how your partner will react to you telling them that you want to spice up your sex life. If you have been in this relationship for a while now and you feel that your sex life is becoming routine, chances are that your partner would agree with you. While this is true, your anxiety about bringing this up has likely increased the longer you have left this unsaid.

It is never a bad time to bring these topics up in conversation, regardless of how long you have been in the relationship or marriage. You deserve pleasure, passion, and lust, and sharing your thoughts with your partner should be a priority. Bringing up your desire for change can be seen as a conversation that will provide you both with benefits, rather than a critique. Letting your partner know that you are not criticizing them, but that you are simply looking for ways that you can both achieve more pleasure will show them that you mean no harm in bringing this up.

Begin by telling your partner that you have been reading about something called the Kama Sutra. They may have heard of this before, but it may help if you explain to them what the Kama Sutra is. As you know by now, many people have ideas about what the text is about, many of which are myths. Give your partner a background about the Kama Sutra, and tell them that you believe it can greatly benefit both of you in the bedroom.

Then, let your partner know that you have been interested in trying some of what you have learned in the bedroom with them. Explain to them what it is that you have wanted to try with them. Explain what it is and how it makes you feel. Whether or not you have tried it in the past with someone else, let them know that you would like to begin exploring it with them.

You can also ask them if there is anything that they have wanted to explore or talk about (that relates to sex) with you. This will open up a dialogue about sex and your sex life in general.

Finally, tell them that your goal is to improve your shared sex life and that you are open to any suggestions or conversations that they would like to share with you. Your sex dialogue should be a two-way street, so be prepared for a mutual exchange of thoughts and feelings.

Beginner Tips for Incorporating Concepts from the Kama Sutra in Your Life

The following subsection includes several tips for incorporating the Kama Sutra into your own sex life. This may be new for you, so follow the tips below to find out how you can get the most pleasure and benefit from this book.

Open Your Mind

Some of the concepts and sexual acts that you will learn about may be very new to you. While you do not have to do anything that you are uncomfortable with, try to read and understand with an open mind. These concepts may lead you to learn more about yourself and your partner.

Rediscover Your Partner

While you may know your partner like the back of your hand- especially if you have been together for some time now, it is important to remember that people grow and change. When it comes to incorporating new things in your sex life, your partner may surprise you with what they are open to and what they enjoy. As you begin to explore the Kama Sutra with your partner, try to view the experience as a rediscovering of each other. Rediscover their pleasure, their body, and their desires. Try to forget what you already know about them and view the experience as if you are learning about them for the first time all over again.

The beginning of any relationship comes with a lot of uncharted territories. You are exploring a new person's entire body- inside and out and letting them explore yours. This stage of discovery is something that we want to return to now and again during a long-term relationship or a marriage. This is because you should rediscover your partner's body as if it is the first time now and again.

People's desires change, and their bodies change. It is important to continue to learn and understand how best to please your partner as they grow and change. You should also expect the same from them in return. Revisiting your partner's body as if you know nothing about it can be a fun and flirty way to re-inject passion into your sex life. Try to remember the first time you had sex with your partner and channel that excitement and curiosity once again.

Trust Yourself

Trust yourself! At the most basic level, humans are animals. Just like any other animal, we are meant to have sex. This means that sex comes wired into our DNA and that we all have some knowledge of how to conduct ourselves during sexual intercourse. This is because our body can take over and follow its pleasure, its arousal, and its instincts. While you don't want to act like a complete animal in bed (unless you and your partner are into it), this is simply useful to keep in mind so that you can keep your nerves at bay. If you let your mind take control, it will get in the way of and inhibit this natural instinct that you came built with. Relaxation and being at ease will make the encounter much more enjoyable for both of you.

If you are able to relax and enjoy the experience, your body will flow much smoother, and pleasure will come much easier to both you and your partner.

Communicate

It may seem like there is an expectation to pretend as you know exactly what you are doing and to seem like you have done it a thousand times before, but this is untrue. No matter who your partner is, they will be happy that you communicated and made sure that they were comfortable all along the way instead of pretending like you knew exactly what they wanted. Being able to communicate in bed is more impressive than not saying anything and guessing the entire time.

While some people may be embarrassed to be vocal and expressive in bed, many benefits can come of it, and many reasons why you may want to consider making a point to do this. By being vocal in the bedroom, you are able to communicate things to your partner without having to worry about ruining the mood or "killing the vibes." What this means is that you don't have to stop having sex or suddenly change your demeanor in order to talk to your partner during sex. By being vocal in the bedroom, you can communicate to them what you like, what you don't like, and what you want more of. This will make your enjoyment of sex better, and it will mean that you can experience more pleasure since your partner will know exactly what you want. You will also be able to please your partner better since you will know exactly what they want if they are vocal as well.

Express Yourself

Expressing yourself during sex allows you to express your pleasure. When you experience the physical bliss that is an orgasm, your body is always shocked at the level of pleasure it is feeling. If you have had an orgasm before, you know that the amount of pleasure you feel is so much that it begs to be let out in some way, usually by grasping something tightly or by screaming out in pleasure. By doing this, it actually enhances the feelings of your orgasm. Think of it this way- if you are experiencing an orgasm and you are holding your pleasure in so that you can remain quiet or because you are embarrassed about expressing yourself, your pleasure can only build to a certain level because there is no release for it. If instead, you let your pleasure out by exclaiming or grabbing onto the bed frame or a combination of the two, your pleasure can continue to build as it has an outlet. With no outlet, there must be a cap on it. Just like when you shake a bottle of soda, and it explodes out the top.

Expressing your pleasure during orgasm is very beneficial for your pleasure and for your sexual experience overall. At first, you may be unsure about how to do this, and you may be a little self-conscious about doing it with a partner. I can assure you, that your partner will most definitely be turned on by your exclamations of pleasure, as it will come as a sort of ego boost to them when they realize how much pleasure they caused you.

The first thing that you can do in order to become more comfortable with this idea is to try it on your own first. When it comes to anything sex-related, trying it first on your own is a great way to get comfortable with it before doing it with another person present. To try this on your own, do so when you are masturbating. This is a great time to try it as you are the person who best knows how to please yourself. Because of this, you can give yourself a strong enough orgasm- to the point where you will want to scream out in pleasure. When you come close to orgasm, open your mouth slightly. When you reach orgasm, allow whatever sounds escape your mouth to come out without holding them back and without judging yourself. You will likely find that you had an even better orgasm than usual because you weren't holding yourself back at all. You let your pleasure come about and let it out, which allows it to grow without putting a cap on it.

When you go to bed with your partner, try this same technique as you did when you were alone, and I guarantee that your partner will become extremely aroused by your orgasm sounds.

Understand Your Body *and* Your Mind

- The Body

The body is responsible for all of our physical sensations.
The body houses all of our erogenous zones and our
sexual centers. The body is our vehicle, and it is what
allows us to feel pleasure at all. The body is responsible
for our deep desires, our lust, our orgasms, our arousal,
and our physical reactions to pleasure. There is something
deep within that is not recognized by our conscious mind
or our heart that moves us toward pleasure and away
from pain. This is responsible for our deepest desires, and
it wants desperately to seek them out.

The heart is the center of our body, and it provides us with our
feelings of acceptance, warmth, comfort, happiness, and love.
The heart is another important part of sex, and it is important
for sexual comfort. If you are making love with someone whom
you really care about, the heart will be where you feel those
deep and intense feelings of inner warmth and connection.

- The Mind

The brain provides us with information about the situation we
are in, allows us to use dirty talk, and makes our decisions,
among other things. If the brain is distracted or tired or
distressed, it will be very hard to know what we want, what we
like, what we want to do, what to do next, etcetera. The brain is
an important part of sex and sexual decision making.

Our emotions also play a large part when it comes to sex. While
sometimes, we can perform the act of sex without emotions
involved, this is not as sexually intelligent as we would like to
be. Having sex with emotions does not mean that we are in love
with every person we have sex with, but that we care for them,
and we care for ourselves. It also means recognizing that we
will have emotions surrounding desire, whether it is happiness,

583

excitement, nervousness, joy. These emotions can all tell us something. Instead of blocking them out, we should be embracing them and listening to them. Being able to observe and read our own emotions, and the emotions of others is part of sexual intelligence. Emotions can also contribute to our enjoyment of sex as when we are feeling happy or in love. We tend to feel more intense pleasure when having sex with the person we feel strongly about.

The brain, the heart, and the body come together to form a sexual being, and this is responsible for all of our sexual preferences, desires, and comforts. It helps us seek out a partner and the activities that we get pleasure from. Being able to get in touch with your body means being able to look to all three of these parts of ourselves and listen to them as a whole and individually. This will ensure that you get the most out of your experiences with the Kama Sutra.

Chapter 3: How to Begin Practicing Kama Sutra

While you probably know how to please each other like it's second nature, rediscovering each other's bodies in a sexy way and learning new ways to please each other is great for couples who have been together for a long time. The Kama Sutra will help you to do this, and in this chapter, we are going to look at how you can benefit from this.

Where to Begin

Before beginning, we will first delve into the topic of the orgasm. We will look at the orgasm from both a male and a female perspective. We will look at the male body and the female body and how to please them, as well as how to give them a wonderful orgasm. This section will be helpful to you no matter how long you have been having sex, and no matter how long you have been with your partner.

Many people are out of touch with their sensuality, their desires, their fantasies, and even their bodies. By learning how to please the opposite sex, you will help your partner to discover their body and their body. This will also help you to become aware of this concerning your own body, and you will know how to get back in touch with all of these parts of your sexuality.

When it comes to sex, we all know that the cherry on top of a great session is the orgasm! There is no denying that an orgasm is the best part of being a creature that has sex for enjoyment and not solely to reproduce.

Understanding the Female Body

To give a woman an orgasm, you will need to understand the female body and all of the places that, when stimulated, will make a woman feel pleasure. Whether you are a female yourself or you are a male with a female partner, both sexes can benefit from learning more about the female body.

- The Clitoris

The clitoris is the place that many people know of as the spot to stimulate that is the easiest way to give a woman an orgasm. The clitoris is located very close to the vagina. It is a small bean-like structure that has many many nerve endings, which is why it can so easily lead to female pleasure. To find it, begin by placing a hand on the pelvic area, with the fingers towards the vagina. A woman can do this to herself, or a man can do this to find the woman's clitoris. Slowly move your hand downward, using your fingers to feel around. As you wrap your

585

fingers underneath her, between her legs, feel around for a small lump-like structure. It is in a slightly different spot, covered by different amounts of layers and of different sizes on every woman, so explore around between the legs to find it. It will be towards the front of her body, right where her vaginal lips begin. On some women, you may even be able to see it with the eyes if there are not as many layers of vaginal lips covering it.

The clitoris is said to be the female penis. This is because it actually enlarges and becomes engorged when a woman is horny. It will be easier to find her clitoris if she is turned on. The clitoris is much larger than it seems, and this is because it extends up inside of the woman's body. Only a small part of it is located on the outside of the body, but the size of it is the reason why there are so many nerve endings located within and the reason why stimulating it will lead to such intense pleasure.

Once you have found the clitoris, you will then be able to stimulate it to give yourself or your woman an orgasm. Begin by gently placing two fingers on it and putting a bit of pressure. Rub it by moving your fingers in small circles- making sure to be gentle. Continue to do this, and she should begin to get more aroused the more you do this. By rubbing the clitoris, you will be able to stimulate the entire clitoris, even the part of it that you cannot see, and this will cause the woman to start to become wet in her vagina.

- The G-Spot

The G-Spot is a lesser-known spot than the clitoris, but a woman can have extreme amounts of pleasure if this spot is stimulated. To find this spot, you will need to insert a finger into her vagina. It is best to try to find this spot after you stimulated the clitoris for a bit because then her vagina will have begun to get wet- as it lubricates itself to prepare for penetration. You can use this to your
586

advantage because it will make penetration more enjoyable for her and will reduce the friction of the entire vaginal area in general. When the vagina becomes very wet, it can lubricate the entire vaginal area, including the clitoris, which will then make it easier to stimulate the clitoris as well. No friction means smooth gliding, which results in pleasure and no pain. When she is wet enough, slide a finger inside of her vagina while she is lying on her back (a woman can do this for herself too) and make a "come here" motion with your finger, so that you are moving it towards her belly button. Feel around in this are, and when you feel a bumpy or rough surface, this is the G-Spot. Just like the clitoris, the G-Spot is slightly different for every woman, but they can all be in the same general area. The G-Spot will be a different size for different women, so be aware of this when trying to find it.

The reason that the G-Spot can give a woman intense pleasure is that it is actually connected to the clitoris. Inside the body, where the clitoris extends up into the woman, it meets the vagina, and this is the spot where the G-Spot is located. This thin wall between them allows for the pressure and stimulation to travel between them so that you are essentially also stimulating the clitoris when you are pleasuring her G-Spot.

To give a woman pleasure by stimulating her G-Spot, you will need to press on it over and over again until she reaches orgasm. This can be done using your fingers, your penis, or sex toys of a variety of sorts. We will talk about sex toys in a later chapter, but for now, we will look at the fingers and the penis. Stimulating this spot with your fingers is quite simple as you will have lots of control, and you will be able to feel around to see if you are in the right spot. When you have found the G-Spot with your fingers, gently press on it with the pads of your fingers and avoid curling your fingers around too much as you don't want your nails to scratch the inside of her vagina. Press with the pads of your fingers on her G-Spot with light pressure, but enough for her to feel what you are doing. Continue to do this, and you should feel her vagina getting increasingly wetter. As you do this, you can increase the speed of stimulation if she wishes. Communicate with her to see what she wants you to do (faster, slower, harder, lighter, deeper, shallower). A woman can do the same to herself in the bedroom. I just the same way, slide a finger inside of your vagina either with lube or after getting yourself a bit wet by watching porn or massaging your clitoris. Then, move your finger towards the front of your body and feel for the spot. Once you have found it, continue to stimulate it by putting pressure on it over and over again. It should feel good and get increasingly better the longer you do this. Eventually, the pleasure will build to a point where it feels as if you are about to orgasm. Continue to do whatever you were doing to get to this point, and orgasm will occur! This type of orgasm will be much more full body than a clitoral orgasm, as it includes the inside of the vagina and is also stimulating the clitoris from the inside.

The penis can also stimulate the G-Spot, but it is a little harder as there will not be as much control as there is when using fingers. Try to choose a position that will have the curve of the penis line up with the front of the vaginal wall, and this will give you the best chance of hitting the G-Spot. We will go into this further in chapter five, where we will look at specific positions. For now, though, knowing where the G-Spot is located as well as how to make a woman feel pleasure in that spot is a great start to being able to give her an amazing orgasm.

- The Anus

The anus is a very sensitive area for women, contrary to the beliefs of some people. While it is well-known that men have sensitive anuses and can receive pleasure here, it is a less well-known fact that so can women. Women have very sensitive anal openings because there are many
588

nerve endings here and a lot of surface area. This means that when stimulated, a woman can feel a lot of pleasure here. Because this is an area that rarely receives stimulation. Therefore, when it does, it can be that much more enjoyable for a woman because she may not be used to the sensations.

The inside of the anus can give a woman lots of pleasure as well when stimulated. When a woman has her anus stimulated, it actually is only separated from the vagina by a thin layer, and similar to the clitoris and the G-Spot connection, she can actually orgasm from being anally stimulated because of the connection between her vagina and her anus. A woman can receive anal sex, and the penis making contact with her anal wall, especially the one toward the front of her body, can give her a very similar feeling to that of a vaginal orgasm.

The anus can also be stimulated with fingers, toys, or orally. Any of these ways can be enjoyable for the woman if she is open to receiving anal pleasure, as they will each give her a slightly different sensation. Think of how a warm tongue would feel vs. a smooth anal toy vs. the rough hands of the man she loves.

Understanding the Male Body

- The Penis

As we know, the male sex organ is the penis. A man can reach orgasm by having his penis rubbed, sucked on, kissed, or stimulated in a number of other ways. While you cannot easily tell when a woman is aroused, it is easy to tell when a man is aroused because his penis will become erect. This happens because then he can have sex with it- think of how hard it would be to have penetrative sex with a limp penis. When a man watches porn, sees a very attractive woman, or is touched in the right way, he will become erect. Then, by sliding his penis into a vagina repeatedly, into a sex toy like a fleshlight, or by having someone stroke it with their hand, he can eventually reach orgasm. Every man's penis is a different shape and a different size, and each man will like something slightly different in order to reach orgasm. There are so many things you can try and ways that a man could reach orgasm, there is lots of opportunity for exploration and trying new things.

We will revisit the topic of sex toys further in this book, so you will get more information on that very soon.

- The Testicles

A man's testicles may seem like they are there only to provide sperm for ejaculation, but they are also very sensitive erogenous zones for a man. If a man's testicles are stimulated, this can make him become very aroused and can make him erect if he wasn't already. A man's testicles can be stimulated during oral sex, during a handjob, or during sex in certain positions, and this will only add to the pleasure he is already feeling from having his penis stimulated in some way.

If you have ever had your testicles bumped in the wrong way, it definitely brought you a lot of pain for those few minutes afterward. Think of that level of pain but in terms of pleasure instead. This is what we want to unlock for you in your testicles. This level of sensation, but in the reverse- intense pleasure instead of intense pain.

Gently stroking the testicles with warm hands will get them used to touch so that they don't seize up and hug the body too closely. Gently rubbing the scrotum and massaging the testicles will add to whatever sexual activity is already happening. They can also be stimulated with the mouth during oral sex. The woman can move
590

down to the testicles and gently suck or lick them to give a different sensation- that of warm moisture on sensitive skin.

A man can stimulate his own testicles while he is masturbating for added pleasure as well. If you are a man and you have never tried this, add it to your next masturbation session. Using one hand to stroke your penis and the other to massage your testicles will add a new dimension to your self-love sessions. Try this in the shower with a partner or without to enjoy the warmth or the water mixed with a massage and penis stimulation. You will never go back.

- The Anus

The anus is a well-known erogenous area of the male body. Males can get intense pleasure and even orgasm from being anally penetrated. This is due to the prostate gland being positioned right sat the spot where whatever is doing the stimulating would make contact with the anal wall. Right on the other side of this wall is the prostate, which happens to be extremely sensitive and leads to intense pleasure when stimulated in the right way.

A man's anus can be stimulated on the outside only, where-like a woman's, it is very sensitive due to a great number of very sensitive nerve endings being located there. This can be done using a tongue, fingers, a vibrating toy, or anything really. Beginning with this will lead the anus to relax and become receptive to being penetrated. Then, a sex toy or fingers can be inserted, and that's when the prostate will get its turn. When they prostate it pressed on over and over in a rhythmic pattern, it will cause a man to feel intense pleasure and eventually to reach orgasm. This is similar to the G-Spot in a woman where it needs to be continuously stimulated to eventually give her an orgasm.

Anal sex for a man is not just reserved for gay couples. Many heterosexual couples practice pegging, which is anal sex from a woman to a man using a sex toy. We will revisit this later, but this point is to say that the pleasure potential of a man's anus is not only reserved for gay couples and should be fully explored by any man or heterosexual couple wanting to unlock the full pleasure that a man's body is capable of.

Understanding Orgasms

We have discussed the female orgasm somewhat in this chapter so far, but in this section, we will look at it in a little more depth.

For a woman to reach orgasm, much of this is dependent on her mindset. She will need to feel comfortable being vulnerable in this space for her to reach her full arousal potential. She needs to reach this point in order for her to orgasm and in order for her to fully enjoy sex. For this reason, mindset and pleasure are very closely linked to a woman.

When the clitoris is rubbed in the right way, it will lead to orgasm, just like the penis of a man. Treating it like this can give both men and women insight into how it works and how to make the woman come. When stimulated physically with someone's fingers or a sex toy like a vibrator, this can lead to an orgasm for the woman. The clitoris is a structure that contains many nerve endings, which is what makes it so sensitive. When a woman is not aroused sexually, her clitoris is still there, but it will not be as enlarged as when she is horny.

A woman's vagina automatically swells when she is sexually aroused because of increased blood flow to her genitals, sort of like how your penis becomes erect when you get horny. What this means for you is that when your penis is inside of her, the walls of her vagina will tighten and swell as the blood flow increases, and you will feel this effect on your penis, resulting in added pleasure for you.

There are different types of multiple orgasms that a woman can achieve. Women are lucky in that they can have both back-to-back orgasms and blended orgasms. They are even able to have back-to-back blended orgasms in some cases! In this section, we will learn more about the different types of multiple orgasms.

We will now discuss blended orgasms. A blended orgasm is achieved when multiple different orgasms are achieved at the same time. This can be two different orgasms at the same time, or in some cases, even more than two! This type of orgasm leads to even more pleasure than a single orgasm and will lead the woman to feel more intense pleasure than ever before. During penetration, there is lots of opportunity for different types of female orgasms to occur. The two most common ways that a woman can reach orgasm are through her clitoris and through her G-spot. We will look at some ways that a woman can have both of these orgasms at the same time, as well as some other options for blended orgasms.

Any combination of these separate but simultaneous orgasms compounds to give the woman a mind-blowing, full-body, blended orgasm. This is especially so if the two locations of stimulation are a larger distance from each other- like the nipples and the clitoris for example. The best type of blended orgasm will vary from woman to woman, depending on her personal preferences and what her most sensitive erogenous zones are. Some of these zones include the clitoris, the anus, the G-Spot, and the nipples. Some women may have others as well, but this is largely dependent on the woman's body.

The first method is a clitoral orgasm during penetration. If the clitoris is stimulated while the man is penetrating the woman, she could have an orgasm through both her clitoris and her G-Spot at the same time. This type of multiple orgasms will make her feel pleasure like never before because these two places are extremely pleasurable even when achieved alone, so together it is a new level of orgasm! There are different ways that you can achieve this, but the most successful way is to penetrate her with your fingers while she rubs her clitoris at the same time. This way, you can feel your way around and stimulate her G-spot while she pleases herself. It may take some practice and will require a lot of communication, but eventually, you will both be able to time it so that she can have both of these orgasms at once. Another way that this can happen is while the man is thrusting his penis into her. While he is doing this, she can touch her clitoris using her fingers or a vibrator, or the man can stimulate her clitoris by using his fingers or a vibrator. Some specific positions will allow for the man's penis to reach the G-Spot when inside of her, and at the same time, the base of his penis or his pelvic region can rub her clitoris, causing both orgasms to happen at the same time. We will look at these specific positions later on in this book.

Another way that a woman can achieve a blended orgasm is through having both an anal and clitoral orgasm at the same time. This is similar to the blended orgasm in which the man is penetrating the woman with his penis while her clitoris is being stimulated, but in this case, it is done while you are having anal sex. The method will happen in a similar way to the vaginal penetration with clitoral stimulation, but the positions used will be slightly different as the positions used in this case would be ones that better allow for anal penetration while giving either the man or the woman free hands to stimulate the clitoris. Either the man or the woman can stimulate the woman's clitoris in a variety of anal sex positions using either their hands or a vibrating sex toy.

Another type of blended orgasm that is possible is a nipple orgasm and a clitoral orgasm. Not every woman is able to achieve a nipple orgasm, but if you are, then this could be a great option for a blended orgasm. If you are unsure whether you are able to reach orgasm through nipple stimulation alone, try this one in order to see if also your clitoris having stimulated leads to more sensitivity in your nipples as well.

One example of a position in which this type of blended orgasm can occur is the following. While you are sitting in a chair with your legs spread wide, your partner will get on his knees in front of you. He will then begin to give you oral sex on his knees. While licking and using his mouth to stimulate your clitoris, he will reach up to your breasts with his hands and massage your nipples with his fingers. Once he has done this for some time and began to please you, he will then switch and using his tongue. He will gently lick, suck and lick your nipples with his tongue, one at a time. While he does this, he will also move his hand down between your legs and stimulate your clitoris with his hand and fingers. Have him alternate back and forth using his mouth on your clitoris and then on your nipples. This will give you pleasure from both of these erogenous zones, and you will likely be able to experience a blended nipple and clitoral orgasm in this way, as long as he keeps stimulating both areas at the same time.

Not only can women have blended orgasms, but they can also have back-to-back orgasms. These orgasms occur one after the other and give the woman immense pleasure because she is able to keep coming again and again and again.

This type of repeated orgasm is only possible for women as the male body is unable to do this. This is because the male body has to wait for a refractory period after every orgasm. What this means is that there is an amount of time after an orgasm during which a man's body is unable to achieve an erection or have another orgasm. During this time, his body is recovering from the orgasm and needs this time to recuperate. The length of this period is different for every man, but it ranges between fifteen to thirty minutes in most males.

The great thing about the clitoris is that after orgasm, it may be very sensitive for a few minutes, but it maintains its "erection" and can be stimulated again a very short time after for a doubly pleasurable second orgasm. This can lead to a third and a fourth and beyond. This is why, as we discussed, it is beneficial to give a woman an orgasm during foreplay as it will increase her chances of orgasm during penetration because of how horny it will have made her. Sometimes, women's pleasure only builds after an initial orgasm instead of going back to zero before climbing again like a man's pleasure would have to. It is important for men to understand this difference because they can then take advantage of it and pleasure their woman to the fullest. While they await their refractory period, they can please their woman in a way that does not involve their penis, give her an orgasm, and then by the time this happens; he will be ready to get hard again and have a second round with her. All the while, she will become increasingly horny and pleased.

Another type of multiple orgasms that may be different from what you had in mind when hearing the words "multiple orgasms" is the simultaneous orgasm." This type of multiple orgasms is great for couples, especially long-term couples. This type of orgasm occurs when both the man and the woman are able to reach orgasm at the same time! The reason why this is great for long-term couples is that it takes practice and excellent communication during sex, but when mastered, it will unlock new levels of pleasure for both of you. When in a long-term relationship, one of the many positive things about having sex with each other is that you know just the right way to make each other orgasm. After having sex with each other so many times, you likely have this down to a science! This comes in handy here as you can use this knowledge to help you both orgasm at the same time. Since you know how to get your partner to orgasm in mere minutes, you can touch each other

596

exactly as you each like at the exact same time in order to reach orgasm simultaneously.

Now, this is a little more difficult than it sounds, but it is entirely possible. To do this, begin with the intention of orgasming together. Both of you will stimulate the other person's genitals in the best way you know, so you will have to figure out a position that allows for both of these ways at the same time. For example, if your partner can make you come very quickly by giving you oral sex while also massaging your testicles and you can make her come very quickly by playing with her clitoris just the right way, then you will have to find a position where you can do both of these at the same time. This position could be one where you are lying on your back on the bed, and she is straddling your chest, facing your feet. She will bend forward so that her mouth reaches your penis, and she will hold herself up with one of her arms on the bed. She can then use her other free hand to massage your testicles. You will then slide a hand between her legs and begin playing with her clitoris, and you can even use your other hand to slide your fingers into her vagina if she wishes.

When you begin, start out slow. This will require a lot of communication between the two of you. Begin pleasing each other and communicating your pleasure with moans or simple phrases like "that feels good" the entire time. When one of you gets close to reaching orgasm, tell the other person. If your partner tells you that they are close to coming, ease up on the pressure or the speed on her clitoris, for example, so that she does not come yet. When, and if you are also close to orgasm, let her know, and you can both continue to stimulate each other's genitals until you both orgasm together at the same time!

One of the benefits of this type of orgasm in a long-term relationship is that when you care about a person deeply, you find pleasure in seeing them pleased. When you please your partner to the point of orgasm, it usually will make you also feel pleasure. Because of this, as each of you comes closer to reaching orgasm, it will make the other person more aroused. For this reason, a long-term couple will be able to do this act of simultaneous orgasms with ease.

Understanding The Female Orgasm Potential
Female ejaculation is a well-disputed concept in modern discussions about sexuality. There is evidence though, that it is possible and actually quite common. While the term *female ejaculation* probably makes you think of something porn-related, it is something that can happen without theatrics and to a much lesser degree in your own sex life. Female ejaculation is often portrayed as a fountain of water spraying across the room; however, this is not the case in real life.

Female ejaculation does not have to occur, and, in many cases, it never does. It is sort of the icing on the cake or the cherry on top so to speak, but it is not necessary in order for the woman to be aroused or to achieve orgasm. Female ejaculation, commonly referred to as *squirting,* is different for every woman and does not have to involve a large amount of fluid like a male ejaculation. It also does not happen every time and does not only happen during orgasm. While it can happen at the time of orgasm, female ejaculation can also occur at any time during sex when the woman is extremely aroused. Thus, ejaculation can be a sign that the woman is feeling aroused regardless of whether she has reached orgasm yet or not. This is a good sign that indicates she is enjoying herself.

Ejaculation does not happen to every woman, but it can be something that can be practiced and learned if the woman would like to experience it. Some people become extremely turned on when they experience or witness female ejaculation, so if you or your partner feel that it would turn you both on, it is possible for the woman to begin trying to achieve this. For some people, it turns them on so much, even to the point of experiencing orgasm.

Female ejaculation has been linked to G-Spot stimulation, so the best way to achieve this is to have your partner stimulate your G-Spot with either his fingers, his penis, or a dildo.

What to Do First

The Kama Sutra text views sex as a spiritual act between two people that, with time, will increase a person's level of spirituality and sexual power. The book aims to help people to get in touch with their desires, which will aid them in reaching the full extent of their sexual power. It aims to liberate people in a sexual sense. These concepts were quite advanced for the time that the book was written, which is why this book is still so widely discussed to this day. Before you begin practicing the concepts of the Kama Sutra, it is important to understand this.

Lubrication

There are many different types of lubricants that you can use to make your sex glide easier and feel more pleasurable. The first type we will talk about is the synthetic lubricant. There are different types of these- water-based and silicone-based lubricants. The type of lubricant you choose will depend on what type of sex toy you are using and what your intended use is. I will go into more detail about the different types of lubrication below, but first, we will look at the benefits of using any lubrication during sex in general. Lubrication has been shown to have sex better in many ways, the first of which is that it makes all body parts glide better and slide easier, which means no painful dry skin on dry skin friction. Lubrication has also been shown to increase the intensity of both male and female orgasms. As I mentioned earlier, in order to have an orgasm vaginally for women or anally for either sex, constant rhythmic penetration is required. Lubrication makes this possible because of the ease of movement it allows for will help with maintaining a rhythm of penetration.

Lubrication can also be used for masturbation with sex toys or with hands and fingers alone for both men and women because it will make toys or fingers move and glide easier, which will lead to more pleasure. Lubrication will make both clitoral stimulation and penile stroking more pleasant because it will eliminate any skin on skin friction that would occur because of a lack of a condom or, in the case of male masturbation the lack of a female's natural vaginal lubrication to act as a lubricant on the penis.

Silicone-Based Lubricant

Silicone-based lube is the type of lube you would want to use if you want to have sex in the bathtub, shower, or any environment involving water since it won't rinse off when it becomes wet. If you are not using it to have sex in a wet environment, the other benefit about it is that it will usually only need to be applied once and will stay thick and doing its job for the duration of your session. This makes silicone-based lube a great choice for activities involving anal sex because it is thicker and longer-lasting than other forms of lubrication. When having anal sex of any sort, ample lubrication is required, and choosing the longer-lasting sort of lube will be best.

The drawback though, is that this type of lubrication is not very easy to clean. This is because it cannot be rinsed off by only using water. This variety of lubrication requires you to use soap and scrub it off of whatever you are cleaning it off of, like a penis or your vaginal area. Silicone-based lubricants aren't ideal on a silicone-based sex toy because it can cause the toy to break down more quickly over time than it normally would.

Water-Based Lubricant

Water-based lubricant is very easy to clean as it can be rinsed off of your body or your sex toys with water alone. The drawback though is that if you enjoy shower sex, bathtub sex, pool-sex, or any sex involving the water, it will wash away immediately and will not provide any lubrication as soon as it gets wet. This is also why this type of lubrication may need to be reapplied a few times in a session. If you do not have much shower or bathtub sex and you use silicone sex toys, then water-based lube would be good for you.

Oils

As an alternative, you can use oil as a lubricant. Oil is beneficial because it is so versatile in its uses. Oil can be used as a massage aid for some sensual foreplay massaging. It can be used without being washed off before oral sex because of its natural roots and its flavor that would not be terrible in your mouth. If you prefer something natural as a lubricant, then oil will likely be your choice. Many people will use coconut oil for this purpose. It can be used as an edible lubricant as it is often seen in cooking and smoothies. The one drawback to oil-based lubricants is that they can't be used with condoms because they will deteriorate the condom and cause it to break.

Gels

There are some gels that are made for sexual encounters that also can be used with versatility. There are some aloe vera scented gels that can be used both as a massage gel for foreplay and as lube for penetrative sex. If you live in a hot place or take this gel with you on vacation, it can also be an after-sun gel for burnt skin. This way, soothing your partner's sunburn could turn into quite the sensual and even sexual experience.

Kissing

There are 16 different kissing techniques outlined in the Kama Sutra. This means that you will never run out of new and interesting ways to show your partner love through kissing them.

- The Normal Kiss
- The Straight Kiss
- The Turned Kiss
- The Throbbing Kiss
- The Touching Kiss
- The Bent Kiss
- The Pressed Kiss
- The Gently Pressed Kiss
- Kiss of the Upper Lip
- A Clasping Kiss
- The Kiss that Kindles Love
- The Turning Away Kiss
- The Awakening Kiss
- Kiss of Showing Intention
- The Transferred Kiss
- The Demonstrative Kiss

Foreplay

Foreplay is generally treated as the time before penetrative sex, where there is some kissing, some touching, and some sensual whispers. What happens during foreplay? In the media, foreplay is often given a bad reputation, as it is portrayed as something that must be done for the woman's body to get ready for sex, or for the woman to feel comfortable enough to begin having sex. While some of this is true, sex is much more than the act of a penis in a vagina. Sex can last much longer than the time between when the man inserts his penis and when he reaches orgasm. The Kama Sutra recognizes that there should be much more importance placed on foreplay, which is why there are several sections of the text which talk about what you can do to share intimate moments with your partner before penetration.

Sex between couples is much more than what happens when the man is inside of the woman. Treating sex as much more than just a physical activity means that we must include all aspects of sex in our discussions about how to have a better sex life. This includes foreplay. That being said, if foreplay is considered part of sex, then the positions in which you engage in foreplay are sex positions.

In this section, we will look at foreplay as a special part of sex, and I will introduce some different techniques for foreplay that focus on your emotional connection and intimacy with your partner.

The Importance of Foreplay

Foreplay is important to ensure that you will be able to have comfortable sex. This is because the man will have to be erect enough, and the woman will have to be wet enough for sex to happen smoothly and without pain. This is the most practical reason that foreplay exists.

Further, foreplay gives you a chance to connect with your partner on an emotional level before you begin connecting physically in such a deep way. This time to connect with one another can make the difference between lovemaking and the physical act of sex. Connecting emotionally while connecting physically will lead to longer-lasting love and more passionate sex.

As we discussed above, foreplay is an important aspect of sex. This is especially true for women. This is because a woman needs to feel comfortable and relaxed to feel sexual pleasure. Foreplay serves to make a woman feel comfortable, letting her hair down, and being vulnerable. This is true whether she is in a long-term relationship or having a one-night stand.

The woman will need to feel comfortable being vulnerable in this space for her to reach her full arousal potential. Further, she needs to reach this point for her body to reach orgasm. Taking some time to set the mood before you have sex will go a long way in terms of a woman's ability to become and stay aroused. This will benefit both the man and the woman because the man will have more fun if the woman is comfortable. Setting the mood also shows the woman that you are concerned with her level of comfort in her surroundings and are invested in her pleasure. Her ability to have an orgasm will depend greatly on her level of ease.

Many times, foreplay involves some kind of stimulation of the genitals, whether it is by oral sex or using your hands. This gets you ready for sex, as your body will respond by becoming more and more aroused. Once in a full state of arousal, you can achieve successful penetration.

There are some benefits to using only your hands to please your partner. When using your hands, you can feel your way around their body. This will mean that you will know exactly what you are doing and where you are touching them at all times. You can control the pressure with which you hold or stroke the penis or rub the clitoris when you are using your hands. For the man, he can feel his way around inside of the woman so that he knows exactly where he is. This way, he can aim for a specific location such as her G-Spot or the deeper areas of her vagina. If he were using his penis, he would not have as much control or as much perception of where he was in relation to her G-Spot.

The other reason why foreplay is so important for the woman is that it is quite difficult for a woman's body to reach orgasm during penetrative sex. If the woman can orgasm during foreplay, she will enjoy penetrative sex much more!

Another reason that foreplay will allow a woman to get more enjoyment out of penetrative sex is the following; The time spent getting each other in the mood for sex will cause the woman's clitoris to become engorged. This is similar to a male erection. The benefit of this is that when you are having penetrative sex, and her clitoris is engorged, it will more easily make contact with the shaft of the man's penis or with some part of his body as he is thrusting into her. What this means is that it will be easier for her to get clitoral stimulation during penetrative sex is her clitoris becomes engorged during foreplay.

Kama Sutra Foreplay Techniques

The first technique we will look at is setting the mood. This may not seem of importance, but it is a very important part of pre-sex behavior that is often overlooked.

As a couple, it is more important to set the mood and environment for your sex than it would be if you were having casual sex or a one-night stand. In a relationship, you have moved past the casual awkwardness of those types of encounters and onto real lovemaking.

When setting the mood, our focus is on creating an environment free of distractions where you can both focus on each other without becoming side-tracked. Another focus is to create an environment that is relaxing and calm. This will allow you to get in touch with your sensations and your deeper feelings to embrace your pleasure and move in ways that feel good to you without your thoughts running too much and getting in the way of your body and its own needs. So, what do I do to set the mood and make the environment relaxing? Read on.

If you are having sex in your bedroom or your home, it is a space that is very familiar to both of you. This may mean that all of your regular distractions are present all over the place, including your phone, your computer, and your textbooks or your work maybe. You don't want these things staring at you from across the room, reminding you that you have to study all night or send a quick email after your orgasm is over, so try to keep the room as free of these things as possible. Maybe leave your phone and laptop in the kitchen or the office, and make sure you put it on silent!

Secondly, we want the environment to be relaxing. Get rid of the harsh lighting of your overhead bulbs and turn on a few lamps with a soft orange glow or light some candles. The candles may seem cheesy, but there is a reason that they became so closely associated with romance. You don't necessarily have to go so far as having rose petals and chocolates, but some candles will be a nice touch for any day of the week.

Setting the mood in this way will allow you both to breathe and focus on each other and yourselves. We all deserve to have some time with our partner and our bodies, where we enjoy the feeling of pleasure. Use this time with your partner as a way to de-stress and let yourself unwind. Have some fun. Now that the mood is set, the next stages of foreplay can begin.

When you begin foreplay, begin by feeling around between your partner's legs slowly. Pay attention to their face to see what areas are most sensitive and responsive to your touch. Remember, this could vary by the day, so what they liked yesterday may not be what they want today.

When you find the spot that is most responsive (or spots, plural), continue to stimulate it, gradually increasing your speed and pressure as they become more excited and hornier. Listen to their audible cues to tell you when you are hitting the right spot, the right speed, and the right pressure and continue with this in order to keep exciting them. They may reach orgasm, or this may lead to some other type of sex. Being able to be sexually intelligent enough to know where to go, where to touch and how, and how to read the person and their cues takes time.

By stimulating a woman's clitoris, you can give her great pleasure if you know how to touch it the right way. During foreplay, try to give the woman an orgasm if possible. This will make her vagina extremely wet, which will lead to better penetrative sex.

How do you know when you have done enough foreplay? The answer to this is the woman's level of pleasure. It also depends on whether you are erect enough of course! If she has an orgasm during foreplay and you are both wanting to begin penetration, then that is an appropriate time to do so. If you want to extend foreplay even longer after she orgasms, by all means do so. If she does not orgasm during foreplay, you will know when you have spent enough time on this part of sex by how wet her vagina is and how ready she is to begin penetration. If she is getting very wet and is telling you she wants you to put your penis inside of her, it is safe to assume she is ready for you. If she is not too wet and she does not seem as passionate about the sex as she is when she is fully aroused, keep the foreplay going a little longer. You can use dirty talk to find out where she is at mentally as well. You can say something like, "do you want me to come into you?" "How wet are you?" or something of the sort. This will allow her to respond in a sexy way, telling you if she wants more in terms of foreplay, or if she is ready to take it to the next step.

Chapter 4: The Kama Sutra Massage Techniques

A great way to begin practicing Kama Sutra sex techniques is to start with a massage. Every couple can have a quick session of sexual intercourse, but this will not provide you with all of the potential benefits that the Kama Sutra contains. By starting with a sensual massage, you and your partner will share intimate moments together, which will have sex that much better once you get to that stage in this book.

The Kama Sutra Classic Massage Technique

The Kama Sutra talks about massages, including the best places to give massages and some techniques for doing so.

Sometimes, giving your partner a massage will lead to penetrative sex, and sometimes it will not. Aside from being part of foreplay, a massage can also be a relaxing gesture of love. Giving your partner a massage at the end of the day is a great way to get intimate with each other.

If you have massage oil, that is a great addition to any massage, but if not, you can use coconut oil. If you don't have either of those, you can use something like lotion to lubricate your hands and avoid skin to skin friction. Warm your hands before you start massaging them so that it feels nice and doesn't send a chill down their spine when you first make contact.

You can let your partner choose what type of massage they'd like- foot, head, back, shoulder, etc. Instruct them to lie in a comfortable position for their massage. Once you have lubricated your hands, put your hands on them lightly. Then you can begin to massage them gently.

The touch of a massage from a lover gives a person a sense of being cared for. It is a great way to deepen your bond. A massage is a great way to show your partner that you care about making them feel good.

After you have massaged their upper body or their feet, begin kissing their body where you just massaged it and then progress to kissing them on the lips. Let this encounter naturally progress, and let your bodies guide you. You can gradually move into touching each other in new areas, and maybe you will even begin touching each other's genitals, though that leads us to the next section of this chapter.

Eventually, all of this massaging could lead to sex, but it doesn't have to. We will discuss this in more detail below.

The Kama Sutra Erotic Massage Versus the Kama Sutra Classic Massage

Above, we saw an example of a classic Kama Sutra massage. This massage technique does not involve sex or massaging of the genitals. This style of massage involves the person's entire body or any specific location that they would like you to focus on. This kind of massage can be done anywhere and does not necessarily require either of you to remove your clothes.

Beginning with a relaxing massage such as the classic massage will help you and your partner to get into a relaxed and connected state of mind. Once you have finished with the classic massage, you may feel the urge to touch your partner and massage them in other places. This brings us to the erotic massage.

An erotic massage is a massage that involves the touching and massaging of a person's genitals. This leads to pleasurable sensations, but not necessarily to orgasm. An erotic massage can lead to orgasm, though that is not the sole intention.

Erotic massages can be given to both men and women, and they will lead to pleasure and relaxation. You can find a sample technique for a female and a male erotic massage outlined below.

The Benefits of Both

In this section, we are going to look at some of the many benefits that massages can provide you with.

- Relaxing

A massage, regardless of which type, is a relaxing way to unwind with your partner.

- Pleasurable

Massages are pleasurable, whether they are massages of the body or erotic massages. They bring a sense of pleasure in the form of human touch.

- Can be Done Man to Woman or Woman to Man

Massages are able to be done by anyone, to anyone. This makes them a great option for any kind of couple or relationship.

- Can be Done Anytime, Anyplace

Since you don't necessarily have to be naked, a massage can be done anytime, anywhere. This makes it a great option for any couple.

The Female Erotic Massage

This type of massage is an erotic massage, which is called the *yoni massage*. A yoni massage involves the woman's entire vaginal area, which is called the *vulva*. The vulva is a broad term for the vaginal area, which includes the clitoris, the large and small labia, the vagina, and the general areas around them. This area is full of nerve endings, so a woman can feel great pleasure from a massage in this location.

A Yoni Massage is done to open up the woman to her sexuality, her pleasure, and her sexual desires. As a partner, you can perform this type of massage for your female partner to unlock her hidden sexual energy and help her to get in touch with it. For this reason, this massage is a great addition to foreplay, though it can also be done independently of sex.

This massage can be done in a variety of ways, such as in a bathtub, in a jacuzzi, in bed or on the floor. The most important factor here is that the woman is feeling comfortable and relaxed, and the environment will play a big role in this.

To help the woman relax before her massage, begin by setting the ambiance. Ensure that you remove distractions so that she can focus on her pleasure.

You can prepare your hands in the same way that you lubricated and warmed your hands for the classic massage, but be sure that you are using lubricant for this type of massage.

Begin by having the woman breathe deeply and focus on her body. Let her know that she can begin getting in touch with any sensations she is having.

Begin by slowly and gently massaging around her entire vulva and her clitoral area. The key to this type of massage is to move very slowly and with intention. Begin to massage her clitoris slowly and do so without the intention of making her come. You are instead trying to give her subtle pleasure. Massage around her entire vulva slowly, including her labia. Do this for a few minutes, being sure to focus on the entire area and not just her clitoris.

When ready, and using lube, slide one finger into her vagina. Begin to gently massage the inside of her vagina.

By lifting your fingers towards the front of her body, you will find the location of her G-spot.

Encourage her to express herself vocally and to release any sounds she naturally makes as a result of this massage. Move your fingers in a circular motion slowly and with your other hand, massage her pelvic area, her vulva, and clitoris. Doing this serves to connect the inner with the outer.

Continue to massage her in this way and let the experience unfold with no end goal in mind. Let her know that if her body reaches orgasm, she should not fight it. If she doesn't reach orgasm, she can simply enjoy the pleasure that the massage is providing her with. As discussed earlier, this massage is intended to reconnect a woman with her pleasure and allow her to focus on herself and her body, so an orgasm is not necessary.

After this massage, she will feel more in touch with her body. If penetrative sex ensues, both of you will feel increased levels of pleasure, and your orgasms will be more intense because of how engorged and activated her vagina and clitoris will be after having been massaged.

The Male Erotic Massage

There are several different options for providing your male partner with an erotic massage. Firstly, you can massage their testicles. This is less likely to lead to orgasm than a penis massage, so it can be a great way to get a man relaxed and in the mood.
Another form of erotic massage for men, which is discussed in the Kama Sutra, is the penis massage. This type of massage can be tricky, as it could lead to orgasm quite quickly. The effectiveness of this massage will depend on the man's ability to last as his penis is being massaged.

The third variety of massage is the prostate massage. Since this type of massage requires the man's partner to insert a finger into his anus, some couples may be less comfortable with this type of erotic massage. If you do wish to try this kind of massage, it can be very pleasing for the man. The *prostate* is a small gland located inside a man's body between the base of his penis and his anus. It is accessed through the anus. This type of massage is similar to anal sex, but it is not the same, as the goals are different, and so is the technique. Keep in mind that this type of massage will require you to use lots of lube for maximum comfortability. Once your fingers are well-lubricated, you can slide a finger or two inside of the man's anus very slowly. As we discussed previously, you will have to go slow so as not to shock the anus into closing tightly. You will need to work your way in gradually. Once in, you will be able to find the prostate by feeling around on the upper (front) wall of the rectum for a small lump that is rough in texture a few inches deep. Once you have found it, you can begin to gently massage it. You can move your fingers in circles and apply light pressure to it. This massage has the potential to feel quite pleasurable for the man. Communicate while the massage is occurring in order to give him the most pleasure possible.

You can perform this type of massage in a number of different positions. The man could be lying down while you straddle his legs, he could be on his hands and knees while you sit or kneel behind him, he could lie across your lap while you sit on a bed, or you could do any position that is comfortable for you.

This massage does not need to lead to orgasm; at least that is not the goal. If it happens, that is fine; however, the aim of this massage is just to provide a relaxing and pleasurable experience for him.

That is the extent to which we will discuss the prostate massage, and we will now focus on the testicle massage. This type of massage is the most common and the most successful for relaxation and pleasure.

You can perform the testicle massage in several different positions. The man could be lying down on the bed, he could be reclining in a chair, be in a sitting position, or you any other position that is comfortable for him. This massage does not need to lead to orgasm- that is not the goal. If it happens, that is fine; however, the aim of this massage is simply to provide a relaxing and pleasurable experience for the man.

Remember from our discussion of the classic massage, if you have massage oil, that is preferable for this type of massage, but if not, you can use coconut oil. If you don't have either of those, you can use a sexual lubricant to lubricate your hands and avoid skin to skin friction. This is especially important when massaging the testicles. Before you touch him, warm your hands by rubbing them together. This will ensure that it feels nice and that it doesn't shock his testicles if you touch them with cold hands.

Begin by cupping your warm hand around his testicles. Gently move your hand in a circular motion. Be sure not to squeeze them too tightly, especially as you are beginning. Allow the testicles to warm up and relax. Massage them in a circular motion and apply gentle pressure to them. You can incorporate your second hand to provide him with extra sensation.

If he can handle it, you can gently touch his penis as you massage his testicles. If he becomes too erect and is about to reach orgasm, focus solely on the testicles. Massage the area around his testicles, including his inner thighs and his lower butt.
Let this massage flow and see where it takes you. Encourage him not to hold back and to let out any sounds that may find themselves escaping his mouth. Try to help him last as long as he can as you massage him.

After completing this massage, you may find that he is extremely horny, and this may lead to sex. If so, there is no problem with that. Enjoy yourselves and the increased pleasure that will come after such a sensual experience together.

Chapter 5: Kama Sutra Sex Positions

Today in pop culture, the Kamasutra's 64 sex positions are often discussed, making it seem like this book is a secret guide to penetrative sex. By this point in the book, you know that this is untrue. In this chapter, we are going to begin looking at some of the sex positions contained within the Kama Sutra to give you an idea of what exactly this book says about sex.

You may have actually performed one or two of these Kama Sutra sex positions without even knowing that they came from this ancient book. In this chapter, we are going to begin our discussion of the Kama Sutra sex positions by looking at the easiest and simplest sex positions that it contains. In the chapters that follow, we are going to look at Kama Sutra positions for intimacy, as well as some of the more advanced sex positions.

Many people wish to try these sex positions for themselves, and they have become quite popular in the mainstream media today. Many variations can be found, which have come as a result of tweaking the original positions of the Kama Sutra. People always push the envelope when it comes to sexual intercourse and physical pleasure, and many novel sex positions have come about as a result. Maybe you will recognize one or two of these!

Easy Kama Sutra Sex Positions

We are going to begin by looking at some of the easier Kama Sutra sex positions. These positions can be done by any couple, regardless of your strength or flexibility.

The Reverse Cowgirl

This position is quite a classic position, though it is one of the positions included in the book of Kama Sutra. This position is great for the female orgasm, as it allows the woman to take control since she is on top.

To get into this position, the man will lie down on his back on the bed. The woman will straddle him, but instead of facing his head, she will face his lower body, as depicted above. From here, the woman can lift her body up and down, using her legs at the speed and depth that feels best. She can also thrust at the angle that she enjoys the most, and she can feel the pleasure build as she moves her body. The man can sit back and relax, as the woman rides him sensually.

Below, you can see another variation of the Reverse Cowgirl Position, in which the woman opens up her body to allow for clitoral stimulation at the same time as penetration. In this variation, the woman will lie back so that she is lying on top of the man, facing away from him- his penis still inside of her. She can plant one of her hands back onto the bed to help hold herself up, while the other hand stimulates her clitoris. She can also use a vibrator on her clitoris in this position.

The Congress of a Dog

This position is called *The Congress of a Dog*. This is a position in which the man and woman are intended to emulate two animals having sex. In this case, they are intended to act as a male dog mating with a female dog. This is similar to the position above, but in this case, this position can be likened to the modern *Doggy Style* position.

This position is a favorite among men and women alike. Both women and men can get intense pleasure from this position because the angles at which their genitals come together creates harmonic pleasure for both parties.

To get into position, the woman gets on her hands and knees on the bed (or couch or floor, this position works anywhere really), and the man kneels behind her. He takes his erect penis and enters her vagina. He starts by slowly sliding it in and gradually begins getting faster and deeper. He does this by thrusting his hips and can control the pace in this way. He grabs onto her hips for a stronger thrust and pulls her body towards his to get himself deeper into her with each thrust. In this position, he has a view of her entire backside and can see it shake and bounce with each movement, making him hornier and hornier. He can talk dirty to her and grab her butt cheeks from here.

Doggy style is a position that women can get a lot of pleasure from. It is no surprise it is most often the favorite position, especially among young people, of both genders. Because of the curve of the man's erect penis and the angle at which it enters into the woman's vagina, her G-spot will likely be stimulated with each thrust. This G-spot stimulation means that it will be very likely that she will reach an orgasm from penetration. G spot stimulation can make a woman feel such intense full-body pleasure for quite a long time before she actually reaches an orgasm. Hitting her G-spot will continue to feel amazing for both the woman and man until finally, one or both of them cannot wait any longer, and ultimate pleasure is reached.

The Supported Congress

This position is a variety of the standing position, but it can be done with more ease than some of the other standing varieties.

To get into this position, the man stands in front of a wall with the woman standing in front of him, facing him. The woman lifts one knee and wraps her leg around one of the man's legs. The man can then slide his penis into her vagina; her leg raised to allow for deeper penetration and easier access. In standing positions, it may be more difficult to get the penetration right away, but with some maneuvering and adjustments because of height differences, you will eventually get into a comfortable rhythm.

This position is a midway point to another Kamasutra position called The Suspended Congress, where the woman has both legs up, and the man is holding them both under her knees and thrusting into her while holding her weight up. This position is quite difficult for the man, but if achieved, it can lead to very deep penetration. The Supported Congress is a great place to start if you want to eventually try it with both legs up, as it is quite similar.

The Mare's Position

This Kama Sutra position is more of a sexual technique than a sex position itself. This sexual technique has the potential to change your sex life forever!

In this position, the man sits with his legs stretched out in front of him and his arms back, supporting his weight on the bed. The woman straddles him, facing away from him and lowers herself down onto his erect penis. Once inside of her, the woman uses her vaginal muscles to apply and release pressure on the man's penis, almost as if she is milking it. This makes for very pleasurable sensations on both the man's penis and the woman's vagina. This creates more stimulation on the man's penis, and also stronger sensations for the woman's vagina. This also strengthens her vaginal muscles, which in time will lead to stronger and more pleasurable orgasms for the woman!

Afternoon Delight

Afternoon Delight is a nice position to try on a quiet Sunday after a long work week when you are both feeling tired and want a bit of lazy sex. You can start this position off with some lazy hand and finger play and then progress it to penetration in the same position if you are already cuddling and don't want to move around too much. This position is optimal for stoners and sleepyheads.

The man lies down on his side, his erect penis poking out in front of him. The woman lies on her back at a 90-degree angle to the man's body, halfway down near his genitals. She then bends her knees, lifts her legs, and drapes them over the man's side, sliding her vagina towards him, so it is close to his penis. He can move forward to meet her and slide his penis in her vagina. The woman can lie back and relax while the man thrusts his hips. This position can be done while you watch a tv show, while you are reading or while you are both half-asleep and want a little bit of Afternoon Delight. If this inspires you to try something more involved once you get into the mood, you can easily transition to Missionary or Doggy Style from here.

The Lap Position

This next position is another that is best for male pleasure and the male orgasm. This position requires strength on the part of the man and the woman and is quite an athletic position, but this is why it is called an advanced sex position. Be careful when trying this one.

To get into position, the man will sit upright in a comfortable chair or on the edge of a bed with his feet planted on the floor. The woman will climb onto his lap and wrap her legs around behind the man or stick them straight out past him. Then, the man can insert his penis into the woman's vagina. From here, the woman will lean back until she is lying straight back, and her body is flat. While she does this, the man will have to hold onto her at her hips or her lower back, depending on your height variations. The man in this position will perform a combination of thrusting his hips into the woman from a seated position and pulling her onto his penis repeatedly. A high amount of upper body strength is required on the part of the man in this position. Place some pillows on the floor underneath the woman when trying this position, just in case. The woman can hold onto the man's arms for support as well here.

This position is great for the male's pleasure because it allows him to control the speed and depth of thrusting.

The Ascending Position

This position allows the woman to take full control of both her body and the man's penis and is good for women who have some trouble reaching orgasm in other sexual positions. The man takes a passive role in this position, with the woman's weight on top of him, which can be a huge turn-on. He can lie back and watch her take control and enjoy the pleasure he is getting from his penis inside of her and from watching the woman gyrate and find pleasure on top of him.

The man lies down on his back on the bed; he can prop up his head on a pillow if he wants a better view of the woman. She sits cross-legged on top of his genital area, her legs crossed over his waistline. She holds onto his penis and puts it into her vagina. She can wait to do this after oral or after giving him a handjob first, or she can get right to the penetration, depending on if they have already done foreplay prior to this. Once he is inside of her, she can lean back and rest her hands on his legs for support if needed. From here, she grinds her hips and can control her hip angles and control the speed of thrusting. In this leaned back position, her clitoris is perfectly accessible to be stimulated with her own hand. The man will be too far to do this for her as he is lying down, and her legs are holding his body down. The restriction of his movement by his naked woman will be sure to make the man so horny and frustrated that his penis will be rock hard. She can change the angle of her hips to reach G-spot stimulation by the man's penis. She may even be able to reach both clitoral and G-spot orgasms at the same time from this position.

The Cross Position

This position is similar to another position of the Kama Sutra, the Half-Pressed Position. If you like this one, you are sure to like the Half-Pressed Position too.

The woman lies on her back with one leg extended straight into the air. The man kneels in front of her, straddling her leg that is extended on the bed and holds onto her other leg, which is in the air. He can then move his body forward between her two legs until he is close enough to insert his penis into her vagina. He can hold her legs spread with his body, straddling one of them and placing the other one on his shoulder. By doing this, his hands will be free so that he can play with her clitoris, massage her breasts, rubbing his hands up and down her body or whatever they please. They can talk dirty to each other while looking at each other in the eyes and tell each other what they want to be done to them or what feels good.

Chapter 6: The Kama Sutra and Intimacy

For a book written so long ago, it is still quite relevant in terms of its discussions on ways to achieve intimacy and how to treat your partner well in the bedroom. In this chapter, we are going to talk about the best Kama Sutra sex positions for intimacy and what the Kama Sutra can teach you about improving the level of intimacy in your relationship or marriage.

What Is Intimacy?

Intimacy is very important between two people when part of a couple, especially in the bedroom. Intimacy is what brings you close and keeps you close. For this reason, we are going to address intimacy in this chapter before moving onto the rest of the concepts related to sex, sex positions, and techniques for you and your partner. Firstly, we will look at what intimacy means and the different types of intimacy that exist.

There are different types of intimacy, and here I will outline them for you before digging deeper into the intimacy that exists between couples. Intimacy, in a general sense, is defined as mutual openness and vulnerability between two people. There are different ways in which you can give and receive openness and vulnerability in a relationship. Intimacy does not have to include a sexual relationship (though it can); therefore, it is not only reserved for romantic relationships. Intimacy can also be present in other types of close relationships like friendships or family relationships. Below, I will outline the different forms of intimacy.

- Emotional Intimacy

Emotional intimacy is the ability to express oneself maturely and openly, leading to a deep emotional connection between people. Saying things like "I love you" or "you are very important to me" are examples of this. It is also the ability to respond maturely and openly when someone expresses themselves to you by saying things like "I'm sorry" or "I love you too." This type of open and vulnerable dialogue leads to an emotional connection. For a deep emotional connection to form, there must be a mutual willingness to be vulnerable and open with one's deeper thoughts and feelings. This is where this type of emotional intimacy comes from.

- Physical Intimacy

Physical intimacy is the type that most people think of when they hear the term "intimacy," and it is the kind that we will be most concerned with in this book, as it is the type of intimacy that includes sex and all activities related to sex. It also involves other non-sexual types of physical contact, such as hugging and kissing. Physical intimacy can be found in close friendships or familial relationships where hugging and kisses on the cheek are common, but it is most often found in romantic relationships.

Physical intimacy is the type of intimacy involved when people are trying to make each other orgasm. Physical intimacy is almost always required for orgasm. Physical intimacy doesn't necessarily mean that you are in love with the person you are having sex with; it just means that you are doing something intimate with another person in a physical way.

It is also possible to be intimate with yourself, and while this begins with the emotional intimacy of self-awareness, it also involves the physical intimacy of masturbation and physical self-exploration. I define sexual, physical

624

intimacy of the self as being in touch with the parts of yourself physically that you would not normally be in touch with. If you are a woman, your breasts, your clitoris, your vagina, and your anus. If you are a man, your testicles, your penis, your anus. Being able to be physically intimate with yourself allows you to have more fulfilling sex, more fulfilling orgasms, and a more fulfilling overall relationship with your body. We will discuss this in more detail later on in this book. Allowing someone to be physically intimate with you in a sexual way is also an emotionally intimate experience, regardless of your relationship with the person. Being in charge of your own body while it is in the hands of another person is very important, and this is why masturbation is such a key element to physical intimacy.

You can think of physical intimacy as something that breaks the barrier of personal space. By this definition, this includes touching of any sort, but especially sexual intercourse, kissing touching, and anything else of a sexual nature. When you are having sex with anyone, regardless of whether you have romantic feelings for them or not, you are having a physically intimate relationship with them. The difference between a relationship that involves physical intimacy alone and no other forms of intimacy and a romantic relationship is that a romantic relationship will also involve emotional intimacy, shared activities and intellectual intimacy is that a deep and lasting romantic relationship will need to include all of these forms of intimacy at once. In this book, we are going to focus on how all of these types of intimacy come together to create a successful and deep romantic relationship between two people in love. We are going to begin by taking the next section to discuss how to maintain and increase the levels of intimacy in your relationship.

The Importance of Intimacy

Feeling awkward when it comes to talking about intimacy is one of the most human experiences a person can have. Sometimes, we fall into a sexual rut with someone, and then we realize that the fiery passion that used to burn at the base of your tummy has dimmed. The way to remedy this is to work on your intimacy.

When it comes to a long-term relationship, you likely have reached a high level of intimacy, and this is often what makes your sex life so rewarding. While you can achieve physical pleasure from having sex with anyone, or from masturbating alone, the connection that you feel when having sex with someone whom you are emotionally intimate with will lead your physical body to be in harmony with your emotions and this leads to great levels of both physical and emotional pleasure, which is exactly where the term "making love" comes from.

When you care about another person deeply, you care about bringing them pleasure in a variety of forms; sexual pleasure is one of them. When you bring two people together who are genuinely invested in the pleasure of each other, this forms a beautiful sexual bond full of pleasure in every sense. This is why intimacy is important in sex and why sex with intimacy is not only a physical act but also an emotional experience.

The Kama Sutra and Intimacy

The Kama Sutra has quite a few things to say about intimacy and how to maintain and restore it. As I mentioned, the Kama Sutra is a guide to love and to enjoy a pleasurable life with your partner. The Kama Sutra can serve as a guide for a long-term relationship or a marriage to keep sex interesting and to try new forms of intimacy.
626

By keeping your relationship new and different, it will keep you both interested in what is to come, which will keep you both engaged in your relationship with one another.

The Kama Sutra text views sex as a spiritual act between two people that, with time, will increase a person's level of spirituality and sexual power. The book aims to help people to get in touch with their desires, which will aid them in reaching the full extent of their sexual power. It aims to liberate people in a sexual sense. These concepts were quite advanced for the time that the book was written, which is why this book is still so widely discussed to this day. Even though it was written so long ago, this book is still quite relevant for couples who wish to improve their relationship or their level of intimacy.

Sex is one part of a romantic relationship, but there are so many other aspects to achieving deep emotional closeness with another person, which can be learned through reading the Kama Sutra. The rest of this book will focus on discussing many of the benefits of the Kama Sutra and the ways that it can help you increase your level of intimacy with your partner.

For example, the Kama Sutra states that taking a bath together is a great way to build intimacy in a relationship.

Taking a bath together is a nice way to unwind after a long day and spend some time together on self-care. Doing self-care together is actually quite intimate, as this is something usually reserved for our time alone. Relaxing in a warm bath, either with bubbles or without, is a good way to set a mood. Sitting together in the closeness of a bathtub with the steam and the cleanliness will get you both in touch with your own bodies, but also in touch with their body. While this doesn't have to lead to sex, it can be a type of foreplay whether you intend for it to be or not. You may get in the bath together to spend some time to relax and share a few kisses. This may turn to making out and progress to much more. You may also get into the bath together to get yourselves in the mood for love and get naked while slowly easing into the sex. In Kamasutra, it is said that washing someone else's hair is a very intimate act. This may not be something that you have thought of before, or may not be something you are interested in. I assure you; it will lead to a greater level of intimacy with your partner if you give it a chance. When these acts of self-care that are usually done in private are shared with our partner, it can create magical moments of connection.

When you get into the bath, you can give each other head massages, back massages, or soap each other up. Begin kissing and making out and gliding your hands over your partner's wet body. Start with their back and arms and face. Let your desires take over both of you. As mentioned above, setting the mood like this will have you both focused on pleasure and touch and forgetting about all of your responsibilities and stressors in no time. This is good! We want to be focused when we have sex as a couple. Begin with one of you lathering the other with soap and shampoo in a slow and caring fashion. Rinse them off in the same way, taking care of their special needs and routines. Then, do the same the other way around. Take your time with this and enjoy the moment. You can do this as an act leading up to making love, or simply as a caring gesture for each other before bed.

It won't necessarily lead here, but a positive aspect of bathing together is that you will both be naked already for wherever you decide to take your sex from here. You will also both be clean, so any type of oral sex can be done without wondering when your partner last showered. As we all know, when we get comfortable with someone, we tend to put less into our image as we don't feel the need to impress them anymore!

How to Increase and Maintain Intimacy

Shared interests and activities are one of the forms of intimacy. This form of intimacy is less well-known, but it is also considered a form of intimacy. When you share activities with another person that you both enjoy and are passionate about, this creates a sense of connection. For example, when you cook together or travel together. These shared experiences give you memories to share, and this leads to bonding and intimacy (openness and vulnerability).

Being able to be vulnerable and open with your emotions is a requirement for intimacy. It is necessary to share oneself with the other person in a relationship. This mutual sharing of yourselves is what will lead to intimacy in the first place or an increase in intimacy.
Sometimes in a long-term relationship, you become so comfortable with each other that you don't have to communicate as much as you used to since you know each other so well. The key here is to continue communicating, even if you think the other person knows what you are thinking or feeling without you having to say it. By doing this, you keep the lines of communication open in your relationship. This avoids any chance of miscommunication or misunderstanding that would be perpetuated by a lack of communication. By having misunderstandings go unresolved, this could lead to resentment and an overall breakdown in communication, which can reduce levels of intimacy in the relationship.

This intimacy and vulnerability include being able to communicate about your desires- be they sexual desires or any other sort of desires. By sharing these with your partner, you will be able to ensure that they know how to please you in every sense of the word. This also leads to boundaries being set and upheld, since your desires include things you are comfortable and okay with, and this conversation will often lead to things which you are not okay with.

By learning these things about your partner, you can begin to work together to ensure each person's intimacy needs are met. For example, if your number one intimacy preference is for emotional intimacy and your partner likes to show their love in physical ways, you can discuss how they can begin to be more vocal about their love for you, and you can be more receptive to their physical displays of affection. Putting these things out on the table for discussion is the best way to learn about each other. You can never stop learning about your partner, and this will only strengthen your relationship.

It is important to communicate about your needs for intimacy regularly since people will grow and change over the course of a relationship. Especially in a long-term relationship, being aware of when a person's intimacy needs change is important to maintaining a good level of intimacy.

Another way that romance is shown and received is through gestures and gifts. This is probably the first thing you think of when you hear the term "romance" for example, bringing your partner flowers after they have a long day, or drawing them a bath when you know they are feeling stressed out. These gifts and gestures are ways of communicating that don't involve words. When you are in a long-term relationship, it is important to be able to show your love and adoration in ways other than saying "I love you," and gestures are a great way to do this. If you and your partner have gotten into a routine way of living with each other, try to spice things up by offering to cook them dinner or by changing something up in order to show them your feelings and bring about some extra romance. This will help you to feel connected in new ways and will keep your spark alive, even if you are extremely comfortable with one another.

Kama Sutra Sex Positions for Intimacy

The Lotus

Arguably the most intimate position of them all is The Lotus. The Lotus position is most intimate because of the closeness of your entire bodies, infinitely pressed against each other at all points from head to toe, while being face to face.

The man sits on the bed cross-legged, his torso upright. His penis is erect and ready to get it on. The woman climbs on top of him and sits in his lap, wrapping her arms and legs around him. He holds her by wrapping his arms around her as well. With some shifting, they slide his penis inside of her. In this position, both people will be grinding more than they will be thrusting or humping. This is also what makes it so intimate. Grinding face to face while she is sitting on his lap with him inside of her, that is about as intimate as it gets.

In this position, you will not be doing any crazy thrusting, so it is ideal for a steamy make-out session, as your mouths will be so close that you can feel each other's breath the entire time. You can look into each other's eyes and whisper sweet nothings to them as you share this intimate experience.

The Position of Indra's Wife

To get into this position, the woman will lie down on her back, and she will bring her thighs to her sides. She will bend her knees so that her legs are bent at her sides. This opens up her entire vaginal area for intercourse. The man will lie on top of her and enter her from the front.

This position may take practice due to the flexibility is requires from the woman, but if she can accomplish this, it will be greatly pleasurable for her. This position opens up the woman to receive the man, which will result in deeper penetration, and thus, greater pleasure for both of them.

Half-Pressed Position

This position is another midpoint to a more difficult Kamasutra position requiring a lot of flexibility, but this one is quite good even at this midway point! The woman's legs are spread wide, and so it is very pleasurable for both of them.

The woman lies down on her back with her man kneeling in front of her. She stretches one leg straight out past him, besides his body and with the other leg, she bends her knee and places her foot on his chest. From here, he enters her vagina. The woman can move her hips up or down to give varying amounts of pressure to the man's penis for added pleasure for him. The stretching of her leg opens her clitoris up to potentially be stimulated by the base of his penis when he thrusts his hips and penetrates deeply into her. Having one foot planted on his chest keeps her legs open wide with every one of his thrusts in order to allow for deep penetration and clitoral stimulation.

The Hinge Position

You may have tried this position before, but may not have known that it was a Kamasutra position. This position is a spin on doggy style, so if you are a big fan of the classic Doggy Style position, give this one a try next time you want to experiment with something new!

The man kneels on the bed with one knee down as usual, and the other leg propped up at a 90-degree angle. The woman is on all fours in front of the man, supporting her weight on her forearms. The man slides his penis into the woman's vagina from behind. Both the woman and the man are able to control the depth and speed from this position as the woman can thrust herself back onto his penis, and the man can thrust his hips forward. With one knee bent, the man has more control over his thrusts and can hold onto his woman's hips for a quicker speed if they want a deeper thrust and a faster and more rough sex session. This is one of those positions where it makes a quick thrusting speed easy because his knee is propped up.

The Closed Door

This position is similar to the missionary position in that both people are lying down face-to-face, and the man is on top. The difference, however, and what makes this an advanced position is that the woman will keep her legs shut tightly the entire time. The man's penis can be inserted while her legs are open, and then once it is in, she will close her legs. What this does is constrict her vagina and make the canal tighter for the man's penis. In addition to this, if she is aroused, her vagina will be engorged, and the canal will be tighter already. Because of this, the man's penis will be hugged closely as it slides in and out of her, and this will make for extra pleasure for him.

The Lock

To get into this position, the woman will lean back and relax on the bed, getting ready to receive her partner. Her partner will then approach her from the front, placing her legs on his shoulders and lifting her buttocks onto his thighs, as he will be sitting on his legs, which are bent behind him. The woman will lift her upper body slightly so that she can wrap her arms around her partner's shoulders or his neck. The man will support the woman's lower back, and then he can thrust into her from his sitting position, and he can use his arms to lift and lower her body onto his penis.

Variation of the Yawning Position

Have you ever heard of the term 'balls deep'?
Have you ever wanted to try it?

The Yawning Position creates the deepest possible penetration of any sexual position. In the classic yawning position, the woman puts her legs in the air and spreads her legs with her knees straight, forming a 'V' shape. The man kneels in front of her and puts his penis inside her from the front. This creates an intense sensation for both partners.

The variation of The Yawning Position that we are going to look at can begin when the woman is fully aroused and wet. The woman lies on her back and lifts her legs into the air with her knees straight. The man lies on top of her in a missionary-like position. She places her straight legs on the man's shoulders. He can then enter her vagina with his erect penis and thrust his hips forward for the deepest penetration. As I said, this position makes for the deepest possible vaginal penetration of any sexual position, and if the woman can manage it, she can slide her legs to the outer edges of the man's shoulders which will make for maximum depth of penetration as her legs will be as far spread as possible.

The Standing Behind Position

In this position, the woman will stand facing a wall and will plant her hands on the wall in front of her. She will then bend her knees so that she can spread her legs. The man will come up behind and below her and come into her from behind. He can grab onto her hips or her shoulders so that he has something to hold onto, and he can use this to thrust deeper into her. This position is good in the shower or in any room of the house as having the woman planting her hands on the wall is both hot and safe when it comes to shower sex. This would be especially useful in the tight space of a stand-up shower. Just be sure to use lots of lubrication!

634

The Crab Position

In this position, the woman will lie on her back, and she will cross her legs. Then, she will hold her legs to her stomach. The man can assist by holding her legs there while he lies on top of her and enters her from the front. This position is quite intimate as it requires the man and woman to work together to hold her body in this posture. They are face to face while doing so, which makes it quite an intimate experience.

The Raised Feet Position

This position needs a little bit of flexibility, but it is also a sort of a stretch, so if you ease into it you should be able to reach it in a few minutes after your body is warmed up.

The woman lies on her back and brings her knees to her chest, wrapping her arms around them, her body forming a small ball shape. The man kneels near her buttocks and enters her vagina from a kneeling position in front of her. Her vagina will be quite easily accessible because her legs are lifted at her chest. If the flexibility is there, the man can now lean forward with his upper body, and with his own chest, he can hold her legs to her chest for her so that her hands are free. With her free hands, she can hold the back of his neck, pull his hair, or caress his face, depending on what direction you want to go with this sexual encounter. From here, the man's penis can very easily meet the woman's G-spot because of its curve, and this will make for an intense orgasm for both parties. The restriction of movement paired with the extreme closeness of their bodies is sure to make for some pent-up arousal that has no other way to be released than through a full-body orgasm.

The Waterfall

This position requires lots of trust between the woman and the man. The waterfall is a position in which the man has complete control. The man will begin by sitting in a chair with his feet on the floor. The woman will climb onto his lap and insert his penis into her. She can wrap her legs around his waist. Then, slowly she will lean all the way back until her head and arms are touching the floor (with pillows underneath). From here, the man will hold onto her hips and can move her body onto his penis at whatever speed and depth he wishes. He can also grab onto her breasts and massage her clitoris in this position if he wishes.

The Sitting Duck

Another position requiring complete trust is the sitting duck. This is a position that allows the woman to have complete control. The man will lie down on the floor on his back. The woman will straddle him and slide his penis into her. Then, one by one, she will cross her legs so that she is essentially sitting on his penis cross-legged. In this position, the man has no freedom of movement, and everything is up to the woman. She can even touch her clitoris in this position if she wishes.

Chapter 7: Advanced Kama Sutra Sex Positions

In this chapter, we are going to continue our examination of the Kama Sutra sex positions by looking at some of the more advanced positions. These positions will require more flexibility and strength from either the man, the woman or both.

While they require more strength and flexibility, they come with great rewards in the form of pleasure if you can get into them.

Advanced Kama Sutra Sex Positions

After reading through this list of advanced Kama Sutra sex positions, try some for yourself with your partner. Challenging yourselves to get into new sex positions will be an intimate and sexy experience that will benefit your relationship.

The Turning Position

The Turning Position is a fun one that you have probably never heard of before. It can add some fun into your stale sex life or some pizazz into a new and youthful relationship. This is one of the more challenging positions to master and requires quite a lot of communication from both parties. It will also require some practice to execute it seamlessly, but don't be intimidated; you will master it in no time and begin to wow all of your present and/or future partners! This position is well suited to couples who would like to try something different and explore new ways of reaching pleasure together at a point in their relationship when they are comfortable with each other and know how to communicate well.

The position begins in the classic Missionary position (as discussed previously in this book) with the man on top of the woman and both of them face to face. The man's legs should both be between the woman's legs, and his penis is already inside of her. This is where it gets more complicated, so listen closely. The man now lifts his left leg over the woman's right leg and then proceeds to lift his right leg over her right leg, keeping his penis inside of her, and continues by moving his upper body in a clockwise direction until he is at a 90-degree angle to her body, essentially lying across her (while still penetrating her). He will then move his legs over her upper body, one leg at a time, continuing to turn around in a clockwise direction so that his feet are at either side of her head, still maintaining the positioning of his penis inside her vagina.

From here, he will complete the turn and come back to his starting Missionary position without ever removing his penis from her vagina. Doing this seamlessly and sensually without accidentally pulling out of her will require some practice and cooperation on both of their parts. When it is done well, it looks like he is turning in a slow and smooth circle around her body.

This position will lead to new sensations for both people as every single angle of his penis inside her vagina will be felt by both of them. It will lead to new challenges for both of them as it is a complex position to try. And it will lead to the exploration of new points of view of the other person's body, all three of these things leading to greater intimacy and closeness between partners.

The Scissors Position

This position is a little difficult to get yourselves into, but once you do, it will be well worth the effort. To begin, the man will sit on the bed with his arms behind him, holding his weight up but leaning back. Then, he will bend one of his knees, so his leg is bent. The woman will lie down on the bed face-down and with her head at the opposite end of the bed as the man. She will spread her legs and move her body toward the man's until their bodies meet. When they meet, their bodies will look like two pairs of scissors crossed into one another. From here, the man will insert his penis into her vagina. The woman can move her body up and down on his penis, and the man can thrust into her. It may take a bit of time to develop a rhythm in this position, but when you do, you will both feel intense pleasure.

The Plow

As the name suggests, this position is designed to make you emulate a human plow, but I assure you, this position is much sexier than it sounds. This position is a great introduction to some of the more interesting and difficult Kama Sutra sex positions. This is a great option if you wish to get acquainted with the world of Kamasutra for the first time and wish to challenge yourselves.

You, as the woman, lie face-down on the bed with your hips and legs sticking off the end and support yourself on your elbows. Your man stands on the floor beside the bed, his body positioned between your legs. He then lifts your lower half up by your hips and thighs and inserts his penis into your vagina, while supporting your legs the entire time. You can take a more passive role in this position, and he can adjust the angle he holds your legs at for maximum pleasure.

The Peg Position

The Peg has a sexy name that implies pleasure and may even have you turned on already. This is a more difficult position, certainly more difficult to get yourselves into, but it comes with the reward of a great all-encompassing orgasm for both parties if it can be done.

The man lies on his side, and the woman lies facing him on her side, with her head towards his feet. The woman will lift her knees towards her chest and place one of her legs underneath the man's legs and have the other on top of his legs. Essentially, she is hugging his legs with her entire body. She slides up so that her vulva is next to his penis. When aligned properly, he can penetrate her and can achieve depth and control as she is positioned perfectly for his penis to enter her. The woman wraps her arms around his legs, and he can use his hands and arms to help with his thrusting, or if she is comfortable, he can use his hands to stimulate her anal area with his fingers or a toy. The woman is positioned like this allows for all of her vulvae to be open and accessible once again, and this is what will lead to a stronger orgasm for her. The man being able to see all of her and to play with her anus will lead to a stronger orgasm for him.

The Posture of Splitting Bamboo

The woman will lie on her back and have the man lie on top of her, sliding his body in between her legs. The woman will lift one of her legs and put it on one of his shoulders, and the other will stretch out past his body. From here, he pushes his hips forward and can easily slide his penis into her vagina, which is open and in a perfect position for penetration. The man will do the thrusting here. After some time, the woman will switch and put the other leg on his other shoulder. She can continue to alternate as they engage in intercourse.

This position requires flexibility in the woman but gives a deep penetration once accomplished and almost rides that line between pleasure and pain due to the stretch.

This position allows for deep penetration as well as varied pressure on the man's penis, which will be extremely pleasurable for him.

If the woman is feeling flexible and wants to try a new position that will have both of them benefitting from a deeper penetration than most of the classics, this position will be a great choice.

The Suspended Congress

To get into this position, the man will stand facing a wall with the woman standing in front of him, her back to the wall. She will then jump into his arms and wrap both her arms and her legs around him. Once here, he can insert his penis into her vagina while holding onto her buttocks or underneath her knees. He can lean her back on the wall in front of him for support so that he does not have to support her entire weight in his arms. If he holds onto her underneath her knees, this will open her up so that her vagina is easily accessible. The fact that she is suspended coupled with this will make it so that there is deep penetration occurring, and this will be pleasurable for both the man and the woman. Deep penetration is great for the female orgasm because there are two places located deep within the vagina that, when stimulated, lead to a very intense orgasm for her. The penis must achieve continuous deep penetration in order for this to happen, and in this position, it is quite possible.

This position is great for the female orgasm because of the angle that the man's penis enters her vagina. It is also quite pleasurable for the woman because the man is in control in this position, so the woman can relax and enjoy the pleasure he is bringing to her body.

Crossed Keys

The Crossed Keys is a relatively simple position but makes for an interesting and new position to try if you have never done it before. This is a great introduction to the world of more complex and acrobatic positions. While this is not quite acrobatic, it will introduce you to this type of sex.

Have your woman lie down on her back at the edge of the bed with her legs sticking straight up into the air, knees straight. She then crosses one leg in front of the other, keeping them sticking straight up. Stand at the edge of the bed and grab a hold of her outstretched legs. Then, with your feet planted on the floor, slide your penis into her vagina and holding her legs as a stable base, you can thrust harder and faster as she likes it. With her legs crossed over each other like this, it tightens her vagina so that it creates a tighter and more pleasurable environment for your penis as well as creating more pleasure for her because the tighter vagina canal will mean more contact of your penis with the walls of her vagina and will lead to G-spot stimulation.

The Toad Position

This position is similar to The Toad (or The Frog) stretch that you may have done in a yoga class before. Facing the floor with bent knees spread wide to get those hips stretched. I bet you never thought that would help you in your sex life... But low and behold, turn that stretch over, and you have The Toad position! I will explain in more detail as follows.

The woman lays on her back, bending her knees towards her chest and spreading her knees open wide. This opens her body up for easy penetration, clitoris access, and maximum exposure of all of her pleasurable parts to her man's body that will be rubbing against them. The woman's entire vulva can be a pleasurable area if it is exposed to touch like the man's pelvis or hips rubbing it. This, coupled with the clitoris being rubbed at the same time, will drive her crazy. The man lies on top of her and slides his penis into her vagina, having lots of space for deep penetration. In this position, the woman's clitoris can easily be stimulated from the thrusting motion of the man's body on top of hers or from the base of his penis when he comes as close to her as possible with each thrust. If the woman wants to take more control, once he is inside of her, she can wrap her legs around his waist and use them to pull his hips towards her along with his movement to increase the pressure and depth of his penetration.

The Widely Opened Position

The name of this position means that the woman's entire body is widely opened to receive pleasure in the form of her man. Her body is in a position that says she is ready for this experience.

As the woman, lie down on a bed on your back with your man on top of you, both of his legs between yours. Have him hold his weight up, so he is hovering over you, allowing you to get into position before he comes into you.

Proceed to throw your head all the way back so you can see your headboard and arch your back at the same time, pushing your breasts into the air. Use your elbows behind you to support you and lift your hips into the air to meet your man's body that is hovering over top of you. Hold onto this position and (in whatever sensual language you feel turned on by) invite your man to put his penis into you. While you hold yourself up in this position, he can then thrust his penis in and out with varying speed and force. If it proves to be too difficult for you to hold up your body weight the entire time, ask your man to help you by holding himself up with one arm, and by wrapping his other arm under your lower back to support you a bit.

So why hold your body in this difficult position you ask? The reason for this is that the woman's raised position allows the man to achieve deep penetration like the vagina is raised up and more exposed to the front where the man's penis is. Further, because she is pressed up in an arched-back position, her clitoris is lifted and exposed more than ever, which will allow for the friction of the man's thrusts against her body to stimulate the clitoris with each pump.

The Standing Position

The standing position may be a little difficult, but with practice, you might just add this one into your regular rotation. Many variations can be done with this position, depending on what feels best for both of you and how your stamina is.

To start, it may be easier to have the man standing against a wall so that he can lean his back onto it for support. The woman then will stand in front of the man, facing away from him. Now for the tricky part, you will need to play around a bit to find the right way for both of you to reach this. The man will now need to insert his penis into his female partner's vagina from behind. This will work best if the man leans back against the wall, lowering his body so that he can push his hips upward toward his partner's vulva. The woman can reach back and hold onto the man if she wishes.

The Fixing of a Nail

This is another position that involves the man on top of the woman in a position similar to the Missionary Position, but this is a more difficult variation.

In this position, the woman will place one of her legs on the man's head, and the other will be stretched out below her. The Kama Sutra states that this position will require a lot of practice to accomplish. Once you are able to do this position, you will benefit from a very deep penetration, as well as a high likelihood of G-Spot stimulation for the woman.

The Pressed Position

This position is a little challenging, but it has great benefits for those who can achieve it. This position requires a little bit of flexibility, but it also acts as a stretch, so if you ease into it you should be able to reach the full position within a few minutes after your body is warmed up.

To get into this position, the woman lies on her back and brings her knees to her chest, wrapping her arms around them, her body forming a small ball shape. The man kneels near her buttocks and enters her vagina from a kneeling position in front of her. Her vagina will be quite easily accessible because her legs are lifted at her chest. If the flexibility is there, the man can now lean forward with his upper body, and with his own chest, he can hold her legs to her chest for her so that her hands are free. With her free hands, she can hold the back of his neck, pull his hair, or caress his face, depending on what direction you want to go with this sexual encounter. From here, the man's penis can very easily meet the woman's G-spot because of its curve, and this will make for an intense orgasm for both parties. The restriction of movement paired with the extreme closeness of their bodies is sure to make for some pent-up arousal that has no other way to be released than through a full-body orgasm.

The Sphinx Position

The Sphinx gets its name from the ancient Egyptian sculptures of women in this type of position, although without the man penetrating her. These sculptures and statues were not erotic! But you can make your own erotic Sphinx at home after you read on about this position.

The woman lies face down, supporting herself on her elbows. She stretches one leg out behind her and bends the other out to the side of her body to spread out and open up access to her vagina. The man lies on top of the woman, and his penis enters her vagina from behind. This may be hard if he has a smaller penis, but he will need to get as low as possible, and it should still work! The weight of the man lying on top of the woman makes for added pleasure for her because it spreads her legs further apart so that her pleasure centers are more accessible. It also increases pressure on her pelvis, which will help in leading to an orgasm, and when it does, an even stronger and better orgasm because the pressure from the outside meets the pressure from the inside and voilà! Full body bliss.

X-Rated

The X-Rated is a position that the man will love if he has not already suggested it sometime in your relationship! You can probably glean this from the name though.

If you are the man, lie down on your back, and the woman will lie on top of you, facing down your body with her head at your feet. She will wrap her arms around your legs and spread her legs so that they are on either side of your hips. She can then slide up or down your body to adjust for ease of inserting your penis into her. If it is easier, start in reverse cowgirl (like we examined earlier in this book) and have her lie forward after you penetrate her so that she is lying on your legs. She can wrap her arms around your legs after this. Either you can pump your hips into her with her lying on your penis, or she can lift her hips up and down on your penis for the magic to happen. She can be in control of the depth and speed of penetration by doing this if you wish. You as the man in this position, will likely want your head propped up by a pillow or three so that you can take in the full view of your woman below the waist with her naked bum in the air, gyrating on your erection in all her beauty.

This position is loved by many men, but also by many women for the same reasons that they love reverse cowgirl. Deep penetration, the ability to be in control of the humping and G-spot stimulation. The trifecta of female pleasure!

Chapter 8: Other Kama Sutra Techniques

Now that you have gained a solid understanding of the sex positions that are included within the Kama Sutra, we are going to look at some of the other topics that the text discusses.

Techniques That Do Not Involve Penetration

As I mentioned in the first chapter of this book, the Kama Sutra contains much more than a list of sex positions. In this section, we are going to look at some of the other demonstrations of love that the Kama Sutra teaches.

These techniques are said to be intended for foreplay. They will help you and your partner to get in the mood by touching and kissing each other. They can also be done anytime that you wish to share some intimate moments with your significant other.

Kissing

The Kama Sutra discusses kissing as one of the many ways to connect with your partner, aside from having sexual intercourse. The Kama Sutra mentions kissing as a way to connect with your partner before sex, during sex, or any other time you wish.

There are numerous places that the Kama Sutra deems the "places for kissing." They are as follows;

- Forehead
- Cheeks
- Eyes
- Throat
- Bosom

- Breasts
- Lips
- Interior of the Mouth
- Joints of the Thighs
- Arms
- The navel

There are also different techniques for kissing. They are listed below.

1. The Normal/Nominal Kiss

A young girl kisses her partner with a small peck on the lips.

2. The Straight Kiss

When two people make contact with their lips.

3. The Turned Kiss

One partner holds the head and chin of the other partner and kisses them.

4. The Throbbing Kiss

When a young girl kisses her partner and moves only her bottom lip.

5. The Touching Kiss

The man and woman touch each other's hands, close their eyes, and the girl touches her partner's lips with her tongue.

6. The Bent Kiss

When the two kissers bend their heads and kiss.

7. The Pressed Kiss

When one partner kisses the lower lip of the other partner with force.

8. The Greatly Pressed Kiss

When one partner takes the lower lip of the other between two fingers and then touches the lip with their tongue using great force.

9. Kiss of the Upper Lip

When a man kisses the woman's upper lip, and she kisses his lower lip.

10. A Clasping Kiss

When one person takes both of the other person's lips with their lips. It is stated that a woman should only have this kind of kiss with a man who has no mustache.

11. The Kiss that Kindles Love

A woman looks at her partner's face while he is asleep and kisses it.

12. The Kiss That Turns Away

When a woman kisses a man while he is fighting with her, or while he is busy with business. This kiss happens when his mind is "turned away."

13. The Kiss That Awakens

When a man comes home late, and his wife is already asleep, he kisses her.

14. Kiss Showing The Intention

When a person kisses the reflection of their lover in a mirror or water.

15. The Transferred Kiss

When a person kisses a child, who is sitting on his lap or a picture while his lover is in the room.

16. The Demonstrative Kiss

When a man kisses a woman's finger if she is standing up, her toe if she is sitting down or while a woman is shampooing her lover's body.

Scratching and Biting

The following list includes several forms of biting which are done to show your partner that you love them. It can also be done as a type of foreplay if this person is turned on by biting.

- Swollen Bite
- Hidden Bite
- Point
- Line of Point
- Coral and the Jewel
- Line of the Jewels

- Broken Cloud
- Biting of the Boar

Striking

The Kama Sutra also talks about something called striking. This may come as a surprise to you, but striking is something that many people find pleasure in. Striking is a form of rough sex, but one that does not involve anything too serious in terms of the acts that it calls for.

Striking can be done in a gentle way, or in a firmer way, depending on what the couple themselves prefer. This can be seen as an introduction to rough sex. In today's world, rough sex is also sometimes referred to as BDSM. BDSM stands for Bondage, Discipline, Dominant and Submissive, Sadism, and Masochism. The four letters in this acronym overlap to mean a wide variety of things. Under this umbrella, there is something for everyone and probably many things that you didn't even know about that turn you on. It is all about finding pleasure without restrictions or judgment and letting yourself explore a different world of sex.

When comparing the striking techniques of the Kama Sutra to modern-day BDSM, many similarities can be drawn. More specifically, this technique could be compared to S&M. Sadism and masochism, commonly known as S&M, is the addition of pain play into your sexual experiences. The thin line between pleasure and pain is ridden here to give extreme pleasure mixed with a little bit of fear. The sadist is the person who gets pleasure from inflicting pain on their partner or rather is turned on by the power it has. The masochist is the person who gets pleasure from being in pain at the hands of their partner and riding the line between pleasure and pain.

Places You Can Strike

When it comes to striking, the Kama Sutra mentions six places that you can strike. They include the following;

- Head
- Shoulders
- Back
- Sides
- Between the breast
- The Jaghana (the buttocks)

The Ways You Can Strike

There are also 4 specific ways that you can strike. They include the following;

- Back of the Hand
- Fingers spread out
- With Open Hand
- With Fist

A Note on Sexual Compatibility

Concerning the techniques above that involves scratching, biting, and striking, one topic that this brings up is sexual compatibility. Firstly, what is Sexual Compatibility?

Sexual compatibility between people means that they share the same beliefs, values, preferences, desires, and expectations related to sex. This can include things like what sex acts you prefer the most, your level of sex drive, the type of sex you wish to have, including any fetishes, and so on. For example, if you have a very high sex drive, meaning that you need and expect to have sex every single day, you will be sexually compatible with someone who also has a high sex drive. If you were in a sexual relationship with someone who had a very low sex drive, this would be incompatible as you would likely become frustrated by their low need for frequent sex. Another example is if you desire a lot of oral sex and you require this in order to become fully aroused during sex, you would be sexually compatible with someone who also enjoys oral sex, especially giving it. If you were with someone who did not feel comfortable with oral sex at all, this would not make for a sexually compatible match.

Your preferences and values do not have to be exactly the same as the person you are in a sexual relationship with, but they must be able to fit together (like yin and yang) for a sexual relationship to be compatible. An example of this is if you enjoy slow and tender sex, but your partner enjoys rough sex. This could mean that you are sexually incompatible, but it could also work if you are both able to meet in the middle. You could start off by having slow and tender foreplay while your arousal builds, and when you are both ready for penetration, the sex can begin to lead towards a rougher style. As long as both people are comfortable with this, this sexual relationship could work.

When it comes to kinks and fetishes, sexual compatibility is quite important. For example, BDSM, including dominance and submission. If you have one partner who is sexually dominant and the other who prefers submission, this works out very well. If, however, you prefer dominance and so does your partner or if both prefer submission, you may have some trouble reaching a place of agreement when it comes to your sexual encounters. The dominant person will not usually become turned on by being told what to do, and the submissive person will usually not be too excited by telling someone else what to do. While these can work on a spectrum and people can enjoy a bit of both, many people are either dominant or submissive.

Taking this into account is important because when trying new things in the bedroom, it is important to ensure that you and your partner are both comfortable with the new techniques that you are introducing.

Double Oral Sex Technique: The Roll

This position is a wonderful oral sex position. Remember, as I mentioned that the book of Kama Sutra includes a variety of oral sex positions, not only positions in which to have intercourse. This is one of those positions.

In this position, the man will be stimulating the woman's anus and/or vagina orally while she gives him oral sex at the same time. To get into this position, the woman will lie on the bed on her back, and she will hold onto her ankles, spreading her legs out to the side as much as possible. The man will come over the woman, facing her feet, and he will place one of his knees on either side of her head, and one of his hands on either side of her hips. He will then lower himself down so that he can stimulate her orally. The woman will pull her ankles toward her head so that her body rolls up into a ball, giving the man more ease of access. She will then take his penis in her mouth and stimulate him orally. This position allows both people to benefit from oral sex at the same time. The man can also use one of his hands to stimulate the woman anally, vaginally, or clitorally while he gives her oral.

Oral Sex for Men

This position is done when the man is standing up, and the woman is on her knees in front of him, giving him oral sex. You may be thinking that this is not an advanced sex position because you have done it many times, and it is quite common. Here, however, we are going to make it an advanced position.

To make this into an advanced sex position, while the woman is kneeling in front of the man and giving him oral sex, she can use one of her hands to hold onto his testicles and gently massage them. This will add to his pleasure quite a bit. She can also (or instead) use her other hand to reach around behind him and stimulate his anus with her finger. She can move her finger around the outside of his anus, stimulating the sensitive skin there, and this will make him feel immense amounts of pleasure. Doing both of these at the same time will make it virtually impossible for him not to orgasm very quickly.

Oral Sex for Women

Similar to the previous position, this one may seem as if it is common and has been done a million times, however, with this position as well, we will be adding some elements that take it from an easier position to an advanced one.

To get into this position, the woman lies down on her back, and the man will lie down as well, but instead of lying down parallel to her with his mouth at her clitoris, he will lie down with his mouth at her clitoris but his body perpendicular to her. This way, their bodies form the letter 'T.' Lying like this makes it so that the woman can have the most pleasure possible from oral sex because it makes it easier for the man to stimulate her clitoris for a longer period without becoming fatigued. It is easier to move your tongue in an up and down motion than in a side to side motion, and when forming a T with their bodies, his tongue can move up and down (side to side on the clitoris) and give her the most pleasure possible. This is because stimulating the clitoris in this way is the most likely to lead to orgasm, whereas moving over it in a top to bottom motion will not lead to as much pleasure or as much chance of orgasm. When lying in a classic oral sex position of the man between the woman's legs, it would be hard for him to move his tongue in a side to side motion for a long time as it would become very fatigued, but if he moves his tongue up and down, it will not be as pleasurable for her. For these reasons, this T position is the best choice for oral sex for a woman.

Chapter 9: The Kama Sutra Theories of Romance

In this chapter, we are going to look at the Kama Sutra in terms of the way it discusses romance. There are a variety of tips that the Kama Sutra contains, which are related to romance, including tips for cuddling and embracing. We will then look at some Kama Sutra theories of relationships. The Kama Sutra outlines various relationships that we will look at in this chapter.

Kama Sutra Cuddling and Embracing

The first embrace we will discuss is called *The Milk and Water Embrace*. This position gets its name from the idea that the two people in this position are enmeshed and become so close that they lose themselves in the other person. Interestingly, this position can be used as a loving embrace after sex or a cuddle before sex.

The man sits on the edge of the bed, his legs planted on the floor. The woman approaches him and climbs into his lap, her face to his. She wraps her legs around his waist and her arms around his neck. He holds onto her by wrapping his arms around her back. The woman is pressed against her man, and this is a great position for cuddling, or she can keep both arms around his neck for a closer embrace.

This position is quite easy to get into and only requires a bit of strength from the man. Both of their bodies are supporting each other in this position, which is what makes it so intimate. Their bodies are touching at every point from head to toe, and they can breathe together and feel each other's heartbeat. This is why this position is said to be two people becoming one, like mixing milk and water when you can't tell where one ends, and the other begins.

From here, if they wish to transition in this position to penetrative sex, the woman can position herself so that her legs are open wide and receive his penis. To begin thrusting, they can work together, with the man using his feet on the floor as support. He can move his hips up and down, and the woman can grind her hips on his lap for pleasurable clit stimulation. If she wants, the woman can touch herself during this movement for extra pleasure.

The Kama Sutra also mentions several positions for cuddling and embracing aside from the Milk and Water Embrace. These other positions can be included after sex or during a time when you and your partner wish to hold each other and share an intimate moment.

Each time you make love with your partner, it is a bonding experience resulting in increased closeness. Each of these experiences of lovemaking contributes to your shared moments and your intimacy. Because of this, post-sex behavior is very important.

After a great orgasm, you probably collapse on top of each other, short of breath and muscles tired. Having made love, you are probably feeling quite close and romantic with each other since you have made each other feel warm and pleasured like no other. Therefore, after collapsing into each other, you will likely want to be as close as possible. We are going to look at some of the closest and romantic positions for that after-sex recovery cuddle.

First is the *head on chest* cuddle. Lie down on your back with your partner lying beside you on their side, their head resting on your chest or in the crook of your neck. In this position, you can hold each other with your arms wrapped around their body, and you can give your partner soft forehead kisses.

Second is the spooning position. Both of you will lie on your sides facing the same direction, with your bodies pressed against each other. Spooning is a position in
658

which you can have sex as well, with the man behind the woman. This position is good for a lazy Sunday morning when you are both sleepily horny for each other. If you have just finished having sex in this position, you can nicely transition to cuddling in this same position right after he pulls out of her. When he finishes, he can then wrap his arms around her and kiss her softly on the cheek.

These cuddling positions are perfect for the after-sex whispered conversation that often happens when you have sex in a relationship. You can tell the person that what they just did to you made you feel amazing, or that they were so sexy when they did that certain thing. You can share words like *"I love you"* and gentle kisses.

If you want a position that allows you to share kisses on the lips and gazes into each other's eyes, this next position will be best for you. Lie on your sides facing each other with your legs intertwined and your faces just inches from each other. From here, you can romantically gaze into their soul and enjoy the after-sex glow on your partner's face.

A common practice after sex is that you may also want to share the intimacy of a nap together. Any of these cuddling positions previously mentioned will be perfect for a post-sex nap. The tiredness that you feel after an orgasm is best accompanied by a cat nap with your lover. The vulnerability of sleeping naked together is something you don't share with just anyone and is a special moment with the person you love.

We are all busy people in this day and age, and sometimes we won't have time to lie around with our partner after sex. So how do we maintain that intimacy of a post-sex cuddle if we have just squeezed in a quickie before breakfast and the kids will wake up soon? The deeper idea here is the connection and making time for our partner. Spending time after sex is a way of showing each other that despite the busy lives we lead, we are still doing life together and share a bond with them that we don't share with anyone else. There are other ways to show this post-sex if you simply don't have time for a cuddle. However, I would encourage you to try to set aside even two to three minutes after sex to get into a close embrace with your partner and to just enjoy their presence without the distraction of life or even of the act of sex. To come together without any sort of action and get quiet together.

Kama Sutra Theories of Relationships

There are a variety of different relationships that are discussed in the Kama Sutra. Some of these relationships are between a woman and a man who are married, some are between a man and his mistress, and others involve group relationships. Below I have outlined some of the different relationships that the Kama Sutra talks about, including how the Kama Sutra says that these individuals should interact when it comes to sex.

Before moving on, note that Kama Sutra discusses sex using the term *Congress*. You will see examples of this below.

The United Congress

The United Congress refers to a sexual encounter involving one man and two women. The Kama Sutra mentions that a man should enjoy sex with two women at the same time, both of whom love him equally.

When a man is having sex with two women at once, this is called the *United Congress*.

The Congress of the Herd of Cows

The Kama Sutra also mentions group sex, though it may not be the type of group sex that you would expect. The type of group sex that is discussed in the text involves many women and one single man.

When a man is enjoying sex with many women, this called *Congress of the Herd of Cows.*

The Gramaneri

Another form of group sex that is discussed in the Kama Sutra is something called *The Gramaneri.*

This kind of group sex involves many men that are having sex with one woman. The woman involved is usually married to one of the men who are present in this group sexual encounter. In this scenario, there are two options. The men could opt to have sex with the woman one at a time, each of the men taking a turn.

Alternatively, all of the men could have sex with the woman at the same time. For this option, the Kama Sutra specifies the following arrangement; One man holds the woman, another man penetrates her vaginally, another man is given oral sex by her, and another holds her "middle part." Then, they will alternate and continue to "enjoy her" in all areas, taking turns at each part of her body.

Keep in mind that the Kama Sutra was written long ago. It was written to be read by men. Further, it was written in a time and place where a man could have multiple women at the same time, even if he was married.

Conclusion

The hope is that this book has given you the tools you need to keep your sex life fresh and ever-changing by introducing you to the world of Kama Sutra. Maybe you have tried some of the positions from the Kama Sutra before, and you needed help to learn more. Maybe you are new to sex, and you wanted to study up on different positions to try for beginners. You now have a whole arsenal of positions to try. Maybe you have tried all of the classics and are looking to get into something completely new and adventurous. Whatever experience you came with, I hope that you are leaving this book having learned a few new things to take with you into your sexual adventures from here forward. I hope this serves as a tool for you to explore and discover yourself and your future partners.

What to Do Next?

As you go on in your sexual life, stay open-minded, and never stop listening to your body. People change, and you will likely change as well. By being open to these changes and being receptive to them in yourself and your long-term partner, you will be able to ensure you are always getting the most out of sex. Don't forget to communicate with your partner to better understand them and sex in general, all communication leads to learning, and this is a great thing when it comes to sex and relationships.

There is something for everyone in this book, so continue to pass it on to your friends and your partners so that we can live in a world of educated and informed sexual beings. The Kama Sutra is a guidebook for love and everything involved in loving another person. It is more than just a book of sex positions, but these days most people only know it for its complex and flexibility-requiring positions for intercourse. The book of Kamasutra includes a general guide to living well in ways other than through sex. It includes a guide to foreplay, a guide to kissing and touching, as well as other ways to achieve intimacy with your partner, such as bathing together and giving each other massages. I hope that after reading this book, you understand and can appreciate this text in a new way.

In addition to the positions enclosed in these pages, I hope that you learned how to focus on your pleasure and the pleasure of your partner, how to be present during sex, and how to become more sexually intuitive, to feel the most pleasure possible. What a waste of pleasure it would be to always have sex in the same positions over and over and never fully reach your potential for orgasm! If you haven't already, try some of the things you've learned through reading this book, and I assure you that your sex life will be much better for it!

You are now ready to go off into the world of sexual exploration and have great orgasms from here on out. Stay curious and keep learning!

How to Benefit from the Kama Sutra for Life

1. New Sex Positions

After reading about the sex positions of the Kama Sutra, you can now incorporate them into your own sex life. Read back through the chapters on sex positions with your partner and try these new positions with them. This will make for a fun and interesting experience for the two of you. Who knows, you may even find a new favorite position for intercourse.

2. New Relationship Dynamics

As I mentioned previously, though it is an ancient book, the Kama Sutra mentions same-sex relations. Within the book, same-sex relations are referred to as *the third nature*. As I mentioned, it also talks about group sex and group relationships. What this means is that although the Kama Sutra was written so long ago, in some ways, it has become more and more relevant over the years. As our modern-day relationships have shifted and changed, the Kama Sutra has stood the test of time. In some ways, it can be said that this book has aged well.

3. New Fantasies and Kinks to Explore

In addition to talking about group sex and same-sex encounters, the Kama Sutra also recognizes that there are many different ways that people find sexual satisfaction. The Kama Sutra allows for the exploration of a person's *kinks*. For example, the Kama Sutra mentions rough sex and how it can bring sexual pleasure and satisfaction to some. As kinks and fetishes have become more widely accepted in our world, this book has begun to show that it has aged well in yet another way.

This book is here to provide you with everything you want to know about the Kama Sutra and so much more! Do yourself a favor, your partner a favor, and everyone that you will ever have sex with favor by reading this book and teaching yourself as much as you possibly can. Give your partner the gift of informing yourself about how to please them like never before using these ancient but ever-relevant positions. All you have to do is click that download button, and you will be able to begin your journey to becoming the best sexual being you have ever been!

Lightning Source UK Ltd.
Milton Keynes UK
UKHW011007241220
375840UK00014B/1628